The Seven Books Of Paulus Ægineta
Vol. 2

by

Aegineta Paulus

Double 9 BOOKS

The Seven Books Of Paulus Ægineta
Vol. 2
by Aegineta Paulus

ISBN: 978-93-59396-44-6

Published by

DOUBLE 9 BOOKS
2/13-B, Ansari Road
Daryaganj, New Delhi – 110002
info@double9books.com
www.double9books.com
Tel. 011-40042856

ABOUT THE AUTHOR

Paulus Ægineta (625-690 AD) was a Greek physician who is best known for his comprehensive medical text, "The Seven Books of Paulus Ægineta". Born on the island of Aegina, he studied medicine in Alexandria before practicing as a physician in Byzantium. His medical text was a synthesis of Greek, Roman, and Arabic medical knowledge, and it became one of the most influential medical texts in the Middle Ages. The seven volumes of the series covered a wide range of medical topics, including surgery, gynecology, and pharmacology, and they were highly regarded for their practical and detailed medical advice. As a physician, Paulus Ægineta was known for his skill and expertise in treating a wide range of medical conditions, including eye diseases, wounds, and fevers. He was also known for his careful observation of symptoms and his attention to patient care.

CONTENTS

BOOK IV

SECT 7

BOOK V

SECT 130

BOOK VI

SECT 203

BOOK IV

SECT

I—ON ELEPHANTIASIS

Well, in my opinion, did Aretæus the Cappadocian say, that the power of remedies ought to be greater than those of diseases; and that for this reason elephantiasis is incurable, because it is impossible to find a medicine more powerful than it. For if cancer, which is, as it were, an elephantiasis in a particular part, is ranked among the incurable diseases by Hippocrates himself, how much more is not elephantiasis incurable, which is, as it were, a cancer of the whole body? But the black bile from which this affection is formed, having a double origin, (for it arises either from the melancholic and feculent part, and, as it were, dregs of the blood, or from yellow bile, both being overheated); the first variety of the black bile produces the reddish elephantiasis, which is the more mild, or to speak more truly, less malignant variety; the others which are more malignant, being accompanied with ulceration of the whole body and falling off of the extremities, are produced by the latter variety, or that from yellow bile overheated. Wherefore, those who are already overpowered by the disease, must be abandoned; but when the affection is in its commencement, so as that none of the extremities has fallen off, nor the surface of the body become ulcerated, nor the hard swellings appeared, and the face merely appears foul, but not altogether unseemly, we must attempt the cure. For not a few, by merely burning the head, have prevented many who were beginning to be affected from being overpowered by this disease. Wherefore, at the commencement of the disorder, we must have recourse to venesection repeatedly, more especially if in spring, when the complaint is most apt to occur, and has its exacerbations. After an interval of a few days, say nine or ten, we may purge them with the pottage of colocynth, not once only but frequently, proportioning the dose of the medicine to its strength. Purging with hiera also suits well with them. After the interval of about ten days again, we must give them the vinegar of divided milk, not in less quantity than three heminæ, nor in greater than five, and on the following days they are to be supported with milk that is not divided into parts, or new-drawn milk; by which means, if the affection yield, the same food may be continued; but if it remains in the same state, after eating acrid things, they must be made to vomit with radishes and frumentaceous articles of food. After these things, purging with white hellebore is proper, twice if possible when in spring, but once only if in autumn. Those, however, who are thoroughly overpowered by the complaint, must be neither bled nor put on a course of hellebore. For neither can a translation of the disease from the superficies to the inner parts, nor a diminution of the offending matter, be any longer accomplished by these means; but the matter is to be determined to the stomach and bowels, and alteratives (metasyncritica), used to dry and constrict the skin. Dry-cupping is also to be applied over the mouth of the stomach and to the hypochondria, and dropaces used to the same places; but after a short interval, the same process is to be repeated, beginning by purging with hiera, and omitting the venesection, which would prove rather deleterious than beneficial. This process is to be repeated three or four times in a year, more especially in the seasons of spring and autumn. The draughts before meals, most suitable for them, are a cyathus of vinegar, with a cyathus of cedria, and two cyathi of the juice of unripe cabbage—they are given mixed together, morning and evening; or, the dried leaves of the herb ironwort, to the amount of a drachm in one cyathus of wine; or, a drachm of hartshorn and a cyathus of the vinegar of squills, is given after the morning walk every day; and other things are to be administered at the same season, such as drs. v of washed squills in honied water, or in honey, as a linctus; or Cyrenaic juice, to the amount of a bitter vetch, mixed with honey and butter; or, dr. ss of the shavings of hartshorn, with two cyathi of wine; or, drs. iij of Æthiopian cumin, with honey, as a linctus. But a more suitable remedy is a drachm of the theriac trochisk, triturated in a cyathus of fine wine, and drunk; and a drachm of the trochisk of squills may in like manner be taken in a draught. And they praise the juice of calamint as a most effectual remedy when drunk, and say that the dose to commence with is three cyathi, which may be increased to six. But of all others the theriac of vipers is the most effectual remedy, both in a draught and when rubbed in externally. But where plenty of these animals can be procured, nothing answers so well as eating the flesh of the vipers boiled in white broth, with much water, salts, leeks, and dill, to the separation of their back-bones, their head and tail being first cut off to the extent of four fingers' breadth, and their entrails and skin taken away. And theriac salts are in the same celebrity when taken with other food. By using them thus, it happens that the scales, or, as it were, the bark, falls off from the skin.

The regimen is to be as follows: After sleep, having been first rubbed, and the bowels evacuated, let the patient have recourse to gestation and vociferation, then to friction and gymnastic exercises of all kinds, partly by leaping, but more especially by using the halcteres and leather bag. Having wiped off the sweat, let him be rubbed with the grease of a boar, of a wolf, of a goat, or of some winged animal, or with fresh butter; and after a short interval let him bathe, having his body anointed with the juice of fenugreek, of ptisan, or with a little ammoniac dissolved in vinegar. After the bath, having got his body wiped, let him anoint with the oil of lentisk, of wild vine, or of myrtles; and with a little wine, containing alum and ammoniac, so as to be of the thickness of the sordes of baths. Having had his body rubbed again with soft rags, let him rest for half an hour, after which, having drunk water, let him make himself vomit by putting his fingers or a feather down his throat. Having vomited, let him drink the wine of wormwood or of marjoram. The food should be barley bread, or a cake of dried barley flour, and of potherbs, the beet, the lettuce, the radish, leeks, and cabbage sweetened in two waters, and capers. Of sea animals, he may take oysters, pelorides, urchin, all shell fishes, limpets boiled with beets, and old pickle in place of medicine. But let him abstain from wine during the whole continuance of the complaint, and from venery; only he may take a little thin watery wine at the time of his recovery from the purging, at which season all acrid substances must be abstained from, except condiments. Give him ptisan, eggs and chondrus, milk and honey, with bread, mallows, dock, skirret, and fishes with tender flesh; and of fowls, those which contain wholesome juices; and of fruits, the fig, grape, and raisins: but of sweetmeats, those which are prepared from pine kernels, toasted almonds, or bastard saffron. He may take food twice a day, as it is injurious to subsist upon one meal. After taking care of the internal parts, let him use detergent ointments (smegmata) in the bath, from the decoction of beet, or of fenugreek with aphronitrum, soap, or myrobolan, and sometimes apply depilatories. Purslain triturated with vinegar is detergent and also the slender houseleek, and the roots of dock boiled in vinegar, and alum with salts, and red arsenic in equal proportions with wine and oil of lentisk. Also the composition for alphos, consisting of alcyonium, nitre, myrtle, sulphur, and the dried leaves of the wild fig, being rubbed in dry with vinegar; and that from the burnt shell of the cuttle-fish, and pumice, nitre, and burnt Cimolian earth, gum, unripe galls in equal quantity, sprinkled dry, or rubbed in with vinegar. And this one is admirable: Of the roots of dock a bunch to the amount of a handful, of natron, dr. xl; of frankincense, dr. xxv; of sulphur, dr. xxv; it is rubbed in with Egyptian vinegar. And this one is efficacious: Of arsenic, dr. x; of sulphur vivum, dr. viii; of costus, dr. xii; of quicklime, dr. iv; of wax, dr. iv; of dried bay berries, dr. xii; these things are mixed with the juice of white poplar leaves, or with a thick decoction, and they are rubbed in, having the consistence of honey.—*Another*: Two fasciculi of the roots of dock are to be boiled in vinegar, pounded in a mortar and triturated, then of alcyonium, lb. j; of aphronitrum, oz. viij; of sulphur vivum, lb. j; of the burnt shells of cockles, oz. iv; of chamæleon with its roots, oz. iv; these things are pounded together until they are of the consistence of the sordes of the baths, and are then rubbed in often in the sun, if summer, but if winter, in the bath, until it occasions sweating. And the dry smegma of Æsculapius would agree excellently with these cases, and all the smegmata about to be described, even unto those for alphos, and also those now mentioned, are applicable for those complaints. And the tumid excrescences, whether inflammatory or ulcerous, are to be rubbed with Indian buckthorn: or horned poppy, or aloe, or the Andronian trochisk, or that of Polyides; and let cataplasms be applied of chondrus with the juice of knot-grass or plantain; or of pellitory of the wall, triturated; and the leaves of the green Melisian herb, when pounded with axunge and applied, are wonderfully efficacious, for they redden the parts, but the redness is easily repressed by the application of bread; or of the cerate made from almond oil. By this means their natural colour is restored. When the parts are ulcerated, plasters are suitable: that from diphryges, and the apple one with wine, that called coracium, that made from oxymel, the Andronian trochisk, pompholyx and calamine. It is a symptom that the whole disease is becoming more moderate when the first ulcers are cicatrized. For the dyspnœa of persons labouring under elephantiasis give a draught of five or six slaters in three cyathi of honied water. And some of the general remedies described for dyspnœa will be applicable for them. Of the natural baths we must select, as being most particularly useful, the aluminous and chalybeate, and if possible, such as are cold. It is also particularly serviceable to drink them. And the use of the sand of the sea-shore has the same effect, and so have all the sudorifics. But since this affection is one of those which are easily communicable, no less so than the plague, they are to be removed as far as possible from cities, and lodged in inland and cold situations, where there are few inhabitants, if this can be accomplished; for so they may descend from thence to surrounding places. This is proper partly on their own account and also on account of those whom they might come in contact with. For they themselves will thus enjoy the use of a more commodious air, and they will not communicate the evil to others.

Commentary. Consult Lucretius (vi, 1112); Celsus (iii, 25); Pliny (Hist. Nat. xxvi, 5); Scribonius Largus (102); Cælius Aurelianus (Pass. Tard. iv, 1); Marcellus (De Med. xix); Serenus Samonicus (11); Octavius Horatianus (i, 32); Isidorus (Orig. iv, 8); Vegetius (Mulom. i, 9); Aretæus (Curat. Morb.

Chron. ii, 13); Plutarch (Symp. viii, Quest. 9); Galen (ad Glauc. ii, 10; de Causis Morb. 7); Oribasius (Morb. Curat. iii, 62; Synops. vii, 5); Pseudo Dioscorides (Euporist. i, 105); Aëtius (xiii, 120); Actuarius (Meth. Med. ii, 11, and iv, 15); Nonnus (Epit. 233); Psellus (op. medicum); Leo (vii); Myrepsus (De Med. comp.); Avicenna (iv, 3, 3, 1); Serapion (v, 14); Avenzoar (ii, 7, 12, 26); Albucasis (Chirurg. i, 49); Haly Abbas (Theor. viii, 15, Pract. iv, 3, ix, 69); Alsaharavius (Pract. xxxi, 2); Rhases (ad Mansor, v, 35, ix, 93, Contin. xxxv, 26.)

We owe the earliest notice which we have of this disease to the poet Lucretius, who briefly mentions it in the following lines:

"Est elephas morbus qui propter flumina Nili

Gignitur Ægypto in mediâ neque præterea usquam."

Celsus says that elephantiasis is a chronic disease, almost unknown in Italy, but very common in certain countries. He calls it an affection of the whole body, even of the bones. The upper part of the body is covered with frequent spots and tumours, the redness gradually changes to black, the skin is thickened, and covered with hard asperities like scales; the body wastes, but the face, legs, and feet swell; and when the disease is protracted, the fingers and toes become buried in the swelling, and a slight fever comes on, which finishes the patient's sufferings. Such is his description of the disease. His treatment consists in bleeding at the commencement, abstinence, then supporting the strength, purging, exercise, sudorifics, and friction. Baths are to be rarely used; fatty, glutinous, and flatulent articles of food are to be avoided, but wine is to be allowed, except at the beginning. The body is to be rubbed with pounded plantain.

According to Pliny, elephantiasis was never known in Italy until the days of Pompey the Great, when it was imported from Egypt, and raged for a time, but soon became extinct. He describes it as affecting the face in particular with hard, rough, black maculæ, which sometimes spread to the bones, the toes and fingers being swelled.

Serenus Samonicus, who is said to have flourished about the beginning of the third century, thus describes the disease:

"Est elephas morbus tristi quoque nomine dirus,

Non solum turpans infandis ora papillis,

Sed cito præcipitans funesto fata venino."

His remedies are the juice of the bark of the juniper, the ashes and blood of the weasel, mint, and various external applications, consisting of ceruse, Egyptian paper, roses, &c.

Scribonius Largus recommends sulphur with common oil for lepra, "et quam elephantiam dicunt," but he gives no description of the latter.

It is greatly to be lamented that Cælius Aurelianus' account of elephantiasis has come down to us in an imperfect state. His description is entirely lost, and his detail of the treatment is in a mutilated state. It appears, however, that his views were similar to those of Celsus, and that he considered it to be a malignant disease, affecting principally the skin. He approves of rubbing stimulant ointments into the skin, and of using medicinal baths, especially the aluminous and chalybeate. When the applications produce ulceration of the skin, he directs us to treat it upon general principles. He makes mention of vomiting by radishes, and latterly by means of the white hellebore. He approves of a sea voyage and change of scene. He says the first author who described elephantiasis was Themison, the same person that is damned to everlasting fame in one of the lines of Juvenal: "Quot Themison agros autumno occiderit uno." (Sat. x, 221.) If this statement be correct, it is clear that Celsus cannot be of so early a date as is generally believed, that is to say, the Augustan age, for Themison flourished towards the end of the first century, p. c. He was the founder of the Methodical sect. Cælius also blames Themison for recommending bleeding and vomiting unseasonably, and disapproves of his directions respecting the applications to the skin. It appears that he also disapproved of the theriac of vipers, and of giving to drink water in which red-hot iron had been extinguished. There can be no doubt, from the circumstances which he mentions, that the disease was thought contagious in his time.

Octavius Horatianus, who lived under the emperor Valentinian, gives a pretty full detail of the treatment, but his description of the symptoms is defective. He makes mention, however, of *maculæ*, which affect principally the face; he contends that the whole system is attacked with the disease, and that the flesh is corrupted. His remedies are much the same as those recommended by the other authorities, namely, bleeding, purging, vomiting, the theriac of vipers, and rubbing with the usual applications for scabies. He also speaks favorably of the natural and the sea-water baths.

Marcellus the Emperic, who is supposed to have flourished in the reign of Theodosius, recommends, like Serenus, mint, juniper, and mezereon, for elephantiasis. He describes it as being attended with hard excrescences of the extremities, eruptions on the face, and disease of the bones. He speaks of its being endemic in Ægypt.

The disease, elephantiasis, according to Isidorus, is so called from its resemblance to the elephant. The skin in it is hard and rough, from which it gets its appellation, because the surface of the patient's body resembles that of an elephant; or because it is a mighty affection, as the elephant is one of the largest of animals.

Vegetius, the great ancient authority on veterinary surgery, describes elephantiasis as it affects cattle. The symptoms are hardness and roughness of the skin, squamæ, eruptions on the feet and head, and a fetid discharge from the nose. He approves of bleeding, and the other means recommended by the regular surgeons.

We shall next give the descriptions of the Greek authorities.

Aretæus gives a most elaborate but surely somewhat overstrained description of elephas, which he paints in colours the most hideous and disgusting. We shall endeavour to convey to the reader an idea of his sketch, stripping his picture of its flowery ornaments, and contracting its bulk. The disease is called *elephas,* he says, from its magnitude, *leontium* or *morbus leoninus,* from the supposed resemblance of the eyebrows to those of the lion; and *satyriasis,* from the venereal desires with which it is attended. The disease is described as escaping notice at first, being deep-seated and preying upon the vitals, but afterwards it is determined to the superficies, commencing sometimes with the face, and at other times with the extremities. The belly is dry, because, as he ingeniously remarks, the distribution of the food is performed regularly, and the vitiated parts strongly attract the chyle to them as a pabulum to the disease. There are large callous eminences on the skin, and the veins appear enlarged, owing to a thickening of the vessels and not to a plethora of blood. The hairs of the head, pubes, and other parts of the body, drop off. The face in particular is affected with callous tubercles or warts, and it is not uncommon for the tongue, and most parts of the body, to be also covered with them. The eyebrows are thickened, stripped of their hair, and hang down like those of the lion. The general appearance of the skin, covered as it is with hard tubercles, and intersected with deep fissures, is said to bear some resemblance to that of the elephant. Sometimes particular members, such as the nose, feet, fingers, the whole hand, or the pudenda, will die and drop off; and it is not uncommon for incurable ulcers to break forth on different parts of the body. Dyspnœa, and a sense of suffocation, are occasionally present. He says, it is dangerous to have any intercourse with persons labouring under the disease, no less so than in the case of the plague, as both are readily communicated by respiration. He directs us, at the commencement, to abstract blood freely, because blood is the *pabulum morbi*. He recommends us to purge with hiera, and to procure vomiting by radishes, but more particularly by the white hellebore, upon which he bestows a glowing and eloquent eulogy. Like our author, he approves of the theriac of vipers. He makes mention of many external applications of a detergent nature, and in particular praises a soap used by the Celts for cleaning their clothes. He also commends natron, alcyonium, sulphur, alum, ammoniac with vinegar, and the like, for the same purpose. When the flesh is livid, he directs us previously to make deep incisions in it. The diet is to be plain and digestible; sulphureous baths are to be used: the patient is to swim frequently in sea-water, to take a sea voyage, and otherwise not neglect suitable exercise.

Plutarch informs us that it was disputed in his time whether or not elephantiasis was a new complaint.

Galen, as far as we can recollect, has nowhere treated very particularly of elephantiasis, but in his work 'De Causis Morborum' he has briefly mentioned that in this disease the nose becomes flattened, the lips thick, and the ears extenuated, the whole appearance resembling that of a satyr: and in his work entitled 'De Curatione ad Glauconem' he ranks elephantiasis with cancerous swellings, and says that the disease is common about Alexandria, owing to the heat of the place and the food of the inhabitants, which consists principally of lentils, snails, pickles, the flesh of asses, and the like, all which things have a tendency to engender the melancholic humour. The temperature of the place likewise, he shrewdly remarks, determines the superfluities of the system to the skin. He recommends the treatment which we have already had occasion to mention, namely, bleeding, purging, and the theriac of vipers. In the 'Isagoge,' the black and white hellebores are particularly commended. Galen elsewhere calls it contagious. (Lib. ii, Simpl. de carne viperæ.)

Oribasius gives no description of the disease, but briefly recommends the theriac of vipers, and in certain cases purging and bleeding for the cure of it.

The account given by Aëtius is principally taken from Archigenes, and is very circumstantial. The disease, he remarks, has been called by the several names of elephantiasis, leontiasis, and satyriasis. Suspicions, he says, have been entertained of its being contagious, and he is of opinion that it is unsafe to hold intercourse with those who are ill of the disease, as the air becomes contaminated by the effluvia from their sores, and by their respiration. The disease, he says, is insidious, for it begins in a concealed manner internally, and does not make its appearance on the skin until it is confirmed. Men are more subject to it than women, and intemperate climates predispose to it. The first symptoms of the disease are torpor, slow respiration, constipated bowels, urine like that of cattle, continued eructations, and strong venereal appetites; and when it is determined to the skin, the cheeks and chin become thickened and of a livid colour, the veins below the tongue are varicose, and eminences are formed all over the body, but especially on the forehead and chin. The body becomes increased in bulk, and is borne down by an intolerable sense of heaviness. Those affected with it become pusillanimous, and shun the haunts of men. Though the disease, when confirmed, is of the most hopeless description, he forbids us to abandon the sick at the commencement. His treatment is almost the same as our author's: venesection at the beginning, purging with colocynth or hiera, and vomiting with radishes or white hellebore. Some, he says, having remarked that eunuchs escaped taking this complaint, have castrated themselves as a preventive. He makes mention of all the medicinal substances recommended by our author, namely, iron-wort, Cyrenaic juice, the theriac of vipers, &c. For the cutaneous affections he recommends a great many external applications, containing white hellebore, sulphur, rue, natron, aloes, and even arsenic. He also speaks of cataplasms, depilatories, and detergent ointments. He is very particular in directing that the diet be light and wholesome.

Actuarius calls elephantiasis a cancer of the whole body, which preys upon all the flesh, and derives its origin from black bile corroding everything like fire. The first symptoms of it are a falling off of the hairs of the eyebrows and chin, tumours on the face, an alteration of the appearance of the eyes, a change of the voice, turgidity of the sublingual veins, and afterwards cutaneous eruptions of an intractable nature. He then states that elephantiasis, lepra, psora, and impetigo are diseases of different gradations of malignity. In another place he has given the treatment, which is exactly the same as that recommended by Aretæus, namely, bleeding, purging with hellebore, detergent and desiccative applications to the skin, &c.

Some applications, seemingly of little efficacy, are recommended for elephantiasis in the 'Euporista' of the Pseudo-Dioscorides.

Nonnus, as usual, abridges our author's detail of the treatment, and omits the description. He says it arises from a melancholic humour, which corrodes the extremities. According to Psellus, the disease is produced by *melancholy adust* and the lees of putrid blood.

The account of elephantiasis given by Leo is brief and imperfect. The disease, he says, is produced by a melancholic humour, which has become putrid, and corrodes the extremities. It is, he adds, almost incurable, but may be benefited by purging with the dodder of thyme, by the theriac, and burning the head at the bregma. The affection, he says, is also called satyriasmus.

Myrepsus merely mentions some of the common remedies for elephantiasis, such as arsenic, turpentine, litharge, &c. He gives no description of the disease.

We now proceed to the Arabians.

Avicenna gives a very circumstantial account of elephantiasis, under the name of *juzam* or *judam*, which his translator renders by *lepra*. He calls it a cancer of the whole body, which arises from black bile, and is sometimes attended with ulceration, and is sometimes without it. The disease, he says, is contagious: it is produced by living upon the flesh of asses, lentils, &c., and is endemic in Alexandria. It is sometimes called *leonina*, because the face assumes the stern appearance of the lion's. He states that, although it begins internally, its first symptoms are manifested on the extremities. He then describes minutely the symptoms, namely, redness of the face, inclining to lividity; falling off of the hairs, enlargement of the veins, affection of the breathing, thickening, and discoloration of the lips; and afterwards ulceration of different parts of the body, corrosion of the cartilages of the nose, then falling off of the nose and extremities, loss of voice, &c. The treatment he gives with great minuteness, but as it is little different from that of the Greeks, we need scarcely enter upon it. Suffice it to say that he mentions early bleeding, purging with hellebore, colocynth, scammony, &c.; the theriac of vipers, the application of the cautery to the head, and so forth. Enough has been said to show that this description applies to the elephantiasis of the Greeks. Considerable confusion, however, has arisen in consequence of his translator applying the term *elephantia* to a very different disease, namely, to an enlargement of the leg with varicose veins, now generally known by the name of the *Barbadoes leg*. This complaint he directs to be treated at first with local bleeding and astringents; but when ulceration takes place, it is to be remedied only by amputation.

Serapion, in like manner, describes the elephantiasis of the Greeks by the name of *lepra*. The face, he says, is swelled, livid, and covered with hard pustules, the hairs of the eyebrows fall off, the whole aspect becomes hideous, the voice is changed, the perspiration becomes vitiated, and ulceration seizes different parts of the body. The disease, he says, takes its origin from the liver, in which the office of sanguification is improperly performed. His remedies are bleeding, hellebore, the theriac, &c.

Avenzoar describes the *lepra* as a cancer arising from contact with other lepers, or from unwholesome food. He recommends to purge away the melancholic humour with scammony, colocynth, black hellebore, &c. The *elephantia* he describes as a disease in which the leg is swelled like the leg of an elephant. He considers it almost incurable.

Albucasis gives an account of the operation of burning the head for *lepra*, i.e. the elephantiasis of the Greeks.

The translator of Haly Abbas, namely, Stephanus Antiochensis, who says he wrote about the year 1127, describes the disease which we have been treating of by the name of elephantia. Like the others, Haly represents it to be a general cancer arising from black bile. He says it proves contagious by respiration. Among the symptoms, he mentions falling off of the ciliary and superciliary hairs, dryness of the nose, which sometimes falls in; in short, he enumerates the same symptoms as the preceding authorities. For the cure he directs us to bleed from the arteries behind the ears, those of the temples, or from a vein in the arm; to give emetics, such as hellebore; to avoid cold; to apply cupping-instruments to the scrobiculus cordis; to administer the theriac, &c. He recommends externally decoctions of beans and vetches at first; and afterwards stimulant lotions, containing arsenic, sulphur, quicklime, and so forth. He also applies the term elephantia, and sometimes elephas, to the swelled leg, which he considers to be a species of varix.

Alsaharavius describes four varieties of *lepra,* namely, the leonina, elephantia, serpentina, and vulpina. The disease, he says, may be contracted, 1st, by an hereditary taint; 2d, by the use of corrupted food, such as the flesh of buck-goats, cows, &c.; 3d, by contagion, through the medium of the respiration. He describes all the gradations of the disease with greater minuteness than any other ancient author. In its last stage, he says, the nose falls in, the hairs drop off, the voice is lost, ulcers break out on the skin, the extremities mortify and fall away, and the breath is fetid. His treatment varies according to the circumstances of the case, but, upon the whole, it is scarcely at all different from that of the others. By the name of elephantia he also describes the *swelled leg,* which he pronounces to be a very intractable disease. He directs us, however, to have recourse to bleeding, melanogogues, abstinence from gross food, emetics, and various external applications of a stimulant nature, among which he mentions burying the leg in hot sand.

The translator of Rhases also applies the term *lepra* to the elephantiasis of the Greeks. The colour of the eye, he says, is changed, the voice becomes rough, the face is swelled, like a bladder, and red with nodes, the hairs fall off, and the extremities at last become swelled and ulcerated. There is nothing peculiar in his treatment. He describes, likewise, the *swelled leg* by the name of elephantia or elephas. He says that, when tubercles arise on it, it is utterly incurable; but that when simply enlarged, it may be remedied by bleeding in the arm, cupping, emetics, attenuant food, and the like. In his 'Continens,' he calls the lepra (elephantiasis) hereditary and contagious. He says, it is a general cancer, arising from black bile. For the *swelled leg* he recommends, as in his other work, bloodletting and emetics, with stimulant applications, containing pearlashes, sulphur, &c., and also tight bandages.

Such is the history of elephantiasis given by ancient authors.

The earlier of our modern writers on medicine, describe elephantiasis as a species of lepra, of which they enumerate four varieties, namely, elephantia, leonina, alopecia, and tyria. This arrangement is evidently taken from Alsaharavius. Such is the account which Platiarius gives of these diseases. In like manner, the Pseudo-Macer ranks elephantiasis with lepra:

"Est lepræ species elephantiasisque vocatur," &c. Upon this passage Cornarius makes the following annotation: "Vulgus medicorum Arabas in hoc secuti lepram cum elephantiasi confundunt. Immo lepram pro elephantiasi accipiunt."

Guido de Cauliaco's account of the disease is also nearly the same as that of Alsaharavius. He states decidedly that the disease is contagious, and recommends bleeding, purging, the actual cautery, the theriac of vipers. (vi, 1.) Rogerius remarks that the disease is contracted *per coitum*. (i, 15.) And here, by the way, we may be permitted to state that we have long been convinced that the syphilis of modern times is a modified form of the ancient elephantiasis. This opinion is maintained by several of the writers of the Aphrodisiacus, and also by the learned Sprengel, who gives a very interesting disquisition on Syphilis in his 'History of Medicine.'

It appears that the disease in its ancient form is still prevalent in certain parts of the world; as, for example, in the Sardinian States, where it is still looked upon as being both contagious and hereditary. It is also endemic in Norway: nay, it is reported to have broken forth with all its ancient character in the province of New Brunswick. In the East, elephantiasis and leontiasis are still considered as aggravated forms of leprosy. (See Heber's Travels, ii, 50; and Niebuhr's Travels, xxvii, 11.) We may be allowed to add, in conclusion, that a great mass of misapprehension has prevailed in modern times regarding the elephantiasis of the Greeks and Arabians. We trust the above sketch will remove the difficulties which formerly beset this subject.

II—ON LEPROSY AND PSORA

Both these affections consist of an asperity of the skin, with pruritus or wasting of the body, having their origin from a melancholic humour. But leprosy spreads over the skin more deeply in a circular form, throwing out scales which resemble those of fishes. But psora is more superficial and variously figured, and throws out furfuraceous bodies. In these cases we must premise venesection when the body appears more than usually plethoric; but, if not, we must by all means purge with those things which evacuate black bile. Externally we may use in common either of the hellebores; and have washed lime dried, and, when going to use it, we may dilute it in water until it attain the thickness of the wrestler's sordes, and anoint.—*Another*: Of sage, of the tears of Æthiopian olive, of each, dr. viij; of the bark of capper's root, of gum, of each, dr. xiij; anoint with vinegar, in the sun. Anemone, when applied, and the root of the white vine particularly, remove psora. But the following are compound remedies: Of the flour of darnel, one chœnix; of the white cardamom, dr. iv; of the scum of natron, dr. j; of copperas, dr. viij; of the middle roots of asphodel, dr. iv; having triturated them in vinegar, and made of the thickness of a cerate, anoint, having first applied nitre to the part; and having removed it, (which do about the third day,) and washed with cold water, again anoint.—*Another*: Of the juice of kings' spears' roots, oz. vj; of sulphur vivum, of manna, of each, dr. x; of natron, dr. viij; anoint, mixing with vinegar. The following simple remedies are particularly applicable for psora: Stavesacre, bitter lupins, cardamom with vinegar, the root of lily with honey, turpentine rosin, sulphur, chick peas, goat's dung; and these compound ones—mix equal parts of chalcitis and misy with wine, and anoint the more humid kinds of psora.—*Another*: Boil the tender leaves of rose-bay in a sextarius of oil until they are dried, and, throwing away the leaves, add to the oil oz. iij of white wax, and, after it is dissolved, cool and sprinkle upon it oz. j of sulphur vivum, and anoint in the sun or in the bath. Some boil also squills with the rose-bay.—*Another*: Of diachylon, oz. ij; of wax, oz. ij; of oil of roses, oz. j; of litharge, oz. iij; of ceruse, oz. iij; of liquid pitch, oz. vj; of the dross of silver, oz. ij; of siricum, oz. ij; of vinegar, what will be sufficient for the trituration of the dry things.—*Another*: Of ceruse, oz. ss; of starch, oz. ss; of lead, oz. j; of red lotuses, or of alkanet, oz. ij; of wax, oz. vj; of oil of roses, oz. ix; boil the alkanet properly with the oil of roses, and then add the other things.—*Another*: Take ten eggs, or as many as are required, and having macerated in the most acrid vinegar until their shell become tender; boil in the vinegar the yelks of them; having triturated with rose-oil and what remains of the vinegar a moderate quantity of litharge, anoint, when of the consistence of the sordes of oil in baths.—*Another*: Three yelks of eggs out of vinegar; of rose-oil, oz. vj; of sulphur vivum, oz. iij; having triturated the yelks of the eggs and the sulphur with the vinegar, add the cerate. And litharge triturated with vinegar and rose oil, until it be of the consistence of a plaster, cleanses the most acrid kinds of psora; and the detergent ointments from dock, and the most of those for elephantiasis, answer well in general with leprosy and psora.

Commentary. See Hippocrates (de Usu Humidorum, Epidem. ii); Galen. (Meth. Med. xiv; de Causis Sympt. iii, 6; et alibi); Oribasius (Morb. Curat, iii, 58); Aëtius (xiii, 134); Actuarius (Meth. Med. ii, 11); Nonnus (Epit. 234); Pseudo-Dioscor. (Euporist. i, 128); Leo (vii, 15, 18); Pollux (Onomasticon, iv,

9); Æschylus (Choeph. 274); Alexander Aphrodisiensis (Prob. i, 146, and ii, 42); Celsus (v, 28); Scribonius Largus; Octavius Horatianus (i, 31); Serenus Samonicus; Marcellus (de Med. xix); Isidorus (Orig. iv, 8); Psellus (op. Medicum); Vegetius (Mulom. iii, 71); Geopon. (xviii, 15); Serapion (v, 2); Avicenna (iv, 7, 2, 9); Avenzoar (ii, 7, 4); Haly Abbas (Theor. viii, 16; Pract. iv, 4); Alsaharavius (xxxi, 1, 2, 3, 4); Rhases (ad Mansor. v, 31 et seq.; Divis. 117, et seq.); Contin. (xxxvi.)

As in the preceding chapter, we shall here give a separate account of the views of the Greeks, Latins, and Arabians, beginning, in this instance, with the Greeks.

Hippocrates makes only casual mention of these diseases, and has nowhere marked their distinguishing characters. In one place he calls leprosy a blemish rather than a disease; and in another he remarks that some varieties of it itch before rain. He speaks of vinegar, and of lime and water as remedies for it. It is proper to apprize the reader that the two works quoted above from the Hippocratic Collection are, most probably, not genuine.

Galen also is very deficient on the subject of lepra, having nowhere given a complete description of it, although he notices it incidentally in many parts of his works. In one place he calls elephas, leuce, and alphos cognate affections. Alphos, he says, is much more superficial than leuce. In another, he attributes these complaints to the melancholic humour which becomes fixed in the skin. In the 'Isagogue,' which, however, seems not to be a genuine work of his, it is said that lepra is an affection of the skin, which becomes whiter and rougher than natural, the roughness resembling that from prominent psydracia. Psora is said to partake more of the nature of ulceration. Both are represented as arising from a saltish phlegm, and as being cured by phlegmagogues, and ointments rubbed into the skin. It is also stated that leuce is distinguished from lepra by there being no roughness of the skin in the former disease. In another place he mentions psora as a disease most inveterate to cure. (Facult. Natur. i, 13.)

Oribasius thus distinguishes leuce, alphos, melas, lepra, and psora from one another. Leuce is occasioned by a pituitous and viscid blood, which, in process of time, renders the colour white. Alphos arises in like manner, but the superficial skin only is affected, and not the whole flesh. When a pituitous humour is the cause of the complaint, it puts on the appearance of alphos, and when the melancholic, of melas. Lepra affects mostly the deep-seated parts, and psora the superficial. For all these complaints he recommends a mixture of lime and water and some other such things.

In the 'Euporista,' generally ascribed to Dioscorides, there is given a long list of medicinal articles for lepra, such as the flour of darnel with sulphur, hellebore with vinegar, verdigris, cantharides, &c.

Aëtius, copying from Archigenes, thus marks the difference between lepra and its cognate diseases. Lepra differs from leuce and alphos, inasmuch as lepra is distinguished by roughness and a sense of itching, and yet the skin only is affected, and when it is removed, the flesh below is discovered to be sound; but in leuce, the flesh below assumes an unnatural degree of whiteness, while the surface of the part is very smooth, and when rubbed it soon becomes red, especially in those who are readily cured; and alphos is altogether superficial, having the appearance of a scale fastened to the skin. Lepra differs from psora, inasmuch as in psora the substances which appear on the skin are of a furfuraceous nature, while in lepra they resemble the scales of a large fish. He omits the constitutional treatment so judiciously stated by our author, but his local applications are little different. They contain hellebore, sulphur, misy, verdigris, liquid pitch, cantharides, natron, copperas, myrrh, galls, vinegar, &c., mixed in various proportions.

Actuarius states that lepra is next to elephantia in malignity, and that it is distinguished from psora by spreading deeper and having scales of a circular shape like those of fishes; whereas, psora is more superficial, and its scales are furfuraceous and of no determinate shape. Both are attended with asperity of the skin, and itching. Leuce holds the same place to alphos that lepra does to psora, that is to say, leuce is more deep-seated, and affects the colour of the hair, while alphos is more superficial, and the hair is in general unchanged. For all these affections he recommends an application containing copperas, black hellebore, arsenic, and cantharides, mixed with oil, cedar resin, or rose oil.

Psellus states correctly that the scales in leprosy assume a circular shape.

Nonnus marks the distinction between these diseases very accurately. Lepra arises from a corroding humour, and hence scales fall from the surface of the skin, and it is attended with pruritus. But lepra is more deep-seated, and affects the skin circularly; whereas psora is more superficial and variously figured. Leuce and alphos albus and niger, he says, are allied; but leuce is deeper seated, so as to change the colour of the hairs, whereas the alphi are more superficial affections.

Pollux, like most of the others, states that in leuce, when the skin is pricked, it does not bleed, and that the disease is difficult to cure. Alphos and melas, he says, are easily cured.

Although Myrepsus has not described these diseases, he gives prescriptions for various compositions to remove them. The most active ingredients in them are hellebore, natron, sulphur, quicksilver, sal ammoniac, quicklime, bay-berries, &c.

Alexander Aphrodisiensis mentions psora among the contagious diseases, but says that lepra and leuce are not contagious.

Chrysostom alludes to the common opinion that psora is a contagious disease. The poet Æschylus gives a short description of leprosy in his 'Chöepheræ' by the name of lichenes. (l. 277.)

Celsus nowhere uses the terms lepra and psora, and therefore there is considerable difficulty in comparing his account of these cutaneous affections with the descriptions of the Greeks. Alphos, melas, and leuce, he describes very intelligibly, connecting them together by the generic term of vitiligo. We shall give his own characteristic description of these diseases:—"Ἄλφος vocatur ubi color albus est, fere subasper, et non continuus, et quædam quasi guttæ dispersæ esse videantur: interdum etiam latius, et cum quibusdum intermissionibus serpit. Μέλας colore ab hoc differt quia niger est et umbræ similis: cætera eadem sunt. Leuce habet quiddam simile alpho, sed magis albida est et altius descendit; in eâque albi pili sunt, et lanugini similes. Priora curationem non deficillimam recipiunt: ultimum vix unquam sanescit." Another class of cutaneous affections he connects by the generic term of impetigo, and it is to be remarked that they are all squamous diseases, and not pustular, like the complaints to which Drs. Willan and Bateman have applied the term. His second species of impetigo (as Bateman remarks) appears to be the psora of the Greeks:—"Alterum genus pejus est, simile papulæ feræ, sed asperius rubicandiusque, figuras varias habens: squamulæ ex summâ cute discedunt, rosio major est, celerius et latius procedit, certioribusque etiam quam prior temporibus et fit et desinit. Rubra cognominatur." His third species bears some resemblance to the lepra nigricans of Willan and Bateman:—"Tertia etiamnum deterior est: nam et crassior est et durior, et magis tumet, in summâ cute finditur, et vehementius rodit, *ipsa quoque squamosa sed nigra*, &c. Nigræ cognomen est." His account of the fourth species seems to refer to the lepra vulgaris:—"Quartum genus est quod curationem omnino non recipit distans colore: nam sub-albidum est et recenti cicatrici simile: squamulas habet pallidas, quasdam subalbidas, quasdam lenticulæ similes: quibus demptis nonunquam profluit sanguis." For all these diseases he recommends a composition containing sulphur, natron, and rosin.

Scribonius Largus describes several compositions, "ad lepram, quæ quasi impetigo est cum prurigine cutis," and for scabies. They contain sulphur, Æthiopian cumin, vinegar, frankincense.

Serenus Samonicus makes mention of a few popular remedies for scabies, prurigo, and papulæ, but he gives no description of these complaints.

Octavius Horatianus recommends for scabies (meaning, we suppose, the psora of the Greeks,) bleeding, purging, frequent baths, and external applications containing natron, frankincense, and sulphur. He does not mention lepra by name, nor does he seem to allude to it at all.

Marcellus recommends for lepra a composition containing equal parts of natron, frankincense, litharge, and sulphur pounded with vinegar.

Vegetius says that the scabies of cattle "contagiosa est et transit in plures." Probably Virgil alludes to the scab of sheep in this line: "Nec mala vicini pecoris contagia lædant." (Ecl. i.) He mentions, as remedies for it, sulphur, litharge, pitch, hellebore, &c. (Georg. iii, 449.) See also Geopon. (xvi, 18, xviii, 15); Columella (viii, 5); and Gratius (Cyneget. 412).

Isidorus gives the following definitions of the complaints we have been treating of: "*Lepra* vero cutis asperitas squammosa lepidi similis unde nomen accepit: cujus color nunc in nigridinem vertitur, nunc in alborem, nunc in ruborem. *Scabies* tenuis asperitas et squammata est. Impetigo est sicca scabies; prominens a corpore cum asperitate et rotunditate formæ. Hanc vulgus *sarnam* appellat."

Justin applies the terms *vitiligo* and *scabies* to the diseases treated of in this chapter. See Hist. (xxxvi, 2.) We now turn to the Arabians.

In the Latin translation of Serapion, lepra and psora are described under the generic term of "impetigines in quibus excoriatur et scinditur cutis;" but they are further distinguished from one another by the specific titles of *albaras* nigra and pruritus. The former is characterized as arising from the melancholic humour, and as casting off round scales. The latter is said to consist of pustules, which appear on different parts of the body, are variously figured, and cast off furfuraceous scales. The leuce is described by the name of *baras,* as arising from viscid, pituitous blood, and being produced by a defect of the assimilative faculty. In it the flesh itself is said to be changed to a white colour. If, when pricked with the head of a needle it bleeds, there is a probability of cure; but if it does not bleed, it is incurable. The two alphi are described by the names of *morphea alba* and *nigra*. The morphea alba resembles the white albaras (leuce) only that in the latter the affection of the skin is more deep-seated, and the hairs in it are turned to a white colour; but in morphea the only change is in the external appearance of the skin. The morphea nigra (melas?) is said to resemble the albaras nigra (lepra nigricans?) only that it is more superficial.

In the Latin translation of Avicenna by Bullonensis, alphos albus and niger are distinguished by the names of *morphea alba* (or *alguada*), and *morphea nigra*; leuce by that of *albaras*; and lepra by those of *albaras* nigra and *impetigo excorticativa*. The specific differences between them are stated with great precision. The morpheæ are superficial affections of the skin, but the albaras affects also the flesh, penetrating sometimes down to the bone. All these diseases are said to arise from a weakness of the assimilative faculty. In the *albaras* nigra, or leprosy, the skin is said to be covered with scales, like those of a fish. Like the authorities formerly quoted, Avicenna states that in *alguada* (alphos albus) the hairs do not change their colour, but that they do so in *albaras*. The puncture of a needle likewise extracts blood from the *guada*, but not from the *baras*.

Avenzoar makes mention of the *morphea* alba and nigra, but has not described them particularly. These authors seem to have treated lepra and psora like the Greeks, by bleeding, melanogogues, and abstergent applications to the skin, such as the two hellebores, lime, lupines, &c.

In the translation of Haly Abbas, leuce is correctly described by the name of *lepra*. It is represented as a whiteness sometimes affecting the whole body, and it is said to be occasioned by debility of the assimilative faculty. When the hairs are white, and the skin does not bleed when pricked with a lancet or needle, the disease is incurable. Alphos albus is described by the name of *morphea* alba, and is distinguished from the former by the whiteness being more superficial, and the colour of the hairs remaining unchanged. In the morphea nigra, that is to say the alphos niger, the colour is said to be black, owing to the prevalence of black bile, and if rubbed a furfuraceous scale falls off, and it becomes red. The lepra nigricans is described by the names of *impetigo* and *sarpedo*, as an asperity of the skin, inclining to blackness or redness, and terminating in round scales, like those of fishes. For the cure of lepra, he directs us to abstain from all articles of food which engender phlegm, to take hiera of colocynth, with pepper, &c., and also the theriac of vipers, and various other internal medicines. He recommends various external applications, containing sulphur, arsenic, hellebore, spurge, &c.

Alsaharavius describes three varieties of *morphea*. 1st. The morphea terrestris, which is attended with furfuraceous scales on the skin, and tingling. This is evidently the psora of the Greeks. 2d. The morphea alba, which consists of a more superficial whiteness of the skin than the *albaras* (leuce): this is the alphos albus. 3d. The morphea nigra, is like the former, only that the colour is black. This must be the alphos niger. All these affections he treats upon much the same principles as the Greeks, namely, by evacuants, and stimulant applications to the skin, such as sulphur, hellebore, &c. *Albaras* he describes as a deep-seated whiteness of the skin, and directs us to prick the skin with a needle, and if it does not bleed the disease is to be set down as incurable. This, of course, is the leuce of the Greeks. He treats it upon much the same principles as the morpheæ. He appears not to make any distinction between the leuce and the lepra.

Rhases describes the lepra of the Greeks by the term *impetigo*; alphos albus by that of *morphea* alba; alphos niger by that of *morphea* nigra; and leuce by that of *albaras*. There is nothing very particular in his treatment of leprosy. It may be worth while to mention, however, that he strongly recommends leeches to the affected part, at the commencement. Scabies, he says, is formed by a salt diet, old wine, and neglect of the bath. For the cure of it, he recommends bleeding, purging, and various external applications, some of which contain quicksilver, nitre, vinegar, and the like. In his 'Continens' he gives a full account of these diseases, upon the authority of preceding writers. He gives the names of *baras* to lepra, and *morphea* alba to alphos. He recommends stimulant applications containing cantharides, nitre, with vinegar, &c. He says that he had found a mixture of sal ammoniac and oil of eggs an excellent application.

It will be remarked that the leuce of the Greeks, the leuce and fourth species of impetigo of Celsus, and the albaras of most of the Arabians, are the same as the *lepra vulgaris* of Drs. Willan and Bateman; that the alphos of most of the Greek authorities and of Celsus, and the morphea alba of most of the Arabians, correspond to the *lepra alphoides* of our English nosologists; that the melas, alphos niger, and common lepra of the Greeks, Celsus' third species of impetigo and his melas, and the morphea nigra and impetigo of most of the Arabian translators, apply to the *lepra nigricans* of our modern arrangement; and that the psora of the Greeks, Celsus' second species of impetigo, and the scabies of Octavius Horatianus, and of most of the Arabian translators, comprehend both the *psoriasis* and *scabies* of Willan and Bateman.

Since many of the ancient authorities speak of *scabies* as being infectious, they must have applied the term to the true itch, with which it is not likely, as Rayer maintains, that they were wholly unacquainted.

The earlier modern writers, such as those of the Schola Salernitana, Platearius, Guy of Cauliac, and Lanfrancus, jumble together the Latin and Arabian names, so as to produce no ordinary degree of confusion. Guy of Cauliac, indeed, maintains that there is little necessity for distinguishing lepra, alphos, melas, impetigo, gutta rosacea, and such like cutaneous complaints from one another, as they are all varieties of the same disease. Lanfrancus, however, is of a different opinion. (i, 3, 6.)

III—ON LICHEN

Lichen is formed by the mixture of a thin and acrid ichor with other gross humours, and passes readily into leprosy and psora; wherefore it requires to be treated by the most desiccative applications. After general depletion, if necessary, the following simple medicines will be proper: chick-peas, hellebore, the urchin which dwells among rocks, pitch mixed with cerate and rosin, the dung of the land crocodile, that of starlings fed solely upon rice. And many have cured the complaint when occurring on the chin, or other parts of the body, by this application alone: take several grains of wheat and place upon a stithy red-hot, and taking the fluid which flows from them while yet warm, anoint the part affected with lichen. The lichen of children is to be rubbed frequently with human saliva. The gum of the plum tree, when rubbed in, is beneficial in these cases. When the complaint is protracted, the leaves of the chaste tree, triturated with vinegar, are to be applied, or the leaves of capers in like manner. The following are compound applications: Dissolve sulphur with rosemary in vinegar, or with ammoniac, and anoint. A trochisk for lichen: Of artificers' glue, dr. iv; of frankincense, dr. iij; of vinegar half a cyathus; dissolve in vinegar, and anoint.—*Another*: Of chalcitis, of gum, of each, dr. viij; of sulphur vivum, of misy, of each, dr. vj; of the flakes of copper, of acacia, of each, dr. ij; anoint with vinegar.—*Another*: Of sulphur vivum, of spuma nitri, of each, dr. iv; of the seeds of rosemary, lx; triturate with vinegar, and anoint only the part which is affected, not touching the sound skin. When dry, wash it away with cold water.—*Another*: Of white hellebore, dr. viij; of the flour of lupines, of burnt shell-fishes called buccina, of natron, of each, one chœnix; rub with it dry. They call that variety of lichen *agrius* which is nowise remedied by moderately desiccative applications, and is exacerbated by more acrid ones. These cases are therefore to be treated by applications which are sufficiently strong, without being pungent, such as this: of horned poppy, of frankincense, of alcyonium, of bitumen, of sulphur, of gum, of each, oz. j; anoint with vinegar. Boil African pitch with vinegar, and, when dissolved, anoint.—*Another*, for lichen and prurigo: Of copperas, of sulphur vivum, of natron, of frankincense, equal parts; use for lichen with vinegar, and for prurigo with wine.—*Another*, for lichen: Of ammoniac perfume, of the flour of bitter vetch, of the flour of lupines, equal parts; add to vinegar.

Commentary. See Hippocrates (de Humor., de Affect.); Galen. (Isagoge, de Med. sec. loc. v); Oribasius (Morb. Curat. iii, 59); Aëtius (viii, 16); Actuarius (Meth. Med. ii, 11); Marcellus (19); Nonnus (236); Celsus (v, 28); Pliny (H. N. xxvi, 2); Serapion (v, 2); Avicenna (iv, 7, 3, 3); Alsaharavius (Pract. xxxi, 7); Rhases (Divis. 117); Haly Abbas (Pract. iv, 10.)

Dr. Bateman states, that the exact acceptation of the term lichen cannot well be ascertained from the writings of Hippocrates; but Dr. Willan affirms that he restricted it to a papular eruption on the skin.

In the 'Isagoge,' usually ascribed to Galen, two varieties are described, the lichen mitis, and the lichen agrius, in both of which scales are formed upon the skin, which appear almost ulcerated when they are removed. They are to be cured by cholagogues internally, and liniments externally.

Galen remarks the tendency of the disease to pass into lepra and scabies. To prevent this, he directs desiccative and detergent applications, for the preparation of which he gives various prescriptions. One of these, which bears the name of Pamphilus, is a powerful escharotic, composed of orpiment, realgar, burnt copper, and cantharides. (Med. sec. loc. v.) He says it affects principally the chin, but is apt to spread over the face.

Oribasius, Aëtius, Actuarius, and Nonnus, treat of the complaint in nearly the same terms as our author. Their translators improperly render it by impetigo. Leo ascribes the origin of the disease to hot and corrupted blood.

Celsus describes the lichen of the Greeks by the name of *papula*, of which he mentions two varieties. In the first, he says, the skin is merely roughened by small pustules, is reddened and slightly corroded; the middle is somewhat smoother, and it spreads slowly, generally in a round shape. This description would seem to apply to the *lichen circumscriptus* of Drs. Bateman and Willan, although the latter author thinks that it possessed a wider signification. The second variety, he says, is called ἀγρία by the Greeks, and in it the skin is more rough, red, and corroded. The more it departs from the circular form the less tractable is it, and, unless removed, it is said to pass into impetigo. From this account it is clear that the lichen of the Greeks, in its original form, was different from impetigo. Celsus recommends friction with the saliva of a fasting person, and also mentions a composition containing natron, frankincense, sulphur, &c.

The translator of Serapion improperly renders the name of this affection by the term impetigo. His remedies are nearly the same as our author's, namely, the saliva of a person fasting, compositions containing hellebore, natron, the ashes of starlings, &c.

In the translation of Avicenna it is likewise described by the name of impetigo. It is called a species of dry achor, by which is no doubt meant papula. It is stated that it has a tendency to pass into lepra or psora. The remedies which are recommended are human saliva, the chaste tree, capers, leeches (which are not mentioned by the Greeks), likewise gum arabic dissolved in vinegar, mustard and vinegar, salt water, the roots of king's spear, &c. Haly Abbas recommends stimulant liniments of a similar kind.

Rhases briefly recommends lotions of vinegar and ammoniac, and, when it becomes inveterate, leeches, strong friction, &c. His translator also misapplies the term impetigo to it.

The lichen appears to be the cutaneous complaint which Alsaharavius describes by the name of *alcoab*. He represents it as a superficial ulceration, and mentions four species of it.

Dr. Willan confirms the statement of the ancient authorities, that the disease has a tendency to pass into lepra and psora. The species called *lichen tropicus* by Dr. Willan, seems to be the *hidroa* of Hippocrates (Aph. iii, 21); the *sudamen* of Pliny (xxiii, 45); one of the *essere* of Haly Abbas (Theor. viii, 17); one of the *alsara* of Alsaharavius (Pract. xxx, 8); and the *hasef* of Avicenna (iv, 7, 3, 8). See also Galen's 'Commentary' (v, 261); ed. Basil. Galen says it is attended with pruritus, asperity, and ulceration. Avicenna and Rhases particularly commend bleeding, cleansing the skin, and the cold bath. Most of Rhases' authorities in his 'Continens,' recommend for the *asaf*, or sudamen, cooling and astringent applications, containing roses, myrtles, galls, sandals, camphor, and the like. They attribute the complaint to profuse perspiration. In certain cases, Rhases directs us to allay the pruritus or tingling, with hot water and the flesh of melons. He also approves of purging with tamarinds and myrobalans. (Cont. xxxvi.) See also ad Mansor. (v, 30). Mercurialis is of opinion that Virgil alludes to the sudamina in the following lines:

> "Verum etiam invisos si quis tentarat amictus,
>
> Ardentes papulæ atque immundus olentia sudor
>
> Membra sequebatur."

(Georg. iii, 565.)

We shall briefly notice in this place the singular disease of the face which prevailed in the Roman empire during the reign of Tiberius, called *mentagra* by Pliny, in his curious description of it, but which he says was named *lichenes* by some. He represents it as a contagious disease, which was readily propagated by kissing. It attacked principally the higher class, the lower and middle ranks and women having generally escaped it. The seat of it was commonly the chin, but it sometimes spread over the whole face, and affected even the neck, breast, and hands. The only means of cure was burning with caustics down to the bone. (H. N. xxxvii; see also Marcellus, 19.) We are inclined to think that it must have been some variety of elephantiasis. Modern authorities have ranked it under *sycosis*, but it would appear to have been a much more intractable disease. The sycosis is distinctly described by Celsus, among the diseases of the hairy parts. He recommends for it elaterium, linseed, or figs boiled in water, &c. (vi, 3.)

IV—ON PRURITUS, OR PRURIGO

The prurigo occurring in old age is not to be thoroughly cured, but may be alleviated by the remedies mentioned below: but that which arises from a cacochymy in other ages, is to be cured by evacuation, being formed by a bilious or pituitous humour that has become putrid, or by a saltish one. It is known by attending to the age, temperament, diet, season of the year, situation, and the like. If, therefore, it appear to prevail in the blood contained in the veins, we must begin with venesection; but if it offend rather by its quality, we must evacuate it by corresponding medicines, and turn our attention to external applications. Wherefore we must use the bath at all times before a meal; and sometimes, after eating a little, it may be used a second time, for the affection is of difficult humectation. They are to be rubbed with the decoction of fenugreek, or of beet, or of barley-meal, or of wild or of garden mallows, or of ptisan; and along with these may be joined the flour of beans, or of lupines, or of myrobalan (ben), or of the detergent ointment called *peponaton*. If it is protracted, we may use the bath in like manner, and foment with the decoction of sage, of tamarisk, of the herb mercury, of marjoram, of pennyroyal, of bay berries, of the root of the wild cucumber, of capers, of strained ley, of vinegar and brine; and then the parts are to be sprinkled with dried natron, or with the lees of vinegar, or with the composition containing of spuma nitri one sextarius, of rosemary, of sulphur vivum, of each, lb. j, of cimolian earth, lb. ss; or this: of aphronitrum, of sulphur vivum, of burnt alcyonium, equal parts; to be used dry, or with some of the decoctions already mentioned; and, if you please, sprinkle some dried hellebore, without grease. But rub in with vinegar and oil, stavesacre pulverized, or sulphur, or red arsenic, or all together; or mustard, with the refuse of expressed myrobalan, and vinegar and oil; or with snails burnt and triturated with honey or the roots of dock, or the detergent ointments prepared from them, as described under the head of Elephantiasis; or with some of the applications for scabies. If the parts become ulcerated, use the plaster called parygron, or that prepared from pompholyx; or melt oz. j of wax in a cyathus of oil of privet, and sprinkle upon it of sulphur vivum oz. j. *Another* application for prurigo: Of large nuts in a rancid state, oz. j; of sulphur, oz. j; triturate with the juice of parsley, and use in the bath with much friction. This alone has proved sufficient for the cure of many cases of scabies and prurigo; and green parsley by itself, when pounded and rubbed in while the patient is in the bath, has been of great service: and in like manner, pellitory of the wall and maple rosin dissolved with rose oil, and rubbed in.—*Another*: Bruise three ounces of pure and very white rice, and, having strained, triturate with strong vinegar until it become of the thickness of the sordes of the oil in baths; and adding separately of sulphur vivum pulverized, oz. j; and mixing properly, use in the bath with much friction. When there is a greater redundance of humours, it will be better to mix the ingredients in equal proportions.

Commentary. See Hippocrates (Aphor. iii, 31); Galen (Comment. et alibi); Oribasius (Morb. Curat. iii, 22); Aëtius (xiv, 20); Actuarius (Meth. Med. ii, 11); Nonnus (237); Alexander Aphrodisiensis (Probl. i, 24); Myrepsus (pluries); Pliny (xxviii, 5); Octavius Horatianus (i, 31); Marcellus (de Med. 4); Isidorus (Orig. iv, 8); Serapion (v, 6); Avicenna (iv, 7, 3, 6); Haly Abbas (Theor. viii, 17, and Pract. iv, 6); Alsaharavius (Pract. xxxi, 5); Rhases (Divis. 121); Avenzoar (ii, 7, 2.)

The prurigo of Dr. Willan is here distinctly described, and a suitable method of treatment recommended.

Hippocrates remarks that prurigo is common in old age. The reason which Galen assigns for this is, that the superfluities of the system are then not properly discharged by the skin. He says in another place, that pruritus may either be produced by external substances, such as nettles, squills, &c., or it may arise from indigestion and the neglect of cleanliness.

Oribasius gives an account of the disease not very different from our author's. Among other applications, he recommends one consisting of opium mixed with liquid cerate.

Aëtius speaks highly of the sulphureous bath for the cure of this disease.

Actuarius characterizes the disease very well, when he says that it is allied to lichen, and that when rubbed either nothing runs from the place, or some slight humidity of various colour and consistence. He assigns, as a reason for its frequency in old age, that the pores of the skin then get constricted.

Alexander Aphrodisiensis assigns, as the reason why the warm bath proves useful in cases of pruritus, that it dispels the phlegm, which is the cause of the complaint.

Celsus gives a particular account of scabies, but says nothing of prurigo.

Octavius Horatianus recommends us, when the patient is young, to bleed, purge, and use baths medicated with frankincense, natron and sulphur. He also says that the cold bath, and friction with the oil of roses, myrtles, &c., will do much good.

Isidorus uses the term prurigo: "Prurigo vocatur perurendo et ardendo." Marcellus also uses this term, and recommends much the same substances as the others.

This affection is clearly described by the Arabians, and is rendered pruritus by most of their translators. Serapion recommends us, if there is a sanguineous plethora, to bleed, and then to purge with myrobalans, colocynth, and black hellebore, and along with these the warm bath is to be used, and the liniments for removing the pruritus, containing vinegar, roses, nitre, &c. The prurigo senilis he pronounces to be incurable. Rhases and Avicenna recommend similar remedies. They treat of prurigo and scabies together, and there is no doubt of their alliance. Hence Bateman says that prurigo, when neglected, terminates in scabies. Haly Abbas says that scabies and prurigo arise from a saltish phlegm. Scabies, he says, consists of reddish pustules, which appear most frequently between the fingers and upon the arms. Prurigo, he adds, is apt to run into scabies. He recommends, as a lotion, vinegar with rose-oil, the use of the warm-bath, and other remedies like those of our author. Alsaharavius says that the disease arises from debility of the expulsive faculty of the body or constriction of the pores. He praises highly the hot bath. Avenzoar states that pruritus arises from bile or a sharpness of the blood.

Our author has omitted to treat of *phthiriasis*, for an account of which see in particular Cælius Aurelianus (de Tard. Pass. iv, 2); also, Aristot. (Hist. An. v, 32); Galen (de Comp. Med. sec. loc. i, 8); Pliny (Hist. Nat. xxvi, 86); Haly Abbas (Pract. iv, 7); Plutarchus (in Vitâ Syllæ.) The authorities quoted by Rhases recommend compositions consisting of stavesacre, white hellebore, arsenic, nitre, sulphur, sublimed mercury, and the like. (Contin. xxxvi.) Antiochus, Herod of Judæa, Philip II of Spain, and many other celebrated personages, are said to have died of phthiriasis. Virey accounts for the disease in the following manner: "Il est, en effet, tel tempérament muqueux, telle dégénération des humeurs lymphatiques, dans le phthiriasis ou la maladie pédiculaire, que ces insectes y trouvent une pâture inépuisable, qu'ils se propagent avec une extrême exubérance sous le peau, pénétrent dans le tissu cellulaire, et établissent d'énormes colonies parmi les ulcères qu'ils y forment." (Hist. des Mœurs des Anim. ii, 207.) Aldrovandi gives a very full history of phthiriasis. (De Insectis, v.)

V—ON LEUCE

Leuce is a change of the skin to a white colour, occasioned by a viscid and glutinous phlegm. Since all the kinds of leuce are not curable, you may form a diagnosis of it in this manner. Pierce the leuce superficially, not deeper than the skin, with a needle, and if blood flow, the complaint may be cured; but if a milky moisture be discharged, it is incurable. Or, rub it with a rough woollen rag, and if the part become red, the complaint may be cured; but if it remain of the same colour, it cannot be cured. And those kinds which attack a great part of the body are to be supposed more difficult to cure than those which are confined to a small space, and old cases than recent. Some, therefore, in leuce, have approved of burning by iron, consisting simply of the application of heat. Others, dreading the pain of burning, and the scar arising from it, as being no less unseemly than leuce itself, have had recourse to escharotic medicines, such as they say will produce a scar of the natural colour. Others rejecting all these things on account of the difficulty of their application, have used dyes (paying more consideration to the deception than the utility which they produce,) which are, of all others, the most to be rejected, owing to the speedy renewal of the affection. We must use, then, the under-mentioned remedial powers: Of adarce, of rosemary seed, of sulphur vivum, of each, equal parts; bruise and strain singly, and then, having triturated together for a sufficient number of days, anoint in the sun, but not in great quantity, lest the skin be ulcerated; and, after some time, a little hellebore and galls may be added in like manner.—*Another*: Macerate the tops of the black fig in vinegar, and having triturated, mix equal parts of aphronitrum, sulphur vivum, and the fruit of tamarisk, and having rubbed natron into the part, anoint and expose to the sun, taking care lest an ulcer be produced. But Archigenes having mixed a sufficiency of quicklime with fig-leaves, used them in like manner: or, he says, having rubbed the leuce with white hellebore until the part perspire and become of the same colour as the rest of the body, anoint with sinopis or melian earth; or, having perforated them with needles until they bleed, anoint with sinopis in vinegar; or, having first rubbed them as formerly said, anoint with the fresh juice of figs, or rub in so much with the leaves of it.

Commentary. In the second Section we have stated so fully the nature of the leuce, and the difference between it and its cognate affections, that it will be unnecessary for us now to resume the subject. It is there mentioned that leuce is Celsus' third species of vitiligo, and the *baras* of all the Arabian translators, with the exception of Stephanus Antiochensis, the translator of Haly Abbas, who applies the term *lepra* to it. It was therefore the white species of leprosy. All the medical authorities represent it as an intractable disease, not only the cuticle being altered in structure, but also the flesh below, and even the hairs, having undergone a change of colour. All direct us to prick the skin with a needle, and, if it bleed, the cure is to be attempted; but if a slight colourless fluid issue from it, the case is to be abandoned as hopeless. They consider it as arising from debility of the assimilative faculty of the part which can no longer convert the nutritive juices into their proper consistence. All recommend nearly the same treatment. The diet is to be regulated with a strict abstinence from gross food; if there be plethora, venesection is to be premised; then drastic purgatives and emetics are to be given, and the parts affected are to be rubbed with stimulant and caustic applications, containing hellebore, nitre, sulphur, misy, red arsenic, &c., or even the actual cautery may be applied. In short, all treat the disease in nearly the same manner as our author. (See in particular Serapion and Avicenna.)

Aristotle, we believe, is the first Greek writer who makes mention of leuce. He calls it a disease in which all the hairs of the body turn white. (Hist. Nat. iii, 11.)

"The snow-white leprosy" of the ancient Jews was the leuce of the Greeks. Moses describes very correctly the method of distinguishing it from the alphos and melas; (Leviticus, c. xiii.) The symptoms of leuce are given in the 3d verse; of the alphos in the 4th; of the melas in the 6th. He calls it contagious, which might lead us to suspect that elephantiasis was mixed up with the leprosy of the Jews. This opinion is further confirmed from what is mentioned by Josephus of its being said that his countrymen were driven out of Egypt because they were affected with leprosy. (See also Justin. xxxvi, 20, and Tacit. Hist. v, 3.) Now we know that elephantiasis was endemial in that country. (See chap. i.) The English translation of this chapter is very inaccurate, the translators having evidently failed to recognize the nice distinction between cognate diseases, laid down by the Jewish legislator.

Leuce is still common in tropical climates. Negroes affected with it are called Albinos. It is merely an aggravated variety of the *Lepra vulgaris*.

VI—ON WHITE AND BLACK ALPHI

The formation of alphos is similar to that of leuce, but the latter produces a deep change of the skin, so that the hairs grow of a similar colour, whilst the alphi affect the skin superficially, except that when continued, they extend more deeply, so that the hairs grow white, owing to the humour which causes it. From the pituitous humour then they are produced white, but black from the melancholic. Wherefore, a common application for both is washed lime dissolved in water, or, the root of dracunculus applied with vinegar; in like manner, either species of hellebore, the decoction of bitter lupines poured on the part, and their flour when applied as a cataplasm with vinegar or oxymel, the bark of the root of capers with vinegar, the root of lily with honey, onions with vinegar rubbed into the part in the sun, the dung of the land crocodile, and in like manner, that of starlings, when they are fed solely upon rice, and the burnt shells of the cuttle-fish. The following is a compound application: of alcyonium, of natron, of each, oz. ij; of white hellebore, of sulphur vivum, of each, oz. j; and some also add the burnt lees of wine.—*Another*: Of sulphur vivum, of the spuma nitri, of each, dr. iv; rosemary seeds, vij; triturate with vinegar. But rub only the part affected with alphos, not touching the unaffected parts, and when dry, wash with cold water.—*Another*: Of the flour of lupines, of buccina, and natron, of each, a chænix; of white hellebore, dr. viij; rub with it in a dry state.—*Another*: Of the flour of bitter vetches, lb. ij; of the seeds of rocket, of bitter almonds, of the root of the wild cucumber, of each, lb. j; triturate with wine and honey and anoint, and after an interval of an hour wipe it away with a sponge. It applies also for freckles, warts, and other spots on the skin.

A tried remedy for white alphos: of sulphur vivum, ii sextarii, of quicklime whitened, oz. iv; five whites of eggs, of nard-oil and vinegar, a small quantity. The sulphur is first pounded, then we add to it the oil of nard, and again triturate; then the vinegar is poured in, and the mixture is again triturated. But the quicklime is to be washed separately, once, twice, and thrice, and then we add it to the sulphur with the white of the eggs and triturate; and we pour out the collected fluid; but leaving a small quantity so that the ointment may admit of anointing, we use it thus.—*Another* tried remedy: Take sulphur vivum, dried fig leaves, aphronitrum, alcyonium, Cimolian earth, and myrtle, use with vinegar.—*Another* of Archigenes: Rub in equal parts of fig leaves dried in the shade, of sulphur, and of alum with vinegar, or of fig leaves, dr. iv; of nitre, dr. ij; of burnt alcyonium, dr. ij; anoint with vinegar in the bath. But red arsenic with one half of sulphur is excellent for removing the black alphos; thus having cleansed the part with natron, anoint with it in the sun. For white alphos: of copperas, of verdigris equal parts, of natron the double, rub without fat: or, of rosemary seeds, of sulphur vivum, of adarce, equal parts; triturate with vinegar, rub, and anoint; but when it is dry, bathe by rubbing. This applies also to the white species.

Commentary. We have again to refer the reader to the second chapter for an account of these complaints, and an exposition of the differences between them and the affections to which they are allied. It will be seen that they are varieties of the genus vitiligo of Celsus, and that they bear a near resemblance to leuce, from which they are chiefly distinguished as being mere superficial affections of the skin. The Arabians treat of them under the names of morphea alba and nigra. Dr. Willan makes them to be varieties of lepra, in which opinion we fully coincide with him.

The description of the two diseases by Actuarius is so precise that we shall give it in lieu of all the others. The alphi, he says, are superficial, but sometimes extend in depth, so that the hairs appear of the same colour.

The white species is tried as to the depth it has spread, by being pricked moderately with a needle; when blood flows though the needle has only penetrated the skin, the disease is curable, but if the discharge be milky it is incurable, inasmuch as the flesh is converted into the disease. Others, he adds, rub the part with rough towels, and if it become red they have good hopes, but if it remain of the same colour they abandon all hopes of recovery. They are of a more aggravated nature when they affect different parts of the body and are inveterate. The alphi, he says, are generally milder than leuce, and can be cured by gentler means, but when they become inveterate they require similar treatment. The difference between the white and the black alphos is produced by the colour of the prevailing humour.

There is scarcely any difference of opinion among the authorities respecting the general plan of treatment. Haly Abbas has correctly remarked, that the alphi are to be cured by the same sort of remedies as lepra (leuce?) only that they do not require so strong applications. The Arabians greatly commend their myrobalans with ginger, mastich, parsley, &c. Their internal applications are powerful detergents and escharotics, such as hellebore, natron, sulphur, vinegar, arsenic, copperas, &c. Celsus says nothing of internal remedies, but recommends external applications of a stimulant nature, containing sulphur, alum, nitre, frankincense, alcyonium, &c. In the 'Isagoge' it is said that all these complaints are to be cured by phlegmagogues, and by abstergent applications externally.

Guy of Cauliac, and the other medical authorities of that age, describe these diseases by the names of *Morphea* alba and *M.* nigra. They recommend applications containing sulphur, alum, natron, arsenic, and the like. As usual they are the mere copyists of the Arabians.

VII—ON STIGMATA, FROM THE WORKS OF ARCHIGENES

You may remove stigmata by rubbing in that which sticks to a chamber-pot, along with the most acrid vinegar, or rub of quicklime, p. j; of red natron toasted, p. ss; with water, in the sun: but when it ulcerates let it be healed like an ulcer. But Crito says, for stigmata, having first scrubbed the part with nitre (soda), cover it with an application of turpentine; then having bound it, let it remain for six days, and on the seventh perforate the stigma with a needle, and having wiped away the blood with a sponge, after a little time rub with some powdered salt. Then, having applied the medicine, allow it to remain for five days. It is this: of frankincense, of natron, of the lye of quicklime, of wax, of each, dr. iv; of honey, dr. viij; having loosed it, you will find the blackness upon the application.—*Another* ointment: Of pepper, dr. ij; of rue, dr. iv; of realgar, dr. iv; of orpiment, dr. j; of honey, q. s. Anoint with it, have previously scrubbed the part with natron, and done otherwise in like manner as for the former. Taking it away after three days, and cleaning away the blackness, anoint with it again; for, he says, it removes the complaint in twenty days, without ulceration or cicatrix.—*Another* called Criticum: Of frankincense, dr. iv; of nitre, dr. ij; of copperas, dr. iv; of wax, dr. vj; of pepper, dr. iij; of lime, dr. iij; of thapsia, dr. iij; of orpiment, dr. iss; of realgar, dr. iij; of honey, q. s; use as the former. Oribasius says, that crowfoot (ranunculus) if applied, or the leaves of capers, take away the marks. But if they be deep seated upon only a small extent of skin, form an eschar by a cold cautery, and thus remove them.

Commentary. Consult Aëtius (viii, 12); Actuarius (Meth. Med. vi, 8); Scribonius Largus (§ 231); Avicenna (iv, 7, 2, 7); Pseudo-Dioscor. (Eupor. i, 116.)

Aëtius explains that by stigmata are meant the marks of injuries on the face or any part of the body. To eradicate them he recommends compositions containing quicklime, natron, arsenic, &c.

The Pseudo-Dioscorides recommends the ranunculus, the juice of the leaves of capers, or that of mandragora, &c.

Actuarius copies from our author.

Scribonius Largus mentions a composition containing garlic, cantharides, sulphur, chalcitis, &c.

Avicenna recommends friction with natron and the other substances mentioned by our author.

Dr. Willan defines the stigma, "a small speck on the skin, occasioning no elevation of the cuticle." The ancient authorities, it will be perceived, apply the term in a wider sense.

VIII—ON EXANTHEMATA

Exanthemata are formed by thick humours impacted in the skin, and more especially if the cuticle be thick. In these cases, then, even if the humours are deep-seated, they must be first purged away; for unless you do this in the first place, before attempting to dispel them, you will only impact them the more firmly, instead of evacuating them by the skin. But if the deep-seated parts be free from crudities, you may evacuate the humours by the skin, and not produce revulsion of them to a distance, which is the case, if you attempt to evacuate them by the belly or emetics. But the cure of humours fixed in the skin, is to be accomplished by fomentations and calefacients, more especially when the exanthemata happen to be broad, for these are formed by a cold and thick humour. Wherefore, take of the tender leaves of bay, of manna, and of rue equal parts, triturate together, and dissolving frankincense in honey, anoint with it; or, having boiled and pounded tender beet, apply as a cataplasm; or, take of wax, dr. viij; of sulphur the same quantity; of salt, dr. vj; triturate them dry, and having poured on them half a cyathus of oil, boil all together, and use the plaster that is formed. But one must attentively sit by while the boiling is going on. It is a very excellent medicine.

Commentary. See Hippocrates (Epidem. et alibi); Galen (Meth. Med. v); Alexander (i, 5); Oribasius (Synops. vii, 7); Morb. Curat. (iii, 21); Aëtius (v, 129); Actuarius (Meth. Med. ii, 11; i, 23); Celsus (v, 28); Pseudo-Dioscor. (Euporist. i, 106); Haly Abbas (Theor. viii, 17; Pract. iv, 8).

As stated in another place, the Greeks used the term exanthema in a much laxer signification than it is applied in Dr. Willan's 'System of Cutaneous Diseases.' Hippocrates in particular may be mentioned as applying it to various classes of these affections. Alexander describes the exanthemata of the head as superficial ulcerations, which are red and rough. Does he allude to porrigo? He recommends for the cure of them a composition of litharge, ceruse, alum, the green leaves of rue, vinegar, and myrtle oil.

Galen says that exanthemata is a term applied by some to all ulcerative and rough affections of the skin, which, according to Archigenes, stand in need of desiccative applications. In another place he mentions the exanthemata as a common symptom of the plague. Aëtius in like manner gives from Herodotus an interesting account of fevers which are accompanied with exanthemata. Both have been supposed to allude to the smallpox, but we agree with Dr. Willan, that this interpretation of their descriptions is altogether fanciful.

Our author follows Oribasius closely.

According to Actuarius exanthemata, properly speaking, are produced by thick humours either formed in the skin or in the whole body, and being detained by the density of the epidermis.

Celsus describes the exanthemata under the generic term pustulæ. His words are: "Earum plura genera sunt. Nam modo circa totum corpus partemve asperitudo quædam fit, similis iis pustulis, quæ ex urticâ, vel ex sudore nascuntur: ἐξανθήματα Græci vocant. Eæque modo rubent, modo colorem cutis non excedunt." For pustules of all kinds he recommends exercise, restricted diet, and abstinence from all things of an acrid and attenuant nature, which regimen is likewise to be enforced upon the nurse, if the child be at the breast. If the patient be strong, he is also to be put into the hot bath, and rubbed with natron and a mixture of wine and oil. If this treatment does not succeed lentils are to be applied, especially if the pustules be large; and after the outer skin has been removed they are to be treated with gentle applications. Such is the plan of cure recommended by the great Roman authority. His directions respecting the diet are particularly important, and appear to be quite in accordance with the practice of the modern physicians, who recommend the *half-starving system* in all such complaints.

For red exanthemata the Pseudo-Dioscorides recommends ceruse with oil of bays and sulphur, pure bark with wax, &c.

The exanthemata are described by the name of pustulæ parvæ in most of the translations of the Arabians. The exanthemata is, we think, the first species of *Serie* described by Haly Abbas.

For the opinions of Alsaharavius and Haly Abbas about the exanthemata of infancy, see Book i, 6.

Dr. Willan thinks that the nettle-rash was comprehended under the term exanthemata. He is also of opinion that the *benat noctis* of Avicenna is the nettle-rash. It would appear, however, that the *benat noctis* was the same as the *sera* or *epinyctis*. See Rhases (Cont. xxxvi, 2). The symptoms of it are said to be itching, roughness of the skin, and small eruptions attacking the patient during the night.

Thucydides, Hippocrates, and Galen mention exanthemata as a common symptom of the plague.

We may take the present occasion to mention that none of the Greek or Latin authorities has given any distinct account of *purpura*. Avicenna has briefly described it in its chronic form. (iv, 3, 1, 8).

IX—ON EPINYCTIDES

Epinyctides are small ulcers breaking out spontaneously on the skin, in the form of bullæ, reddish, and when broken, discharging a bloody ichor. These are not very troublesome during the day, but at night, they are more painful than the smallness of the ulcer would bespeak. Wherefore, having dissolved the juice of laserwort in water, apply it; for it is desiccative without being pungent; or, having levigated hemlock, apply it; or crude cabbage with water, or triturate parsley with polenta, and apply; or, triturate the leaves of henbane with honey, and apply; or, strychnos by itself, and with the green coriander; or, use the leaves of olives boiled with water; or, having triturated raisins deprived of their stones, and spread them upon a splenium or oblong pledget, apply; or triturate maiden-hair with honey. They must avoid all acrid, acid, and saltish things, also fomentations, baths, and insolation.

Commentary. Celsus (v, 28); Aëtius (xiv, 61); Oribasius (Morb. Curat. iii, 54); Actuarius (Meth. Med. ii, 11; vi, 8); Pollux (Onomasticon iv, 24); Avicenna (iv, 3, 1, 13); Serapion (v, 8); Haly Abbas (Theor. viii, 17); Pract. (iv, 8); Rhases (Divis. i, 122.)

Celsus describes the epinyctis as a bad species of pustule, somewhat livid or red, about the size of a bean, very painful and inflamed, and coming on principally at night, whence it derives its name. Persons of all ages, even infants at the breast, are subject to it, and in treating them he directs the regimen of the nurse to be properly attended to. In laying down the rules of treatment he puts particular stress upon the hot bath.

Aëtius, Oribasius, and Actuarius treat of it as our author. Pollux defines it to be a vesicle of a palish colour, somewhat humid and bloody, and forming about the legs and feet in the night.

The Arabians give a similar account of epinyctis, under the names of Sare, Serie, and Essere. Thus Serapion recommends bleeding if required by the general symptoms, purging with myrobalans and prunes; and external applications, containing sumach, savin, &c. Haly Abbas, who describes it as one of his serie, approves of much the same treatment. Avicenna and Rhases in like manner recommend bleeding, gentle purgatives, cooling lotions, and the tepid bath. Rhases, in his 'Continens,' applies the directions given in this chapter by Paulus to the treatment of the cutaneous disease, which he calls sera. This establishes their identity (xxxvi, 6.) As stated in the preceding chapter, the epinyctis is also the "benat noctis," i. e. "filia noctis" of the Arabians. Marcus Aurelius Severinus, therefore, is mistaken in distinguishing between the epinyctis and the benat noctis. Ingrassius admits their identity.

Fracastorius gives the following account of this affection: "Si inflammata et accensa sit cholera, pustulam illam facit, quæ ἐπινυκτις vocatur, quod sæpissime noctu nascatur, Arabes Essere appellant." (De Morb. Cont. ii, 15.) Both Lorry and Rayer confess themselves unable to determine what the epinyctis of the ancients was. It would appear to have been some peculiar species of eczema, now extinct. It must have been a more formidable disease than the nettle-rash, which certain modern authorities have taken for the *epinyctis* of the ancients.

X—ON PHLYCTÆNÆ OR BULLÆ

As Bullæ when they burst spontaneously are attended with acute pain, it is proper to perforate at their under part with a sharp needle, and then to squeeze out the humour gently, suffering the skin which covers it to remain. And if the wound should close up and the bullæ fill up, it is to be evacuated again in like manner, and pressed out; and the incumbent skin is to be kept pressed down until the ulcer below be healed. Before the bullæ break, apply boiled lentils triturated with water; or, the shoots of pomegranate, having been warmed upon hot coals, are to be applied, so as to burn the parts. But if they burst and form an ulcer, having melted axunge, and mixed levigated litharge, put into a linen cloth, and apply; or, having boiled the root of lily in water, triturate it with cerate, and apply.

For epinyctis and phlyctæna. Having triturated equal portions of litharge and sulphur vivum with vinegar and myrtle-oil, until it become of the thickness of the sordes of baths, rub with oil and wine. For hot eruptions, warm papulæ, achores, incipient furunculus, and burns, the composition of plumbago, and that from eggs is applicable.

Commentary. See Aëtius (xiv, 63); Oribasius (Morb. Curat. iii, 23); Actuarius (Meth. Med. vi, 8); Avicenna (iii, 3, 1, 11.)

This appears to be the pompholyx of Drs. Willan and Bateman. Aëtius remarks, that the disease principally attacks women whose menses are obstructed. (Bateman says, "it seems to affect only women.") He recommends emmenagogues, laxatives, and diuretics, and forbids all acrid things.

Our author copies the whole from Oribasius. Actuarius recommends nearly the same applications.

Celsus describes the phlyctænæ as a variety of the pustulæ. There is nothing particular in the treatment recommended by Avicenna.

Thucydides mentions small phlyctænæ and ulcers among the symptoms of the plague of Athens. (De Bello Pelopon. ii.) Hippocrates gives the name of *pemphyx* to the cutaneous eruption, by which the plague of Athens was distinguished. (Epidem. vi.) See Galen's Comment. (v, 453, ed. Basil.) Procopius also takes notice of black phlyctænæ among the symptoms of the great plague which raged in the reign of Justinian (Pers. ii.) See also Diodorus Siculus (Biblioth. xiv.) Some suppose, however, that by phlyctænæ were meant petechie. See Prælect. Marc. p. 301.

XI—ON BURNS

Burnt parts require applications which are moderately detergent, without being decidedly heating or cooling. Wherefore, Chian, Cimolian, Cretan, and every light earth, when rubbed in with vinegar not very acrid, or mixed with water, are excellent applications, and prevent blisters from forming; also a whole raw egg immediately applied upon soft wool, for it cools moderately, and dries without being stimulant. And anoint the part with black ink, or with frankincense dissolved in water, or use a cataplasm of boiled lentils, or of tares. For burning with hot water, before blisters arise, pour frequently on the part the brine of pickled olives, or apply olives themselves triturated with polenta; or, triturate stone-alum with vinegar, and rub it in; or, anoint with bull's gall dissolved with much water; or, pour on the part strained ley with sauce of pickles, or brine; or, triturate the bulbous roots of lilies, hyacinths, or narcissi with rose-oil, and having made it of the consistence of the sordes of oil in baths, anoint with it. But Marcellus gives the following composition: having smeared a rag with honey, and wrapped it around barley, burn it, and mix of the ashes, dr. viij; of ceruse, dr. iv; of butter, dr. viij; of wax, dr. xvj; of goat's fat, dr. xvj; of rose-oil, dr. xvj. For burnt parts already blistered, having triturated sumach and polenta with vinegar, apply it; or, mix quicklime with cerate, put it on a rag, and apply. And the medicine called Sphæria is applicable in such cases. The parts which are ulcerated, may be covered with pounded leeks; or, triturate purslain with polenta, and apply; or, put pigeon's dung into a rag of linen, burn it, and mix the ashes with oil, and use; (this is an excellent application:) also the bark of pine and of spruce fir, or dried maiden-hair levigated, or the burnt leaves of myrtle, are to be triturated and sprinkled upon the part. Each of these things answers well, when applied with cerate. But a good application is formed by triturating together of the dried roots of the red alkanet, oz. iv; of white wax, oz. ix; of rose-oil, oz. xviij; and also that made of ceruse, with a small quantity of stag's marrow.

Commentary. See Hippocrates (de Ulceribus.) Celsus (v, 27); Galen (de Simpl. Med. et alibi.) Aëtius (xiv, 64); Pseudo-Dioscor. (Euporist. i, 178); Actuarius (Meth. Med. vi, 6, 8); Nonnus (240); Serapion (v, 11); Avicenna (iv, 4, 2, 12); Haly Abbas (Pract. 4, 25); Alsaharavius (xxix, 2, 8); Rhases (Antid. i, 27); (ad Mansor. vii, 18); (Div. i, 136.) The author of the Hippocratic treatise referred to above, recommends various applications to burns, such as old axunge rubbed into the part, and the root of squills applied above; or a mixture of old axunge, rosin, and bitumen, spread upon a rag and heated at the fire; or the roots of the ilex boiled in white wine at a gentle fire until it be of the consistence of a liniment.

Dioscorides, Avicenna, and Galen, agree in praising Cimolian earth as an application to recent burns. Galen says that copperas, especially when dissolved in vinegar, forms an excellent application for the ulcers occasioned by burning.

Aëtius treats burns upon nearly the same principles as our author. When blisters rise he forbids an early opening to be made in them. As an application to them he recommends alum with water and the white of an egg. Some of his applications can only be supposed proper for the foul ulcers left by burning. Such is that consisting of verdigris and litharge, pounded with wine and oil. For healing ulcers he recommends a composition containing ceruse, litharge, toasted barley pounded, wax, and rose or myrtle oil.

In the 'Euporista' Cimolian earth, litharge and oil, and many other applications are recommended.

Actuarius recommends a composition of litharge, ceruse, wax, turpentine, and some other articles of less importance. We need scarcely mention how much the oil of turpentine has been used of late in such cases. He praises such things as are moderately astringent, such as alum dissolved in vinegar, &c.

Celsus recommends at first such things as are, "mediocriter exedentia reprimentiaque," and afterwards articles of a soothing nature. To the former class belong the farina of lentils and honey; myrrh with urine, or the Cimolian chalk, with the bark of frankincense; and to the latter belong all fatty applications, and such things as contain the dross of lead and the yelks of eggs. He also mentions turpentine rosin, as an application to foul ulcers from burning.

Serapion, like our author, recommends applications which are moderately detergent, and neither very calefacient nor refrigerant. He gives the following directions for making a preparation from lime. Take of lime, seven times washed in sweet water and dried, oz. viij; of wax, oz. ij; of oil of roses, oz. vj: let the wax be melted along with the oil, and well mixed with lime. This is to be rubbed into the part. He also gives a prescription for preparing a mixture of lime-water and oil, exactly similar to that which is now used in cases of burns. (vii, 28.) Avicenna, with his usual accuracy, lays down very particular rules for the treatment of burns. To prevent blisters from rising he recommends cooling things; when the burning is occasioned by hot water, he directs us to apply sandals, rose-water, and camphor: or a cloth dipped in congealed water is to be kept constantly applied, and it will prevent blisters from rising. Most of the applications recommended by our author are also mentioned by him. Haly Abbas directs us to apply a cloth cooled in rose-water. He also speaks of the ointment of lime and rose-oil, mentioned above. When the burning is not severe, Alsaharavius directs us in the first place to wash the part with vinegar and salt, and then to sprinkle upon it the flour of barley or of oats. Then if blisters do not rise, but there is a sensation of burning in the part, he recommends us to apply cloths dipped in cold water, rose-water, or snow-water, which are to be changed frequently. Afterwards some emollient applications, such as the white of an egg, with gum arabic is to be used. When the burning is more severe, he recommends us to bleed and use a cooling application, such as the brain of a sheep, the white of an egg mixed with rose-oil, or an ointment made of white wax and rose-oil. He also makes mention of the application from lime. Rhases recommends an ointment containing ceruse, camphor, opium, &c. Like Avicenna, he directs us to apply at first a cloth wetted in cold water, or in rose-water, which has been cooled with snow. If the burning be extensive he recommends venesection, with a cooling and attenuant diet. When the pain is great he directs us to apply the yelks of eggs mixed with rose-oil. When a large ulcer is formed, he directs us to dress it with the ointment of lime, described above. He also approves of a white ointment, consisting of ceruse, oil of roses, and wax. In his 'Continens,' he relates a case of severe burning, which he treated with liniments composed of sandals, camphor, and roses; a cloth wetted in snow-water being applied externally to it. He approves of opening the blisters. To prevent them from forming, he recommends strongly an astringent collyrium of galls. Like many of the other authorities, he recommends Cimolian earth very much. The applications recommended by Haly Abbas are of a refrigerant and cooling nature, such as Armenian earth in vinegar, the white of an egg, ceruse, &c.

The earlier modern authors treat burns upon the plan laid down by the ancients, more especially the Arabians. Thus Guy, of Cauliac, recommends us in cases of extensive burning to have recourse to venesection, along with a cooling and attenuant regimen. As a local application, he recommends a cloth wetted in rose-oil congealed in snow, and afterwards cooling ointments containing ceruse, litharge, and the like. He approves of opening the blisters, of afterwards dressing the part with desiccative remedies, such as the ointment of lime, seven times slaked. (Tr. vi, Doct. C. 6.)

XII—FOR THOSE BEATEN WITH SCOURGES

Take of ceruse and litharge equal parts, of wax four parts, use as a plaster with the oleum susinum, or rose-oil; but on the first day use the susinum separately; or, of saffron, dr. j; of tragacanth, dr. j; unite with them a whole egg, without the shell, and use. For those who have been scourged, the skin of a sheep newly taken off, when applied while yet warm, of all remedies cures the soonest, effecting this purpose in a day and a night.

Commentary. See Aëtius (xiv, 62); Avicenna (iv, 4, 2, 7); Haly Abbas (Pract. iv, 26); Alsaharavius (Pract. xxxi, 2, 1); Rhases (Contin. xxviii.)

Aëtius gives similar directions. The following is said to be an excellent application for the stripes of a whip: mix washed lime with raw eggs, and add some rose cerate. Aëtius, Galen, Nonnus, Avicenna, Rhases, Haly Abbas, and Alsaharavius join our author in recommending the fresh skin of a newly-killed sheep as an application in such cases. Alsaharavius recommends an ointment containing white wax, rose-oil, and ceruse, when the wounds are deep; when there is any apprehension of heat and inflammation, and more especially if the patient be plethoric, he approves of venesection. When on the other hand the patient is weak, and is in danger of falling into a state of syncope, he recommends musk and wine to be administered. When there is much appearance of ecchymosis he speaks of scarifying the part after the heat is gone. Rhases recommends a composition of ceruse, litharge, wax, and rose-oil, as a general application.

Most of the applications recommended by Bertapalia contain litharge, ceruse, tutty, wax, and oil. (De Ulceribus, 16.) The other earlier medical authors of modern times likewise follow the ancients in this case.

XIII—TO MAKE HAIRS GROW ON A PART THAT HAS BEEN BURNT

Hairs grow on a burnt part if you apply fig leaves boiled in a pot with cerate, in the form of a plaster; or, of dried fig, dr. viij; of marjoram, dr. j; triturate with oil to the thickness of a cerate, and use; or, of gypsum, dr. *c*; of squama æris, dr. j; form trochisks with water, and keep. When going to use, mix one part with eight parts of cerate.

Commentary. The Arabians mention various things which were supposed to be possessed of the property of making hairs grow; such as turpentine, spikenard, thapsia, &c.

XIV—FOR EXCORIATIONS

For excoriated surfaces and superficial ulcers, at first use astringents, such as wine, or vinegar and brine, and afterwards such plasters as contain fat and promote cicatrization, and the most delicate of the white plasters. This is particularly applicable: of ceruse, p. j; of ammoniac, p. ss; of myrtle-oil, q. s; having triturated the ammoniac in water, mix the ceruse, adding the myrtle-oil, and use in an oily state: or, mix the squama æris with gypsum, and having triturated with myrtle-oil, use: or, having triturated Cimolian earth and litharge with wine, and the oleum ricini, or myrtle-oil, use.

For excoriations, intertrigo, chronic ulcers, and old and tender skin. Of golden-coloured litharge, dr. lx; of wax, dr. xx; of dried pitch rosin, dr. xij; of oil, iss cyathus: having boiled the litharge and the oil, add the other things, and having agitated it with a spatula, or softened it in a mortar, use. Skin which has been torn away, ought not to be cut from the sores, but it ought to be laid on, and the medicine applied; for thus they coalesce, even if it is black. When stripped of the skin, the cicatrization is difficult, the ulcer being irritated and rendered foul. Excoriated parts are preserved from inflammation by the application of red sumach, triturated with honey, or with the hair of sweet flag burnt and applied with honey.

An anodyne for excoriations, sores from stripes, and contusions of the joints. Of litharge, of ceruse, of each, oz. j; of wax, oz. vj; of pure oil or rose-oil, lb. iss; of starch, oz. ij. The composition called pelarium, from the dross of silver, produces the same effects, and that from eggs in like manner.

Commentary. See Oribasius (Morb. Curat. iii, 18); Aëtius (xiv, 66, 67); Scribonius Largus (88); Marcellus (De Med.); Avicenna (iv, 4, 2, 9); Haly Abbas (Pract. iv, 10); Rhases (ad Mansor. vi, 18.)

Our author copies closely from Oribasius.

Aëtius recommends as a good application for intertrigo occasioned by the friction of shoes, the warm liver of a pig or lamb, or unwashed wool. Here he follows Dioscorides (ii, 37.) He also makes mention of several cooling applications, containing ceruse, litharge, the dross of lead, &c.

Scribonius Largus recommends an ointment containing litharge, ceruse, the flour of frankincense, alum, axunge, old austere wine, roses, and sour oil.

Marcellus also recommends litharge for intertrigo.

The Arabians treat these cases similarly. Thus Avicenna agrees with Aëtius in recommending the liver, and the ointment containing ceruse, &c. For bruised parts he recommends astringents; such as galls, acacia, &c.

To relieve the heat and irritation occasioned by riding, or any such cause, Rhases directs us to apply a cloth dipped in rose-water properly cooled, he means, perhaps, with ice. After the heat and pain have been removed, an ointment of ceruse, or litharge is to be applied. Blisters produced by walking are to be opened and then washed with rose-water; and afterwards they are to be dressed with an astringent application, containing Armenian bole, galls, pomegranate flowers, or the like.

XV—FOR MYRMECIA AND ACROCHORDON

Each of these is a small rising of the skin, of a callous nature, and for the most part circular; but the myrmecia have a broad base, and when rubbed, convey a sensation like the bites of ants. But the acrochordon has a narrow base so as to seem to hang, resembling the extremity of a cord. Wherefore, elaterium with salts, when applied, removes these swellings; and frankincense with vinegar, green figs with vinegar, flour and natron, the juice of the fig rubbed in, and in like manner, that of the spurge, the pickled head of picarel burnt, verdigris burnt with sulphur vivum, the leaves of basil with copperas; that which flows from green vine shoots when burning, sheep's dung with vinegar, a buck-goat's gall when rubbed in, the fruit of the large sun-flower, when applied with wine, rue with natron and pepper, natron with the urine of a youth not come to puberty, the dung of an ox of the herd in vinegar.

Commentary. See Celsus (v, 28); Galen (Meth. Med. xiv); Aëtius (xiv, 4); Oribasius (Morb. Curat. iii, 55); Actuarius (Meth. Med. vi, 8); Pollux (Onomast. iv); Avicenna (iv, 3, 1, 6); Rhases (Divis i, 131, *et seq.*; ad Mansor. vii, 15, 16.)

Celsus defines these tumours in the following terms: "Ἀκροχορδόνα Græci vocant, ubi sub cute coit aliquid durius, et interdum paulo asperius, coloris ejusdem: infra tenue, ad cutem latius: idque modicum est quia raro fabæ magnitudinem excedunt. Vix unum tantum eodem tempore nascitur; sed fere plura, maximeque in pueris; eaque nonnunquam subito desinunt; nonnunquam mediocrem inflammationem excitant; sub quâ etiam in pus convertuntur." He then describes the θύμιον to be about the size of an Ægyptian bean, and of the colour of thyme. He adds: "Μυρμήκια autem vocantur humiliora thymio durioraque: quæ radices altius exigunt, majoremque dolorem movent: infra lata, supra autem tenuia; minus sanguinis mittunt; magnitudine vix unquam lupini modum excedunt. Nascuntur ea quoque aut in palmis aut in inferioribus partibus pedum." The acrochordon, he says, if cut out, leaves no roots, and does not grow again. This is not the case with the myrmecia. For it he recommends an application consisting of alum and red arsenic.

Galen describes minutely the method of extracting these tumours; but that belongs more properly to the surgical part of this work.

Applications containing arsenic, chalcitis, quicklime, elaterium, sulphur, and alum are mentioned by Oribasius and Aëtius. See in like manner the 'Euporista' of the Pseudo-Dioscorides.

The myrmecia is generally rendered *formicaria* by the Latin translators of the Greek medical authors, and *formica miliaris* by those of the Arabians. Avicenna seems to confound the myrmecia with the herpes.

Pollux defines the thymus, or thymium, to be an excrescence about the pudenda, anus, fingers, or face, of a red colour, rough, bloody, and not difficult to remove. The acrochordon, he says, is white at the root, and it gets enlarged at the extremity. The myrmecia he defines to be a hard, rough excrescence of a callous nature, but bloody at its extremity.

The acrochordon is thus described by an intelligent modern author: "Est verruca subcutanea durior et asperior, callosa, atque plerumque teres, cute concolor, in basi tenuis, summitatis vero latioris, fabæ magnitudinem raro excedens, juniores maxime infestans." (Mangeti Bibl. Chirurg. i, 72.) The terms thymus, myrmecia, and acrochordon, have now fallen into disuse.

XVI—ON GANGLION

Ganglion is a round tumour of a nerve (tendon?) arising from a blow or pressure, in many parts of the body, but particularly in those parts which are moved, such as the extremities of the hands and feet. In this case, says Archigenes, apply quick lime with the grease of geese and turpentine. But Poles uses the medicine from agate stone, and Oribasius the following: of ceruse, of pine rosin, of old oil, of each, oz. j; of ammoniac perfume, of galbanum, of each, oz. j; of wax, oz. iv; or, he says, apply a thick plate of lead, like the vertebræ, and larger than the ganglion, and bind it on; for by its weight this dissolves it in process of time. This we have used.

Commentary. See Hippocrates (De Artic. xxvi); Galen (Comment., de Med. Simpl. ix); Celsus (vii, 6); Oribasius (De Virt. simpl. ii, in voce Plumbum); Aëtius (xv, 9); Actuarius (Meth. Med. ii, 11); Avicenna (iv, 3, 2, 6); Albucasis (Chirurg. ii, 50); Rhases (ad Mansor. vii, 15: Contin. xxviii.)

Hippocrates points out the danger of opening these tumours indiscriminately. They consist, as Galen remarks, of a viscid and mucous fluid. Galen and Oribasius agree with our author in directing a piece of lead to be bound upon the ganglion. Nearly the same plan of treatment is recommended by Aëtius, who directs us to bind a piece of lead upon the tumour, and after some days to remove it, when the ganglion will be found much softened; it is then to be squeezed firmly between the thumb and the fingers, by which means it will be speedily dissolved. Albucasis approves of extirpating the tumour, unless it be seated near a joint. Rhases as usual collects the opinions of all preceding authorities. Antyllus, he says, directed the surgeon to break the sack, or to bind a heavy plate over it, or to extract it by the knife. When an operation is attempted, he recommends that the surgeon be sure that he has removed the whole sac. He relates a case in which the swelling was dissolved by an application containing mustard.

XVII—ON PHLEGMON

In general, we call all those swellings phlegmons which are red and painful, and accompanied with heat; some diversity of their nature arising from the cause which occasions them. For when good blood and of moderate consistence rushes abundantly to a part and from its quantity becomes seated in it, the disease is that which is properly called phlegmon; but when yellow bile is seated in a part, it is called herpes; and when blood and yellow bile together are collected in a part, erysipelas is formed; but when in this case the blood is hot and thick, it usually gives rise to carbuncle. Wherefore, we shall begin with what is properly called phlegmon, which occurs in many cases, being a swelling which is red, painful, elastic, and hot, deriving its origin, as I said, from good blood which is sometimes collected from the whole body, and sometimes is formed abundantly in the part itself, so that it cannot be contained in the vessels, but escapes from them in the form of vapour into the surrounding cavities. And this affection supervenes upon wounds, fractures, ulcers, and many other causes. When therefore a part becomes inflamed without any obvious cause preceding it, the whole body sending a defluxion to the part, we must evacuate the general system by venesection, and apply to the part embrocations and cataplasms, not such as are of a heating and moistening nature, but such as are calculated to repel the fluid, which is flowing to the part, and evacuate that which is already contained in it. Apply, therefore, a cataplasm of house-leek, and of the bark of the pomegranate tree boiled in wine, with sumach and polenta: when the pain is not violent, this or such like applications are to be used; but when there is a defluxion to the part with greater pain, then cataplasms of hot water and oil, or of polenta, must not be applied (for all these are inimical to such defluxions); but the vehemence of the pain is to be allayed by that which is composed from musk, rose-oil, and a little wax, with unwashed wool containing much grease: these things are to be prepared and applied cold in summer, but tepid if in winter, so that the parts above the affected places be covered with a sponge soaked in austere wine or cold oxycrate. But we must add to the cataplasms such herbs as are proper for the purpose required. Pellitory of the wall, therefore, is applicable to every phlegmon at the commencement, and while on the increase; and in like manner, horned poppy, orach, mallows, lettuce, and gourd, when applied on hot parts. Both kinds of caltrops (tribuli) are applicable to inflammatory defluxions, and the cabbage to such as are hard. When a change is thereby effected, and no pus falls into the part, you may accomplish the cure by means of the plaster from chalcitis, or some of those plasters of a similar nature, which apply to defluxions; but clean wool soaked in austere wine is to be put externally to the medicine. In this manner you may cure phlegmons from defluxion. But such as are occasioned by any external cause will not be injured by moistening and heating applications, and if necessity require, you may scarify them with advantage. But in phlegmons arising from defluxion, scarification, more especially at the commencement, may become the cause of much mischief to the patient.

Commentary. See Galen (ad Glauc. ii); de Different. Morb. (12); Meth. Med. (xiii, 2); Celsus (iii, 10); Oribasius (Morb. Curat. iii. 41); Aëtius (xiv. 31);

Leo (vii, 4); Actuarius (Meth. Med. ii, 12); Avicenna (iv, 3, 1, 2); Serapion (v, 22); Haly Abbas (Theor. viii, 9; Pract. iii, 27); Alsaharavius (Pract. xxix, 2); Rhases (Divis. 126, and Contin. xxvii.)

Galen explains that the term *phlegmone* is used either to signify inflammations in general, or a red, resisting, and painful tumour in particular. It is here used in the latter acceptation. He says, when a defluxion of blood of good quality and of moderate consistence takes place to a part, and from its quantity becomes fixed in it, the person is seized with a violent pain, unless the part be very insensible; it is also accompanied with a deep-seated throbbing; it seems stretched and broken; there is a sensation of increased heat, so that the part feels as if it were burnt and desires cooling; there is a florid redness as in those who have been in the bath, or have been warmed at the fire, and by other means. This affection, he says, gets the generic appellation of phlegmone, or inflammation. He enumerates many causes of it, such as bruises, fractures, and dislocations; but even without these, he adds, it may arise from the veins being immoderately distended with humours, and the superfluity being cast off upon a part fitted to receive them at the time. Such a part, from some cause or other, happens to be weaker, or more lax, or more calculated to attract, or is more inactive than the other parts of the body. He lays it down as a general principle, that the cure of such affections is to be accomplished by evacuation. Reason and experience, he adds, teach us that the general system is to be evacuated by the suitable means, and the inflamed part by embrocations and cataplasms of a repellent nature, and such as are calculated to give tone and strength to it. Such are his general principles of treatment. His particular remedies we need not mention, as in fact our author's are entirely borrowed from him. Oribasius, Aëtius, Actuarius, and Nonnus, in like manner, borrow from him everything which they advance upon this subject.

Celsus does not treat of phlegmon in particular, but he has given an excellent account of inflammation in general. His definition of inflammation is singularly appropriate: "Notæ inflammationis sunt quatuor, rubor, et tumor, cum calore et dolore." Isidorus attempts the same not so successfully: "Phlegmone est fervor cum extensione et dolore; sive est inquietudo cum rubore, et dolore, et extensione, et duritie, et vastitate: quæ quum cæperit fieri, inquietudo et febris insequitur."

Avicenna gives a clear and comprehensive exposition of the doctrines of the Greeks, but supplies no new information. He is at pains to explain that the term phlegmon applies generally to every inflamed part; and also to a hot aposteme in particular. He joins Galen in recommending a free incision when it is apprehended that the member in which it is seated will become corrupted. Serapion's treatment is nowise dissimilar. A phlegmon, says Haly Abbas, is a sanguineous collection, arising either from an external cause, such as a bruise, a blow, a wound, or the like, or from an internal cause, namely, a defluxion upon the part. He attributes the collection which takes place in a part to its debility, which makes it unable to cast off the load which is thrown upon it. When seated in a vascular part, phlegmon, he says, is attended with a throbbing pain. He approves of free and bold incisions. Alsaharavius treats of phlegmon at great length, but there is nothing original in his views. Rhases recommends at first bleeding, purging, and applications of a cooling and astringent nature. But when suppuration has commenced he properly forbids depletion, lest it only protract this process. He remarks that phlegmons are often occasioned by disorder of the stomach, and the use of too much food and drink. He recommends in general maturative applications, to which, if necessary, narcotics may be added.

XVIII—ON EXTERNAL ABSCESSES

If it appear to you impossible to prevent suppuration, boil bread in water and oil, and apply it as a cataplasm; or apply barley flour prepared in like manner; and bathe the part with an infusion of marshmallows. But when the swelling is difficult, either to convert into pus or to dissipate, you may use a cataplasm of dried figs. But sweet and fat figs are to be dissolved by boiling in water, and made like thin honey, and barley flour added to it. And if the swelling is resolved but imperfectly, you may boil with the figs hyssop or marjoram; or, if you wish to increase its strength, add salts to the decoction. But you must attend that the part be not dried too much, for thus will it be rendered hard. If you perceive any such thing, you must boil with the water the root of wild cucumber, or of marshmallows, or of bryony. But the root of the dracunculus is stronger than these and more discutient; and the medicine formed from the dracunculus itself is very discutient. Sometimes, therefore, you may apply decoctions of these things alone; but at other times you may add dried figs, and mix polenta with fat. And the oil of dill is discutient, and adapted for concocting crude humours, and unconcocted swellings. And pitch, more especially the liquid, concocts all hard and unconcocted swellings, when added to the cataplasms. A compound medicine for procuring the discharge of the concocted matter of abscesses, so that often the pus is found on the pledget; and for thoroughly discussing what is not concocted: of pyrites, of levigated ammoniac, of each, dr. xij; of the flour of beans, dr. vj; add to liquid pitch, and spread upon skin, and apply. But do not take away the pledget until it fall off spontaneously. The medicine must not be prepared long beforehand, as it soon becomes dry. When the tumour is no wise dissipated by these means, and matter falls into it, it is to be opened, and the matter evacuated, taking care not to apply to it water or oil; or, if it be necessary to clean the sore, it must be done with honied water, oxycrate, wine, and wine and honey; and if it become inflamed, the cataplasm of lentils is to be applied; but if it is not inflamed, we may use some of the plasters to such openings, more especially that from chalcitis; but apply to them sponge or wool soaked in austere wine. But to the wound itself, do not apply any of the oily ointments, such as the tetrapharmacon, for it stands much in need of being dried.

Those things which open abscesses. Since some persons will not endure to have abscesses opened with iron, we must endeavour to have recourse to epispastic medicines. Having triturated the root of narcissus in honied water, boil it with oil of iris, and apply; or, having triturated the tender root of calamus, and if it be hard, boil it in honied water, and apply; or, use a cataplasm of birthwort and honey. But equal parts of dry pitch and Cretan bee-glue, produce the rupture of abscesses and promote cicatrization.

The Dionysian plaster, a wonderful epispastic application for abscesses, to the breasts and to buboes, dissipating by the insensible pores. Of old oil, of water, of each, lb. j; having boiled the oil and water for a little time, add of aphronitrum, oz. vj; of misy, oz. j or ij; and boil until it does not stain the finger; then add of the manna of frankincense, of wax, of turpentine, of each, oz. vj.

For abscesses of the nervous parts. Of wax, of colophonian rosin, of butter, of each, lb. j; of dry pitch, of honey, of each, lb. ij, oz. vj; of verdigris, oz. iij; of bird lime, q. s.—*Another,* an epispastic: Of ammoniac perfume, oz. vj; of wax, of turpentine, of each, oz. iv; of sulphur vivum, oz. iij; of natron, oz. iij; and the application called smilium, and that from garlic are strongly calculated to promote the breaking of abscesses already formed. But that which consists of the juice of linseed dissipates, changes, and bursts abscesses most aptly. For the milder sorts of abscesses, those also which were mentioned for parotis will apply. These observations apply to an abscess following phlegmon. But, Galen says, that an abscess will sometimes take place without being preceded by inflammation, in which case, it has its origin from good blood. For at the commencement, he says, owing to some humour, excoriation takes place, and in process of time, the containing parts are separated from those below. And, therefore, when opened, they appear to contain within them all kinds of fluid and solid bodies. For, bodies resembling dung, urine, thrombus, a honey or mucus-like humour, bones, nails, and hairs, have been found in abscesses. And even animals have been found very like to those which derive their origin from putrefaction. Nay, they affirm that, more particularly in chronic abscesses from metastasis, bodies have been formed resembling stones, sand, shells, wood, coals, clay, the sordes of the oil of baths, the lees of oil, and the lees of wine. Wherefore, we shall now give a succinct account of abscesses, more especially such as are seated in the external parts of the body, and those which do not admit of resolution by medicines. An abscess, then, is a corruption and change of the flesh or fleshy parts, such as muscles, veins, and arteries. Of them, some are contained in a cyst, as atheroma, steatoma, and meliceris, and others are formed without a cyst, and are properly called by the generic name, and of them we have now to treat. The formation of an abscess then is most commonly preceded by inflammation, as we have stated, but sometimes it arises at once originally, as we have just now mentioned. An abscess, then, is attended with strong heat of the place, the swelling becomes greater and more red than formerly, and is hard, with a pungent pain, throbbing, and weight, so that it seems as if something were suspended from the part. And if the part be a vital one, fever supervenes with irregular rigors, and the pain and fever are greatest at night. Sometimes too a bubo is formed in the neighbouring glands. When the abscess is fairly formed, the most of these symptoms are diminished, the pungent pain becomes itchy and somewhat dull, the swelling is more sharpened into an acute point, is soft and yielding to the touch, and the skin at the top is separated; I speak with regard to those that burst externally. If therefore, it has burst spontaneously, or from medicines, it is to be cured by means of pledgets spread with ointment, the pus being evacuated by degrees; but if not, it is to be opened in the manner to be described in the surgical part of the work.

Commentary. All the writers referred to in the last Chapter may be consulted on the treatment of abscesses. See especially Aëtius. He recommends when suppuration is not taking place properly to apply barley meal, or bread boiled in the decoction of figs, to which if necessary may be added nitre, turpentine, or the like. When suppuration takes place, the abscess is to be opened where the skin is thinnest. (See Book 6.) The incision is to be made long and narrow, and if any putrid substance appear it is to be cut out. The opening is to be sprinkled with frankincense and suitable pledgets applied. When the neighbouring parts are inflamed a cataplasm will be the most proper application. When the ulcer is foul, turpentine and honey will serve for cleaning it; or applications containing verdigris may be used for the same purpose. After the ulcer is cleaned, first incarnants and afterwards incrassants are to be applied. For producing rupture of the abscess, he recommends various applications, such as ammoniac, and nitre triturated with vinegar, and the like. This account, however, is mostly taken from Galen.

The treatment recommended by Celsus is nearly the same in principle. At first if the part be soft he recommends applications of a repellent and cooling nature: but if it is hard he directs us to use applications which digest and produce resolution, such as dried figs pounded. To such applications may be added equal proportions of ammoniac, galbanum, bees-glue, and birdlime, with somewhat less than one half of myrrh. The plasters and malagmata for this purpose are likewise to be applied. When these applications do not produce resolution, we must conclude, he says, that the abscess will ripen. The symptoms of an unripe abscess are strong motion of the arteries, weight, distension, pain, redness, and hardness; to which are to be added horror and fever if the abscess be large. When there is a remission of these symptoms, and the part becomes itchy, and somewhat livid or white, the suppuration is ripe, and the matter is to be let out by medicines or iron. Unless the opening be large he properly forbids tents or pledgets to be put into it. When these are used, however, lentils and honey, or pomegranate rind boiled in wine are to be applied over them. Whatever is applied must not be tightly bound.

The Arabians mention a variety of applications for producing the rupture of abscesses. (See in particular Avicenna and Rhases.) Thus, they recommend a plaster consisting of cantharides and old oil. Some of their applications contain nitre, quicklime, and arsenic. Such a composition, by producing a slough, would no doubt effect the purpose for which it was intended. Haly Abbas recommends a poultice made of leaven, boiled figs, and the seeds of rosemary. He speaks of onions as an application to indolent abscesses. Alsaharavius treats of abscesses at great length.

By abscesses of the nervous parts it will be readily understood that our author does not mean that they are seated in what are now properly called nerves, but in tendinous and membranous parts, for all these were comprehended under the name of nerves by the older writers, namely, Hippocrates, Plato, and Aristotle. Galen pointed out clearly the distinction between these parts, but the term is often used in its old and popular acceptation by the writers subsequent to him.

The account which our author gives of deep-seated abscesses is highly interesting, but is mostly borrowed from Galen (ad Glauc. ii.) Rhases, in his 'Continens' (xxvii), gives an interesting outline of the opinions of all preceding authorities, with some ingenious observations of his own. When there is any hope of producing resolution he approves of scarifications. When the pain is violent he recommends hot and humid applications with the addition of narcotics. After the abscess has been opened with the knife, he says that desiccative applications are indicated, and not ointments containing wax or oil. He describes the leaven cataplasm, and others of a similar nature. He gives Antyllus' directions for opening abscesses. Abscesses in the limbs are to be opened by a straight incision, but those about the ancles by a circular, as they are apt to terminate in fistulæ. He recommends it to be made at the lower part of the abscess, but mentions that Galen prefers the thinnest part.

XIX—ON GANGRENE AND SPHACELUS

When the inflammation is neither resolved nor converted into pus, it often passes into gangrene and sphacelus, of which we shall now treat. Wherefore, we give the name of gangrene to mortifications arising from the violence of the inflammation, when they are not yet formed but forming; and if such a state is not speedily cured, the affected part readily dies, and the disease seizing upon the surrounding parts, kills the person. But when the parts thus affected become totally insensible, the affection is no longer called gangrene, but sphacelus. This affection happens also to the bones when the flesh that surrounds them engendering noxious humours impregnates the bones therewith, and causes them to putrefy. When, therefore, the part is completely mortified, it must be speedily cut away, where it joins the sound part. Gangrene is to be cured by evacuating as much as possible of the blood in the affected part; and we may either procure the discharge of the corrupted blood by opening a vein, when the vein of the part is large, or we may divide the whole skin by many and deep incisions, so that the blood may be permitted to escape; and we may apply some of the medicines suitable to mortifications. These are, the flour of tares, or of darnels, or of beans with oxymel. When wishing to apply stronger ones we may add salts, or use the trochisk of Andron, or the like. Old walnuts are good applications for gangrene. The nettle also cleans them, and the juice of spurge, when applied in season and in proper quantity. The decoction of bitter lupines, poured on the part, is also beneficial. Some after the incision, for the sake of security, apply the cautery, in which cases we must use salt with leeks: afterwards, in order to remove the eschar, we may apply a cataplasm of bread, or of barley, or of wheaten flour boiled in water and oil; or the dry cephalic powder with honey, and the tetrapharmacon; and that called the Macedonian may be used. The eschars may be properly removed by bread triturated with parsley, or basil, or by iris, panacea, or birthwort, or by the sweet-flag with honey, or by frankincense. And the medicine of Machærion takes away the eschars in a proper manner, and the iris spread upon pledgets with honey; but in soft bodies the flour of tares, with honey, is sufficient.

From the works of Oribasius, for gangrene. Of scraped verdigris, of vermilion, of stone alum, equal parts; triturate in water and anoint. The flour of darnel, with radish and salts, and sometimes with vinegar, will, when applied as a cataplasm, be proper for the scarified parts; also dried grapes deprived of their stones with the bark, and with salts and oxymel;

the inner parts of walnuts, and myrtle leaves boiled in wine and triturated with honey. Radish, with vinegar, breaks the eschars even to the bone.

Commentary. See the authors referred to in the 17th Section.

Paulus copies freely from Oribasius (Synops. vii, 27.) Upon comparing Oribasius with our author we have ventured to give an interpretation of the last sentence not justified by the text as it now stands, and at variance with the translation of Cornarius. Oribasius does not say that the flour of darnel will scarify the parts (how could he?) but that it will be a proper application after the parts are scarified.

Galen (ad Glauc. and Comment. in Hippocr. App. vii. 50,) is the great ancient authority on mortification, and from him Oribasius, Aëtius, Paulus, and all the subsequent writers on this subject have copied. He lays it down as the great rule of treatment, to evacuate the blood which is impacted in the part and prevents the diastole of the arteries. To accomplish this end he directs free incisions to be made, after which the actual cautery is to be applied, at the line of separation between the sound and diseased parts.

Celsus is a strong advocate for this practice, which has been revived lately and is much used in France. (See Encyclopédie Méthiodique, art. Gangrène, and Cross's Sketches of the Medical Schools in Paris.) He states, however, that when the disease goes on spreading, amputation of the mortified limb is the "auxilium unicum." At the commencement he approves of venesection, if the strength permit, and of a restricted diet; and, afterwards, astringent food and drink are to be given. He also recommends, for gangrene, applications containing arsenic, quicklime, chalcitis, and the like (v, 22.)

The practice of the Arabians is little or nothing different from that of the Greeks. Avicenna at the commencement approves of Armenian bole and terra sigillata with vinegar; but if these have not the effect he directs us to empty the part by scarifications, leeches, or opening the veins which lead to it. He then recommends us to apply the flour of beans and the other remedies mentioned by the Greeks. When the disease proceeds, free incisions and the actual cautery must be had recourse to. Alsaharavius recommends us to bleed at first, if the strength permit; then to use powerful caustics and escharotics such as arsenic, quicklime, and sublimed quicksilver; or if these do not succeed, the actual cautery. He approves of early incisions, and of amputation, if the mortification spread. He describes a species of gangrene which seizes the hand and spreads upwards; and relates a case of it in which he refused to amputate for fear of hemorrhage. The same case is related by Albucasis, which certainly amounts to a strong presumptive proof that Alsaharavius was the same person as Albucasis. Rhases inculcates in the strongest terms that when an inflammation threatens to terminate in mortification, it is to be treated by scarifications, stimulant applications, and the cautery.

The earlier modern surgeons followed the ancient practice of applying the cautery in cases of gangrene.

XX—ON HERPES

When yellow bile, unmixed with any other humour is fixed in a part, the affection is called herpes: but if it is thicker and rather acrid it ulcerates the whole skin as far as the subjacent flesh, and is called herpes exedens; but if it is thin, less acrid and hot, it raises small blisters on the surface of the skin like millet-seeds, and hence has been called herpes miliaris. According to Oribasius, a mixture of phlegm, with yellow bile, produces the herpes miliaris. Wherefore we may evacuate the whole body with cholagogue medicines, and apply cooling and desiccant things to the affected part. At the commencement, therefore, we may apply cataplasms from vine shoots, bramble, and plantain; but afterwards we may add lentil to them, sometimes with honey and polenta. And the cataplasm recommended for phlegmons from defluxion may be applied without the house-leek. But ulcerated parts are to be rubbed with trochisks dissolved in must, or in a thin and austere wine, not very old, or in a watery oxycrate. Administer also horned poppy, and similar things in water; and when these do not prove effectual, vinegar may be added. But wine diluted with the juice of plantain or strychnos is of great service, or linseed bruised and boiled in wine and oil may be applied; or Cimolian earth, mixed with the juice of strychnos may be applied by anointing: and take of litharge, oz. iv; of the juice of leeks, vij cyathi, and of the juice of beet an equal quantity, triturate and anoint. But when these ulcers have become chronic, the trochisk of Musa and that of Andron will be convenient applications.—*Another*: For herpes phlyctænodes: having triturated the dross of lead in austere wine and anointed with it, apply above it beet leaves boiled in wine, or of wax, oz. iv; of myrtle oil, oz. xvj; of the dross of lead, oz. iv; anoint with one half of wine. When it has stopped from spreading, use the cerate from the dross; or apply boiled lentil with honey. For herpes, under the skin, mix the dross of lead with the juice of levigated rue, or myrtle cerate, instead of the rue.—*Another*: Of old unwashed wool wrapped round a dead pine and burnt, dr. xij ss; of wax, dr. xxv; of the dross of lead half an acetabulum; of goat's tallow cured and washed in water, dr. xxxj; of myrtle oil, oz. v.—*Another*: To those which spread rapidly: of the rind of the sweet pomegranate, dr. vj; of litharge, dr. vj; of unwashed wool about a dead pine and burnt, dr. iij; of wax, dr. xij; of ceruse, dr. viij; of fissile alum, dr. j; add to wine and myrtle oil.

Commentary. The writers on phlegmon treat immediately afterwards of herpes and erysipelas. Fabricius ab Aquapendente, Dr. Bateman, and most of our modern authorities on this subject, are of opinion that the *ignis sacer* of Celsus and the other Latin authors was herpes. Scribonius Largus, however, distinguishes the ignis sacer from zona, which, he says, was called herpes by the Greeks. The ignis sacer of Octavius Horatianus likewise appears to be erysipelas. And Isidorus states decidedly that the ignis sacer was erysipelas:—"Erysipelas est quam Latini *sacrum ignem* appellant, id est, *execrandum,* per antiphrasin. Siquidem in superficie rubore flammeo cutes rubescunt. Tunc mutuo rubore quasi ab igne vicina invaduntur loca ita est etiam febris excitatur." (See a learned dissertation on the ignus sacer in Burman's edition of Serenus Samonicus, 'Poet. Latini Minores.' ii, 335.) Having thus stated the doubts which prevail respecting the ignis sacer of the ancients, we shall return to Celsus's account of it, which certainly, as already mentioned, seems to apply to herpes. He describes two varieties of it. The first is reddish, or a mixture of redness and paleness, and in it the skin is covered with a great number of small pustules. The disease spreads, the part first affected either healing, or becoming ulcerated from the rupture of the pustules and discharging a humour intermediate between sanies and pus. The breast and sides are mentioned as being frequently the seat of this complaint, and hence Bateman concludes that it is the herpes zoster. The second variety is described as consisting of a superficial ulceration of the skin, broad, somewhat livid, but unequal; the middle part healing as the extremities spread, and the part about to become affected becoming swelled, hard, and of a colour compounded of black and red. It affects principally old and cachectic persons, especially their legs. We cannot understand what could have led Dr. Bateman to think that this is the same as the herpes circinatus of his arrangement. Rayer rather supposes it to be the *dartre squameuse centrifuge* Alibert. His general treatment consists of abstinence, opening the belly, food intermediate between the glutinous and saltish, and if there is no fever, exercise, austere wine, and the like. The ulcers (vesicles?) are to be washed with hot water, or, if they spread, with hot wine; they are then to be opened with a needle, and dressed with applications for eating away putrid flesh. When the sore is cleaned, gentle applications are to be used.

For the zona or herpes, Scribonius Largus recommends applications containing alum, galls, chalcitis, misy, quicklime, &c.

Pollux defines herpes to be inflammatory and pungent pustules, which spread most commonly about the neck, but sometimes affect also the hands and feet.

Galen gives a very full account of the nature and treatment of herpes. According to him the complaint arises from yellow bile separated from the blood and fixed in a part. When it is thickish it ulcerates the skin down to the bone, and forms the disease called by Hippocrates *herpes exedens.* But if thinner, it only burns as it were the surface, when it is called by the generic term of herpes. Of the other two varieties, the one, as has been said, is called *exedens,* and the other *miliaris,* because it is attended with many small bullæ (phlyctænæ) like millet-seeds. As our author's treatment is entirely derived from him we shall not enter into any detailed exposition of his practice. We may mention, however, that he decidedly recommends purgatives for proper herpes. When the ulceration is of a malignant nature and attended with putridity it requires the most acrid medicines, and such as in power resemble fire, namely, misy, chalcitis, arsenic, quicklime, and sandarach. For, he adds, these medicines burn like fire, and often when they fail, we must have recourse to fire itself.

Aëtius gives an accurate account of herpes, but it is professedly borrowed from Galen. Like him he divides the disease into three varieties, the herpes proprius, the herpes exedens, and the herpes miliaris, the last being characterized by an eruption of vesicles (phlyctænæ). We shall here notice what Dr. Bateman says respecting this division of herpes:—"The ancient division of herpes into three varieties, miliary (κεγχρίας), vesicular (φλυκταινώδης), and eroding (ἐσθιόμενος), may be properly discarded, for there appears to be no essential difference between the first two, which differ only in respect to the size of the vesicles." This is evidently an incorrect account of the ancient division, in which no distinction was made between the herpes miliaris and the herpes phlyctænodes.

Palladius makes mention of only two varieties of the disease, namely, the proper, and the eroding herpes. (De Febribus 2.)

Leo briefly refers to Galen's account of the disease (vii, 3.)

Actuarius mentions only the proper herpes, and the herpes miliaris. This is, perhaps the best division of any, as the herpes exedens is evidently a disease of a very different nature from the other varieties.

The Pseudo-Dioscorides recommends strong stimulant applications containing sori, misy, sulphur, onions, &c.

Avicenna seems to confound herpes with myrmecia, which detracts from the value of his account of it. (iv, 3, 1, 7.)

Rhases describes separately the formica miliaris or herpes miliaris, and the herpes esthiomenos or exedens. For the former he recommends astringent applications, for the latter strong caustics. In his 'Continens' he directs the herpes miliaris to be treated with cholagogues and astringent applications.

Serapion in like manner describes two varieties of the disease, but his account of it contains nothing particularly interesting.

Haly Abbas adopts the division laid down by Galen (Theor. viii, 10.) His treatment also is quite similar (Pract. iii, 29.)

In the translation of Alsaharavius the three varieties are described by the names of formica or erysipelas muscina, formica corrosiva (herpes exedens?), and formica miliaris. He describes the formica corrosiva as being a dangerous complaint, spreading deeper and deeper. His treatment, although amply detailed, contains nothing remarkable (Pract. xxix, 9.)

The earlier modern writers on medicine being the servile copyists of the Arabians, describe herpes by the name of formica, as a disease nearly allied to erysipelas, and like it arising from corrupted bile. See Guy of Cauliac (ii, 1), and Theoderic (iii, 16). For the herpes esthiomenos or lupus they recommend the application of arsenic or the actual cautery.

XXI—FOR ERYSIPELAS

Galen, giving the name of erysipelas, more especially to the swelling formed of a hot and thin blood, to that which is formed of both blood and bile, he applies an appellation from the prevailing humour, calling it erysipelatous inflammation when blood prevails, and inflammatory erysipelas when yellow bile prevails. But in general the swelling formed of hot blood and bile is called by him erysipelas. Whatever division we adopt, it will make no great difference as to the treatment. But it is proper to know that erysipelas is a most dangerous disease, more particularly about the head; so that if active treatment be not resorted to, it will sometimes prove fatal to the patients by suffocation. At its first appearance then we must open a vein at the elbow, especially the humeral, or, if it cannot be seen, any one that appears. But if any thing prohibit venesection we must have recourse to purging by cholagogue medicines. The same treatment may be applied to erysipelas of other parts, or we may administer strong clysters. And we are to rub the parts affected by erysipelas with cooling things, in order to repel the defluxion, and with moderately heating and moistening things so as to dissipate that which is collected, before the parts become livid or black; but the parts which are anointed are to be kept constantly in a wet state, by frequently changing the applications, which may be done by cleansing them with soaked sponges: for the heat of the part by converting them into vapour soon renders it dry. As I have said, erysipelas at the beginning requires such things as are cooling and moistening, without astringency; such as house-leek, purslain, and fleawort; the marsh lentil, endive, and gourd; the nightshade, henbane, lettuce, and horned poppy. And parsley, and the leaves of rhamnus by themselves, and made into a cataplasm with bread, are proper applications; also cerates used with very cold water; but we may mix with them some opium, the juice of poppy, cicuta, and mandragora, and thus form them into compound applications. And a cerate may be made of white wax mixed with four parts of rose-oil, prepared from the oil of unripe olives without salts, the ingredients being pounded in a mortar, and as much cold water poured in as it can receive. But if you add a little thin and transparent vinegar, you will render the medicine still better: but polenta, with some of the aforementioned cooling herbs, cool very properly, and fat dates with any of them. And the part may be anointed with ceruse, Cimolian, or potter's earth, with the juice of strychnos, or litharge with rose-oil, or chalcitis with oil and must; or ceruse, with vinegar and buckthorn; or acacia, with vinegar. When the effervescence subsides we may use these simple applications, native sulphur and mint, with vinegar and rose-oil; or rue with worm-wood; vinegar and oil, or litharge with the juice of leeks and beet; or compound ones, as this trochisk, more especially to the head: of litharge, of ceruse, of saffron, of native sulphur, of opium with must; and in common, for all parts, of Sinopic vermilion, of chalcitis, of roasted misy, of verdigris, of copperas, of fissile alum equal parts, use with vinegar.—*Another*: Of native sulphur, of ceruse, of opium, of acacia equal parts; use with vinegar. A cataplasm for erysipelas, herpes, abscess, parotis, and burning: of the tender leaves of fresh marsh-mallows, lb. j; having boiled in water and oil, triturate properly, and adding of rose-oil, oz. iv; of litharge, of ceruse, of each, oz. iiss; triturate again with the juice of coriander, or of house-leek, or of strychnos, then adding crumbs of bread so as to form a plaster, apply it. And use this plaster: of oleum cicinum, i. e. castor-oil, lb. j; of oil of myrrh, lb. j; of wax, oz. v; of litharge, oz. iv; of scraped verdigris, oz. ij; the verdigris and litharge are to be triturated with vinegar. A cerate for erysipelas and burns: of white wax, oz. iv; of rose-oil, oz. iij; six eggs, of pellitory of the wall, oz. iv. When the inflammation ceases or becomes chronic, before the part becomes livid, apply a cataplasm of raw barley-meal; but if it has already become livid, incisions must be made in the part, and cataplasms moreover applied, and hot sweet water poured on it, and sometimes sea-water or brine; and sometimes these ingredients are to be mixed with the cataplasm, and then we must use the aforesaid compound medicines with caution: for should these symptoms continue, a transition to suppuration or mortification takes place.

Commentary. Hippocrates in his 'Prognostics' has stated the danger of an erysipelas being translated to an internal part. He also states that gangrene supervening upon erysipelas is dangerous. He has not, however, given any very particular account of the disease. In one of his aphorisms he states that cold is useful in erysipelas when not ulcerated, but prejudicial when it is ulcerated. His commentators, Theophilus and Damascius, confirm this statement. (Scholia in Hip. et Galen, ii, 456).

Celsus recommends bleeding if the strength permit, and then repellent and refrigerant applications, especially ceruse with the juice of solanum (nightshade), or Cimolian earth with river water, and the like. When refrigerants fail to produce the effect, sulphur, ceruse, and saffron are to be pounded with wine and applied. If the part become putrid he directs us to use corrosive applications or the actual cautery. Afterwards the sore is to be cleansed with honey and rosin, and treated upon general principles.

We have stated in the preceding Section that the ignis sacer of Scribonius Largus is not herpes. That it was erysipelas seems probable from the similarity between his applications for it and those which Celsus and the other authorities recommend for erysipelas. Thus for ignis sacer he recommends Cimolian chalk, diluted with the juice of solanum, or the solanum by itself, or with bread; or a mixture of sulphur vivum, ceruse, and litharge.

We may remark further in this place that the *ignis sacer*, or St. Anthony's fire of the middle ages, would appear to have been some variety of erysipelas.

Galen's account of erysipelas is particularly deserving of attention. In the 14th Book of his 'Meth. Med.,' he is at pains to state the nature of the disease, and the difference between it and phlegmon. The common symptoms of both are heat and swelling. But they differ, first and principally in colour, which is red in phlegmon, but pale or yellow, or a compound of both, in erysipelas. Throbbing is also a characteristic symptom of a great phlegmon, for it is deep-seated, whereas erysipelas is rather in the skin. Erysipelas, he pointedly inculcates, is occasioned by a bilious humour. This humour being thin, readily passes the fleshy and rare parts, and flows to the skin, where, unless it be particularly watery, it is unable to pass the pores, and, consequently, is retained. When things, indeed, are in their natural state, this bitter bile passes through the pores of the skin by the insensible perspiration, but when it is either too abundant or thicker than usual, it is retained by the skin, which it inflames and causes to swell: hence the reason why erysipelas chiefly affects the skin or the prolongation of it which lines the internal cavities. He states that the great indication of cure is refrigeration or cooling, but that there is danger of carrying this plan too far, lest the humour should be driven to some vital part: wherefore cooling applications are to be used until the part change its colour, but are not to be continued until it become black or livid. It is necessary, therefore, as soon as a change of colour in the affected part is remarked, to exchange them for those of a contrary nature. His cooling applications consist of strychnos (solanum?) and the other articles mentioned by our author. When the part becomes livid, he directs us to make incisions, and afterwards to apply cataplasms and fomentations with hot water, to which salt or vinegar may sometimes be added. It is only at this time that quicklime may safely be added to the applications; for it would prove highly prejudicial at first. With respect to the general treatment, he approves strongly of cholagogues, but does not think bleeding necessary in ordinary cases. When erysipelas arises from ulcers or any obvious causes, he recommends scarifications and cataplasms of barley flour. He recommends much the same plan of treatment in his 'Therapeut. ad Glauc.' ii. He speaks highly of early incisions.

Aëtius, as he professes, merely copies from Galen.

Oribasius recommends, at first, such things as are cooling without astringency; namely, henbane, nightshade, &c. When the inflammation subsides, he directs us, before the part becomes livid, to apply a cataplasm of barley flour; but when it does become livid, he recommends free incisions, and afterwards cataplasms and fomentations with fresh water, or water with salt and brine.

Actuarius states the danger of carrying refrigerant and repellent applications too far, and recommends something discutient to be added to them.

Octavius Horatianus approves of bleeding (unless contra-indicated by the want of strength), and of cholagogues, with free incisions and fomentations.

Avicenna states that bleeding in general does no good, unless the humour be seated between the two skins. He approves most of cholagogues and of applications strongly refrigerant; only he cautions us not to carry this plan too far, lest the disease be determined to an internal part, or terminate in gangrene.

Serapion treats of the disease very accurately by the name of *al massire*, but in nearly the same terms as Galen. He approves decidedly of cooling and repellent applications at the commencement. Serapion and Avicenna notice the eruption of bullæ in erysipelas.

Haly Abbas directs us, when erysipelas is not attended with swelling, to use cooling and repellent applications to the part, and to administer gentle cholagogues, such as myrobalans, tamarinds, and prunes. But if swelling be present, and if there is nothing to contra-indicate venesection, he recommends us to bleed and apply cataplasms.

Alsaharavius describes three varieties of erysipelas; namely, the erysipelas properly so called, the ignis Persicus, and the erysipelas inflativa. The first variety, he says, is attended solely with redness of the cuticle. It is to be treated by bleeding, purging, and local applications of a cooling and humid nature. In the ignis Persicus, the heat and redness are strong, and black blisters rise on the part. It is to be treated by bleeding at the commencement, and scarifications. The erysipelas inflativa arises with a sudden swelling, and blisters, like those produced by fire. It is to be treated by bleeding and cooling applications, containing ceruse, litharge, &c. The *ignis Persicus* would appear to have been some variety of anthrax, or the malignant pustule.

None of the ancient authorities express themselves so decidedly favorable to bleeding as Rhases. Like the others, he attributes it to heated bile. He, and most of the authors quoted by him in his 'Continens,' approve of cooling applications, but he cautions against carrying this practice too far. He remarks that vesicles like those from burning often arise on the part.

Fabricius ab Aquapendente is a strong advocate for the ancient theory, of which he gives a full explanation. The system, he says, being loaded with vitiated bile, the more important organs cast it off: it is, therefore, sent outwardly, and is detained by the cuticle when its pores are obstructed. He attempts to reconcile the contrary opinions of the ancients with regard to venesection. He himself approves decidedly of bleeding when the disease is seated in the head or neck.

None of the ancient authorities seem to have entertained the same apprehensions as most of the moderns do against liquid applications in cases of erysipelas. When this prejudice became general we do not exactly know. Heister mentions that, in his days, some surgeons disapproved of liquid applications, but, as he thought, without any good reason. He himself recommends camphorated spirit of wine. The earlier modern surgeons, as, for example, Brunus and Theodoricus, decidedly recommend cold applications at the commencement. When the disease is not thereby resolved, they direct us to have recourse to leeches and scarifications. They approve much of cholagogue purgatives, but do not recommend bleeding unless inflammatory symptoms run high.

XXII—ON PHYMA, BUBO, AND PHYGETHLON

According to Galen, phyma, bubo, and phygethlon, are affections of the glands: bubo being an inflammation of a gland; phygethlon, an inflammatory erysipelas, or an erysipelatous inflammation of a gland; and phyma, an inflammation of a gland passing rapidly into suppuration. But, according to others, all tumours of the nature of apostemes, which arise in any part of the body, are called phymata. For Hippocrates says, "Those in whose urethra phymata form are relieved when they suppurate and burst." Wherefore those buboes which are occasioned by accidents, either ulcers or pains, are not dangerous; but those which occur in fevers, more especially in the pestilential, are of a very bad description, whether they are formed in the groins, the armpits, or neck. But those of the first kind, as is the case in every other inflammation, we must endeavour to put back with cooling and astringent applications, either applying a sponge out of oxycrate, or wool out of wine and raw oil, or oil of roses, or oil of apples, or oil of lentisk, or oil of myrtles; and then we are to apply diaphoretics. But if the whole body is plethoric, it is to be evacuated. If free from superfluities, we must manage the ulcer arising from it in the manner to be described when treating of ulcers. When the gland is in a state of inflammation, it is to be mitigated by wool soaked in some of the emollient oils, and the whole limb is to be wrapped therewith. When the tumour has suppurated, we must not be in haste to open it, but endeavour to dissipate it by the medicines in the form of cerates, such as that prepared from apyranon, and that from herbs called botanica. When resolution is not thereby accomplished, we must forward the rupture as in the other abscesses, and cure it in like manner as them. In those buboes which arise in fevers or from a collection of humours, we must abstain from all repellents, lest the matter should be repelled and regurgitate to the deep-seated parts; but we must begin at once with discutients. When nothing prohibits, such as the age or strength of the patient, venesection from the arm is to be had recourse to, and fomentations applied to the part, either from the decoction of camomile, or of dill, or of some such; but the materials of the other applications may be transferred from our account, in the Third Book, concerning parotis, and from what has been lately delivered, more especially respecting phlegmons. And in like manner the cure of phygethlon may be learned from what has been stated respecting them and erysipelas. But the herb aster atticus, which, on this account, they call bubonium, not only in the form of a cataplasm, but also when bound round the part as an amulet, is believed to be of use for buboes. Phymata may be discussed by the following applications in particular: maiden-hair; orache; pellitory of the wall; the root of marsh-mallows, boiled in wine; ammoniac, softened with honey, and applied; birdlime, with the rosin cerate. But bee-glue, bitter lupins applied with vinegar, the root of the wild cucumber added to turpentine, and in like manner root of capers, and nitre with leaven, or figs, promote the rupture of these tumours.

Commentary. The account here given of these glandular inflammations is taken from Galen (ad Glauc. ii.) See also 'de Tumoribus' and 'Comment. in Hippocrat. Epid.' vi.

Celsus describes phyma as resembling furunculus, but as being larger, and turning to pus. According to Rayer, his description of phyma applies better to the boil than his account of anthrax. (Malad. de la Peau, p. 229.) The phygethlon, he says, is a tumour not high, but broad, and containing something resembling a pustule. It occurs mostly in the armpits, neck, or groins. He proposes applications of a repellent and refrigerant nature; but if the swelling is hard, digestives must be had recourse to, such as dried figs bruised, &c. He also recommends a composition of sal ammoniac, galbanum, bee-glue, and mistletoe, with a small proportion of myrrh. His treatment is considerably different from our author's. When matter is formed, he directs us to let it out by medicines or the lancet, but he decidedly forbids the use of cerates. In another place, however, he recommends an application containing lime, spuma nitri, round pepper, galbanum, and salt mixed with rose cerate.

Scribonius Largus recommends a malagma containing pitch, aphronitum, pine-rosin, wax, bay-berries, axunge, ammoniac, Illyrian iris, galbanum, and white pepper, for discussing phygethlon.

Oribasius and Actuarius mark the distinction between these affections in the same terms as Galen, and direct us to treat them with emollient, concoctive, and discutient applications. For concocting phymata, the Pseudo-Dioscorides recommends southernwood, boiled with raw barley flour; figs, boiled with yeast, &c.; and for breaking them, the juice of thapsia, with sulphur; cantharides, mixed with turpentine, &c. (Euporist, i, 156.)

Nonnus' account is mostly abridged from our author's. Thus, he recommends at first venesection, and sponges squeezed out of oxycrate and the like; then digestives are to be applied; and afterwards cataplasms and such things as will favour the rupture of the abscess, namely, compositions containing bee-glue, bitter lupins, vinegar, nitre, yeast, or figs and pitch.

Avicenna describes these affections by the name of *althaum*. It is remarked by his translator that the Arabian recommends the same medicines as Paulus, but neglects the distinction which the latter properly makes between the bubo when attended with pestilential fever and when without it.

The phyma seems to have been merely an acute inflammation of a gland, terminating in suppuration. The phygethlon was an erysipelatous inflammation of a gland. These complaints are well defined and described by Fabricius ab Aquapendente (1, i, 23.) Dr. Willan uses the term phyma in a different sense from that of our author. The term occurs in Marcus Antoninus (ii, 16), where see the note of Gataker.

XXIII—ON FURUNCULUS

Furunculus is an apostematous swelling, formed of thick humours in the fleshy parts of the body most especially; being mild when it is formed in the skin only, but of a malignant character when it rises up from a deep-seated part. Furunculus may be discussed and concocted by wheat, chewed and applied; by Egyptian mastic; by raisins, deprived of their stones, and triturated with salts, and applied—(this either discusses or breaks the swelling); or apply dried figs boiled in hydromel; or rosin may be mixed with the figs and applied; or the figs themselves, when they are fat, may be split open and applied; or leaven with nitre; or linseed with honey; or the leaves of henbane, triturated with butter: of compound applications, that which is prepared from leaven and fine flour, and that which is particularly named Dothienicon, are very applicable. Foment with soft sponges frequently dipped in hot water, and then apply the medicines.

Commentary. In this and the two following Sections, see the authorities on phlegmon.

The furunculus, according to Galen, is an inflammatory affection which is of a malignant nature when deep-seated, and differs from phyma only in hardness. (De Tumoribus.)

Furunculus, says Celsus, is an acute tubercle, attended with inflammation and pain, more especially when converted into pus. After it has been opened, and the pus discharged, there appears part of the flesh below converted into pus and part corrupted, of a whitish or reddish colour, which they call the ventricle or belly of the furunculus. He says that the disease is not attended with danger, and that medicines are necessary solely for removing it the more expeditiously. For this purpose he particularly commends galbanum. If repellent applications do not succeed, suppurative ones may be used; and, failing these, rosin or leaven. When pus is formed, no further treatment is required. According to Rayer, Celsus' description of furunculus applies to the malignant pustule and not to the boil. (Malad. de la Peau, 233.)

The simple remedies recommended by our author are borrowed from Oribasius.

It is to be remarked that Galen, Celsus, Pliny (Nat. Hist. xxiii, 7), Octavius Horatianus, and Avicenna concur in recommending figs for furunculus or the boil. It was with a lump of figs that the prophet Isaiah cured Hezekiah's boil.

Avicenna and Rhases treat furunculus judiciously by bleeding and purging, which prevent the formation of a large abscess. When there is throbbing in the tumour, they direct us to use maturative applications. When it is ripe, and does not break readily, they recommend us to open it. Haly Abbas says, that boils arise from gross and depraved humours. (Theor. viii, 11.) Alsaharavius also ascribes them to a full and unwholesome diet. He mentions that he often succeeded in stopping the formation of the furunculus by cauterizing it with a piece of myrtle or any other wood. When the pain is violent, he recommends an application of the leaves of henbane and poppies with the yelk of an egg. When the boil is indolent, he approves of a stimulant plaster. (Pract. xxix, 4.)

XXIV—ON TERMINTHUS

Oribasius says, that terminthus is a species of phyma, but that a dark bulla lies over it, which having burst, the part below appears as if excoriated, and when it is divided, the pus is found. But Dioscorides of Alexandria says, "Terminthi are eminences formed in the skin, round, of a dark green colour, like the fruit of turpentine." These, therefore, are to be cured like other phymatous swellings, by applying the remedies there described.

Commentary. Aëtius gives the same account of terminthus, which is a species of phyma. See Hippocrat. (Epidem. ii, 11; de Humor. xi, 1); Galen (Comment. in Epidem.); Oribasius (Synops. vii, 136.) Avicenna describes these affections by the name of *albothin* (iv, 7, 3, 1.) He says that they are ulcers produced by black bile; that they appear upon the leg, and are of the same nature as varices.

The terminthus would appear to have been the cutaneous disease to which Willan applied the name of ecthyma.

XXV—ON CARBUNCLE OR ANTHRAX

When the blood having become more melancholic than natural, ferments and fixes in a part, the diseases called carbuncles are formed, which are sloughy ulcers, for the most part beginning with bullæ, like burnt parts, but sometimes without them; and the patients at first rub the part for its itchiness, whether one bulla is formed or several small ones, like millets, which, having burst, a sloughy ulcer takes place, resembling those occasioned by cauteries, the eschar being sometimes of a cineritious colour and sometimes black, along with its being fixed to the base, and in a certain manner nailed to it, and it spreads at the same time, the surrounding flesh is in a fiery state, black in the colour, and shining like bitumen and pitch. Such is the true black bile. But carbuncles that form in the flesh are speedily circumscribed; whereas those which take place in membranes or nerves remain long, and affect sympathetically the parts below, so as to give origin to erysipelatous inflammations. Not a few terminate in suppuration, and most cases are attended with fever.

Carbuncles also sometimes arise from epidemic causes. We must treat them, unless they are very small, by venesection, carrying evacuation as far as to occasion deliquium animi; and after venesection it will not be improper to make deep scarifications in the part, on account of the thickness of the humour. To the affected part we may apply such things as are moderately repellent and discutient, as the cataplasm of plantain and boiled lentil, receiving the tender part of bread baked in an earthen pan, neither very fine nor foul; and above the ulcer we must put some of the strong applications, such as those of Andron, of Polyides, and of Pasion, mixing them with must, until they are of the consistence of the sordes of oil in baths. And so also the dry Massaleotic powder, which may be diluted in like manner. And the root of dracunculus, or of birthwort, or the juice of laserwort, or the Cyrenaic juice may be properly rubbed in, each of these with vinegar. Cases of an erysipelatous nature may be anointed with the applications for erysipelas; but those parts which are suspected of being sympathetically affected are to be wrapped in unwashed wool, out of wine and oil. When the inflammation abates, we must apply to the carbuncles the cephalic cerates spread upon pledgets. That from herbs is an excellent one, and that from natron, and the dry application for spreading ulcers, separately and with rose-oil. When the hardness remains, we must use the one from apples ascribed to Serapion. But we must hasten the suppuration of the carbuncles as much as possible, by changing the cataplasms and medicines twice during the day, and once during the night. In order to root out the carbuncles, and free them from their attachments to the surrounding parts, having divided sour pomegranates, boil in vinegar, and when softened, triturate, put into a linen rag, and apply. When dried, let them be moistened with vinegar. The carbuncle is made to suppurate and burst, by the inner part of old walnuts, or even of that which is not old, and by the leaves and shoots of cypress, or by its young and tender balls (pilulæ), with barley-flour; by raisins deprived of their stones; by dried figs boiled in wine; by the flowers of horned poppy; by the juice of laserwort, with rue and some honey; by liquid pitch with raisins and axunge.

An excellent application for carbuncles. Of litharge, lb. j; of old oil, lb. j; of arsenic, oz. j; boil the oil and litharge until they do not stain, and taking them off the fire, add the arsenic, and then boil it until it become black, and having levigated it in a mortar, use upon pledgets.

For gangrene, old ulcers, those called chironia, strumous ulcers, and the gout: it is a most admirable application for carbuncle, particularly in the eyelids. Of opium, of acacia, of toasted misy, of flakes of copper, of each, dr. ij; of copperas, dr. j; of the seed of henbane, dr. j; triturate in water, and use. They say also that the ointment called tetrapharmacon, having a fifth part of frankincense, is an excellent application. But for carbuncles in the pudenda, take of chalcitis, of copperas, of each, dr. viij; of aphronitrum, dr. ij; triturate with water, and use. Sheep's dung roasted with honey is also a good remedy. In Alexandria they use the green serapias, which is also called orchis and triorchis, with crumbs of bread, as a cataplasm for carbuncles and all sloughy ulcers; and when the eschar falls off, they cure them as a common ulcer.

Commentary. The carbuncle is briefly treated of by Hippocrates (Epidem. ii, 1), and is frequently mentioned by him as a symptom of the pestilential fever. (Epidem. iii.)

Celsus gives a very minute description of carbuncle. With regard to the treatment, nothing, he says, answers so well as immediate burning, which produces no pain, as the flesh is dead. The sore is to be treated like other burnt parts. Under the use of eroding applications a crust is formed, which, being removed from the living flesh, carries all the corrupted parts along with it, and leaves a clean cavity, which is to be filled up by incarnants. When the disease is superficial, corrosive or caustic substances may be substituted, of such a degree of strength as to produce a separation between the dead and sound flesh. But if these applications fail, recourse must be had to burning. He recommends abstinence from food and wine at the commencement, and directs water to be given freely, especially if fever be present.

Pliny gives an indistinct account of an epidemical anthrax, which, he says, prevailed in the province of Narbonne. (Nat. Hist. xxvi, 4.)

Galen ascribes the carbuncle to a defluxion of hot, black, and thick blood, which gives rise to blisters, ulcers, and eschars. He directs us to apply to the eschars those medicines the properties of which resemble fire, such as misy, chalcitis, arsenic, quicklime, and sandarach. His particular remedies are quite similar to our author's. (Meth. Med. xiv), and (ad Glauc. ii.) He mentions the carbuncle as a very unfavorable symptom of the plague. (Epidem. iii, and de Diff. Febr. i, 6.)

The account of the carbuncle given by Aëtius is full and accurate, but is entirely derived from Galen. Oribasius, Actuarius, and Nonnus also repeat his doctrines. Actuarius says that the disease is occasioned by melancholic blood overheated. This is much the same as Galen's theory.

Octavius Horatianus recommends bleeding at the commencement, and external applications of an acrid and caustic nature, or the actual cautery itself. When danger is apprehended from a hot cautery, he directs us to use a cold one.

In the Latin translation of Avicenna the carbuncle is described by the names of pruna and ignis Persicus. It was called pruna from a black slough which is formed in it, resembling a burnt coal. His account of the disease is ample, but mostly copied from Galen and his successors. Rhases approves of venesection at the beginning, and of the actual cautery. He also recommends an application containing mustard and figs. Alsaharavius describes the varieties of anthrax by the names of *alcubam* and *alcoasat*. (Pract. xxix, 12.) At the commencement, he approves of general bleeding and leeches, and afterwards of refrigerant and analeptic medicines, to obviate the tendency to sinking. When these things do not succeed, he directs us to use powerful caustics or the actual cautery. Serapion, like Avicenna, describes it under the name of the ignis Persicus.

Procopius mentions the anthrax as one of the symptoms of the great plague which he describes. (Persica, ii.)

For the carbunculus or anthrax, Brunus and the other writers of that age recommend, at first, bleeding and restricted diet, with maturative applications, such as figs and mustard, or the yeast cataplasm, with oil and salt. When the part becomes black, Theodoricus directs us to have recourse to the actual cautery. (iii, 12.) Municks rather disapproves both of purging and bleeding, but strongly commends the actual cautery, which he greatly prefers to the potential. (Chirurg. i.) Vigierius, however, prefers a paste made from quicklime and soap. V. Manget. (Bibl. Chirurg. i, 374.) The learned Schelhammer speaks favorably both of the potential and the actual cautery. (De Humoribus.)

XXVI—ON CANCERS

Cancer occurs in every part of the body; for it takes place in the eyes and uterus (as we have stated when treating of those parts), and in most other parts of the body; but it is more particularly frequent in the breasts of women, because owing to their laxity, they readily admit the thick humours which occasion it. For cancers are formed by black bile overheated; and if particularly acrid, it is attended with ulceration. On this account, they are darker than phlegmons, without being attended with the same degree of heat. The veins are filled and stretched around like the feet of the animal called cancer (crab), and hence the disease has got its appellation. But some say that it is so called because it adheres to any part which it seizes upon in an obstinate manner like the crab. Owing to the thickness of the humour which occasions it, cancer is an incurable disease, for it can neither be repelled nor discussed; not yielding to purging of the whole body, resisting the milder applications, and being exasperated by the stronger ones. It may be possible, however, to prevent incipient cancers from increasing, by evacuating the melancholic humour before it becomes fixed in the part. We may evacuate, first, if nothing prohibit, by venesection, and afterwards by purging at the commencement, with the simpler purgatives, such as giving dodder of thyme to the amount of oz. ivss; in whey or honied water, and afterwards hiera, containing the black hellebore.

The juice of strychnos may be applied to the ulcerated parts without exciting pain, a linen rag being folded and wetted in it, and laid on; but externally to this, we must apply soft wool, which also has been soaked in the juice, and care must be taken that they do not become dry, by frequently pouring on some of the juice. In all carcinomatous ulcers of a chronic nature, one may use the preparation from pompholyx; and those remedies which were mentioned in the Third Book for cancers in the womb may be applied with advantage.

For carcinomatous and malignant ulcers, for rugose ulcers on the fundament, and for inflammations on the pudenda, testicles, and breasts. In a leaden mortar, and with a leaden pestle, having triturated the Lemnian earth with oxycrate and honied water or milk, so that it become black, or having triturated rose-oil, or the oil of unripe olives, or the juice of house-leek, or that of wall-pennywort, or of lettuce, or of fleawort, or of unripe grapes in like manner, anoint with them. The patient's diet should consist principally of the juice of ptisan and the whey of milk, and from among pot herbs, of mallows, orache, blite, and gourd, of the fishes which live among rocks, and of all kinds of fowls, except those that live in marshes.

From Archigenes, for carcinomatous and malignant ulcers. Levigate equal parts of burnt river crabs and calamine, and sprinkle or apply the ashes of crabs with cerate; or apply the seed of hedge mustard triturated with honey.

Commentary. See Hippocrates (Epidem. v); Galen (de Tumoribus; Meth. Med. xiv; Therap. ad Glauc. ii); Celsus (v, 28); Scribonius Largus; Aëtius (xvi, 43); Oribasius (Morb. Curat. iii, 28); Actuarius (Meth. Med. iv, 16); Avicenna (iv, 3, 2, 15); Serapion (v, 24); Alsaharavius (Pract. xxix, 1, 16); Avenzoar (ii, 7, 27); Haly Abbas (Pract. iii, 32); Rhases (ad Mansor. vii, 9; Contin. xxvii.)

Hippocrates relates a fatal case of cancer in the breast, attended with a sanious discharge, but he does not explain the nature of the treatment.

Our author's description of cancer is abridged from Galen (de Tumor. l. c.) The treatment is derived from the 14th Book of the 'Meth. Med.' He recommends melanogogues to remove the material cause of the disease. In external applications he places little confidence, but prefers those prepared from metallic substances which have been burnt and washed. The only chance of a radical cure consists, he says, in making a complete excision of the part; but in doing this he forbids us to secure the arteries with ligatures, as they will occasion a recurrence of the disease. The part, he says, is loaded with a thick, black, or recrementitious blood. When the cancer is ulcerated, he disapproves of cutting and burning.

Celsus describes carcinoma as an immovable and unequal tumour, attended with swelling of the veins, which are pale or livid. His account of the treatment is so important that it deserves to be given in his own words: "Quidam usi sunt medicamentis adurentibus; quidam ferro adusserunt; quidam scalpello exciderunt: neque ulla unquam medicina profuit; sed adusta, protinus concitata sunt, et increverunt donec occiderent; excisa, etiam post inductam cicatricem, tamen reverterunt, et causam mortis attulerunt: cum interim plerique nullam vim adhibendo, qua tollere id malum tentent, sed imponendo tantum lenia medicamenta quæ quasi blandiantur, quo minus ad ultimam senectutem perveniant, non prohibeantur." In another place, however, he recommends compositions containing arsenic, copperas, cantharides, galls, &c. (v, 22.) He makes a distinction between the *cacoethes*, or malignant tumour, and the true carcinoma, but says that the difference between them is to be recognized only "tempore et experimento." He marks the gradations of malignant disease with singular precision: first, there is cacoethes; then carcinoma without ulceration; and last, there is the fungated ulcer. (The reading in the edition of Milligan is a great improvement.) In doubtful cases he directs us, first to apply caustics or heating medicines, and, if the disease is alleviated, to proceed to the scalpel or burning, according to circumstances; but if it is exacerbated, we are to conclude that it is of a carcinomatous nature, and must abstain from all acrid and vehement applications.

Scribonius Largus recommends for all malignant ulcers, even such as are cancerous, an application consisting of arsenic, p. vj; of squama æris, p. iij; of elaterium, p. j; of burnt paper, p. iij.

Aëtius gives from Archigenes and Leonidas an interesting account of the disease, which he divides into ulcerated cancer, and cancer without ulceration. He describes the disease in the female breast as consisting of a large tumour which is unequal and resisting, extending its roots far, and being attended with varicose veins: its colour is either cineritious, verging to redness or livid; it appears soft, but is in reality very hard; is accompanied with a pungent pain, and gives rise to malignant phlegmons in the armpits. The pains shoot to the clavicle and scapula. An ulcerated cancer, he says, goes on corroding and spreading deeper, nor can it be stopped; it discharges a sanies of an abominable smell, and is aggravated by medicines and handling. The disease he considers as generally incurable. His surgical treatment will be stated in the Sixth Book. He recommends purging with hiera and the theric, Mithridatic antidote, &c. Apparently, in order to mitigate the violence of the pains, he directs us to make an application containing equal portions of plantain, poppy heads, the seed of the wort, and other things of the like kind. For ulcerated cancer he recommends emollient epithemes, such as the one containing litharge, axunge, white wax, oil, and the yelks of eggs.

Oribasius and Actuarius supply nothing of importance that is not to be found in our author. Nonnus, according to Sprengel, is the only ancient author who attributes cancerous ulcerations to acrimony of the bile. But Nonnus merely copies the words of our author.

The Arabians agree with the Greeks in representing the disease as being produced by black bile. They were, no doubt, led to form this opinion from remarking that the blood in the part is thick and black, which they considered owing to its not being properly purged of its recrementitious sediment. The moderns deride this theory, but they have substituted nothing satisfactory in its stead. Van Swieten thinks more favorably of the ancient doctrines. (Comment. § 485.) Avicenna speaks highly of a milk diet. Serapion likewise approves of milk deprived of its butter, and of a vegetable diet. He speaks of no other treatment as being likely to prove remediable, with the exception of excision and the cautery. Haly Abbas rather approves of excision when the disease is seated in a part which admits of this operation. However, like Galen, he disapproves of tying the arteries. The characteristic symptoms of the disease, he says, are a stony hardness and distension. The account given by Alsaharavius is nothing different. Rhases has little confidence in excision. After ulceration has taken place he approves of using a cooling application, containing ceruse, tutty, rose-oil, the juice of nightshade, and some other such things of a cold nature. He mentions a case of cancer of the breast, in which the whole mamma was extirpated, but the disease returned on the other side. One of his authorities, Antyllus, describes the cancerous sore as having a tendency to spread inwards, its edges being thick, large, and everted, and the discharge thin and acrid. When the disease cannot be got completely extirpated, he forbids us to meddle with it.

Theodoricus and all the earlier modern writers on medicine, call the cancer by the name of apostema melancholicum, and recommend the same treatment for it as the Greeks and Arabians.

XXVII—ON ŒDEMA

Having treated of swellings formed by hot humours, we shall now treat of those from the opposite, beginning with the œdema. For as erysipelas is formed by a bilious humour, so is œdema by a pituitous, being a loose swelling devoid of pain. We are aware also, that œdematous swellings occur in the feet, in dropsical affections, in phthisis, and in cachexia, but in them the œdema is a symptom of the complaint under which the person is labouring, and requires no very particular treatment; for it will be sufficient in general to rub the limbs sometimes with vinegar and rose-oil, and sometimes with oil and salts, or the salts may be added to the vinegar and rose-oil. When the œdema is occasioned by a pituitous humour being determined to the part, a sponge soaked in oxycrate may be properly applied with a bandage loosely put on, beginning below and terminating above. The sponge ought to be new, but if such a one is not at hand, that which is may be cleaned with natron, or more especially with what is called strained lye. If the swelling do not thereby subside, we may mix some alum. And a very convenient application is a tender wick of a lamp, soaked in such a fluid, and applied. A good remedy also is horned poppy. When the œdema has become chronic, having first anointed the part with oil, and then applied a sponge out of lye, bind it firmly, and you will effect a cure. Every kind of earth discusses and represses œdematous swellings, more especially the Ægyptian, and also the matured woad.

Commentary. See Galen (ad Glauc. ii; de Tumoribus); Aëtius (xv, 1); Oribasius (Morb. Curat. iii, 51); Leo. (vii, 5); Actuarius (Meth. Med. iv, 16); Nonnus (251); Serapion (v, 23); Avicenna (iv, 3, 2); Haly Abbas (Theor. viii, 11; Pract. iii, 30); Alsaharavius (xxix, 13); Rhases (ad Mansor. vii, 12.)

Our author's account of this disease is taken from Galen, Oribasius, Aëtius, and, in fact, all the Greek, Latin, and Arabian authorities adopt his views, without any material alteration. They all concur in recommending cooling and astringent applications, with suitable bandages; and, in certain cases, friction. Rhases recommends that the limb should be buried in heated sand. He also approves of various cooling and astringent applications with bandages. In the translation of Alsaharavius, the œdema is described by the name of *apostema flegmaticum*; in those of Avicenna, Haly Abbas, and Serapion, by that of *undemia*. The celebrated Paracelsus used the term undemia for œdema. In some late works we have seen it stated that the undemia was a species of erysipelas, but this is evidently a mistake.

XXVIII—ON EMPHYSEMA

Emphysema is formed by a flatulent spirit, collected sometimes under the skin, sometimes under the periosteum, or the membranes which surround the muscles. And it is also sometimes collected in the stomach and intestines, or between them and the peritoneum, in those kinds of dropsy which are called tympanitic; and it differs from œdema in this, that the parts do not pit upon pressure like it, and that it sounds like a drum. The density of the body co-operates in preventing the flatus from being dissipated, at the same time that the flatus also is of a thick nature. Wherefore, the indication of cure is to rarefy the body, and attenuate the thick air; which is to be accomplished by means of attenuant and heating remedies. When the complaint is seated in the stomach and intestines, this is to be brought about by a fine oil, having rue, cumin, or parsley seed boiled in it. And sometimes a large cupping instrument without scarificators, applied two or three times to the navel, will discuss it. When the muscles from contusion are inflated, so as to sound like an emphysema, the parts will not bear very heating and acrid applications. Wherefore, at the commencement, we must use paregorics liberally, and, when the disease is on the decline, discutients. Thus we may use sodden must with a small quantity of oil, applying them warm upon unwashed wool, or mixing the cerate of unwashed wool. And we must take care that the heat be preserved, for it is not expedient that the part be cooled. When the patient has been soothed, we are to mix vinegar and nitre or aphronitrum, and afterwards some lye; and lastly, we may use discutient plasters, for the removal of the complaint such as the following: having boiled the sordes of the oil used in baths, strain it first, so that it may become pure, and again throw it into the pot, and having triturated slaked lime like flour, sprinkle until it become of the consistence of clay, and use. A still more effectual application is the compound medicine from sycomores.

Commentary. See Galen (Meth. Med. xiv); (Therap. ad Glauc. ii); Aëtius (xv, 2); Oribasius (Synop. vii); Actuarius (Meth. Med. ii, 12); Nonnus (252); Scribonius Largus (§ 119); Avicenna (iv, 3, 2, 20); Serapion (v, 23); Alsaharavius (Pract. xxix, § 1, 14); Rhases (Divis. 127, Cont. xxvii.)

Our author has copied closely from Galen. The great indications of cure, as laid down by him and acknowledged by all subsequent authorities, are to rarefy the containing parts and attenuate the spirit. By *spirit*, as we stated in another place, the ancients meant a thick air or gas. The indications which we have mentioned are best fulfilled by friction with oils, in which calefacient medicines, such as cumin, parsley, anise, and the like, have been boiled. When, however, any inflammation is suspected, he properly forbids us to use acrid or heating medicines. When the pain of the bowels is violent in cases of tympanites, he allows medicines containing opium, which are to be given by the mouth if the small intestines be affected, but are to be administered in a clyster if the large intestines be the seat of the disease. When the disease is in a muscular part, he directs us to use a combination of attenuants and emollients. In certain cases he recommends dry-cupping. Oribasius, Aëtius, Actuarius, and Nonnus, adopt the views of Galen, without any alteration.

For tympanites, Scribonius recommends cumin internally.

Avicenna, like our author, in ordinary cases recommends combinations of attenuants and calefacients, dry-cupping and the like, for dispelling the spirit; but when the disease arises from contusion of the muscles, he directs us to use resolvents and paregorics. Serapion approves of similar treatment. Alsaharavius recommends attenuant and calefacient remedies externally and internally. In the translation of his works, the disease is called inflatio. Rhases recommends friction with calefacient oils; he remarks that the disease occurs most commonly in the stomach and intestines. He calls it by the name of apostema inflatum.

XXIX—FOR SPRAINS AND CONTUSIONS

Sprains of the joints and contusions are remedied by unwashed wool, or a sponge soaked in vinegar and oil, and applied; by the tender parts of boiled bulbous roots with honey, by the leaves of the chaste tree, salts, and roasted nitre, triturated with cerate. The affusion of sweet water, or of hot sea water, may be used. But after the inflammation and pains have subsided, apply rubbing to the sprained parts.

Commentary. See Aëtius (xiv, 71); Oribasius (Synops. vii, 14); Actuarius (Meth. Med. ii, 35); Scribonius Largus (§ 209); Rhases (Divis. i, 140.)

Aëtius makes mention of all the remedies recommended by our author, with the exception of the affusion of water; which, however, is a method of treatment deserving of attention. Oribasius mentions particularly the affusion of hot sea water. Scribonius Largus recommends a plaster containing litharge, alum, ærugo, ammoniac, &c. Rhases directs us to use attenuant ointments, sedative plasters, and loose bandages, with rest.

XXX—ON CONTUSIONS OF THE FLESH AND ECCHYMOSIS

The flesh being bruised by some weight falling upon it, and the small veins in it being ruptured, blood is poured out from them by exhalation, and collecting under the skin, is called ecchymoma. When the skin is not divided, a soft yielding tumour is the consequence; it is pale, and for the most part unattended with pain. Our object, therefore, is to discuss the contained blood, and that quickly, before it become black; and at first, astringents are to be mixed with the discutients, because the bruised coats of the veins stand in need of condensation. After these things, we must use those applications which are merely discutient without astringency. And by scarifying the ecchymomata at the commencement, we may thus apply the subsequent treatment. For chronic cases of ecchymoma, radish in the form of a cataplasm is a suitable remedy, but it must be taken away when it becomes pungent; or a cataplasm of the juice of radish with crumbs of bread, may be applied. The diseases called hypopion and hyposphagma, are species of ecchymosis, and also the effusion of blood below the nail from a blow; of these, the first two are treated of in their proper places in the Third Book; and the affection of the nail will be handled in the Surgical part of the work.

Commentary. This is taken almost word for word from Oribasius (Synops. vii, 14); Aëtius directs us to scarify the part affected with ecchymosis, and then to apply to it the inside of citrons (xiv, 68.)

Avicenna approves of scarifications, provided the extravasated blood cannot be got otherwise removed. (iv, 4, 2, 3.)

XXXI—ON RUPTURE AND TEARING OF THE FLESH

Rupture is altogether attended with ecchymosis. It is cured by medicines which are moderately heating, as the acopon from black poplars, and such as resemble it. But when the rupture is deep-seated, we must have recourse to such remedies as are more acrid and cutting. The use of the cupping instrument is likewise beneficial to them. Should therefore the whole ecchymosis be discussed, the separated flesh readily unites; but if it continue a long time, and sordes form under it, the ruptured flesh can no longer unite; and we must only apply the lips together, so that a small occasion may readily separate them, and that the intermediate space may be filled with some moisture, and in a certain manner an ecchymosis may be formed as at the commencement, except that it is sooner discussed, as containing a thin humour, whereas that at the commencement was formed of blood. Vulsion takes place when certain fibres are torn asunder, and it only requires soothing applications until the pain is removed; for they cannot be made to coalesce. Wherefore, the round birthwort, if any, is a convenient application to ruptured and torn parts; and in like manner, the root of the large centaury, and the juice of it, rhubarb, costus, and bdellium, drunk with oxymel.

Commentary. These remarks are taken from Aëtius (xiv, 69, 70); or Oribasius (Synops. vii, 14); and they are copied by Nonnus (Epit. 254); and Actuarius (Meth. Med. iv, 16.)

The Arabians treat these accidents upon exactly the same principles. See in particular Avicenna, as quoted in the preceding section.

XXXII—ON SCIRRHUS

Genuine scirrhus is a preternatural swelling, hard and devoid of sensibility; but that which is not genuine is only attended with diminished sensibility. That which is wholly insensible, then, is utterly incurable; but that which is attended only with diminished sensibility is not incurable, and yet it is not easily cured, for it is occasioned by a viscid and thick humour, which is fixed in the hardened parts, so as to be difficult to get discharged. Sometimes, then, the scirrhus is the original complaint, and goes on to increase; but for the most part, it is occasioned by the physicians applying too cooling and astringent remedies to erysipelas and phlegmon.

If one, therefore, apply strongly discutient medicines to indurations of the body, one will indeed produce a visible diminution of the scirrhus in a short time, but will leave the remainder of the complaint in an incurable state; for the thin moisture being dissipated, what remains is rendered dry and hard as a stone. The discutient application, then, ought to be in a certain degree emollient, without possessing manifestly heating and desiccant qualities. Such are all kinds of marrow, more especially that of a stag or of a calf, and the grease of a lion, of a panther, or of bears, or of a bull, and among birds, that of geese, of domestic fowls, or of pheasants: but that of bucks and he-goats is drier. And to these may be added, ammoniac perfume, bdellium, more especially the Scythian, the humid and fatty storax, and the Egyptian mastich. To all other parts of the body, when in a scirrhous state, these things may be applied singly, and in composition; but for tendons and ligaments, we are to dissolve in the strongest vinegar some stone that has been heated in the fire. If possible, the one to be used should be pyrites, or if not it, the lapis molaris or millstone. In this, therefore, the affected part is to be moved, so that it may receive the vapour which arises from it; and afterwards, an emollient medicine is to be applied. A thin oil then, and not water, is to be poured on the part, by all means once a day, and sometimes one may boil in the oil the root of marshmallows, or of wild cucumber. The patients ought to abstain from the use of the bath, at least from the frequent use of it. But when the scirrhus is moderately softened, the softest ammoniac is to be dissolved in very strong vinegar, and the part rubbed with it for several days in succession; after which, we must again have recourse to an emollient application, having the fattest galbanum and opoponax added to it. Such are that from bacon, that ascribed to Amythaon, and those which we are about to describe for scrofula.

Commentary. See Galen (De Tumoribus; Meth. Med. xiv; Therap. ad Glauc. ii); Oribasius (Synops. vii, 34); Aëtius (xv, 3, 4); Leo (vii, 4); Actuarius (Meth. Med. iv, 16); Serapion (v, 23); Avicenna (iv, 3, 2, 12); Haly Abbas (Pract. iii, 31); Alsaharavius (xxix, 1, 15); Rhases (Antid. i, Cont. xxvii, Antidot. i.)

This section is entirely taken from Galen (Ther. ad Glauc. l. c.) Galen's account, however, is somewhat fuller than our author's, and contains a case treated upon the principles which he lays down. It was a case of hard swelling in the thigh, arising from an erysipelas which had been improperly treated by astringent and cooling applications. Galen informs us that he began by pouring upon the limb an attenuant oil, namely, the Sabine; after which he caused it to be rubbed with marrows and fats medicated with bdellium, mastich, ammoniac perfume, and the like. After this he bathed the whole limb with a solution of ammoniac in very acrid vinegar. When the swelling had been lessened, but not completely removed by these means, he afterwards applied one of the pitch medicines, and at length effected a cure. In another place he states that scirrhus is sometimes allied to cancer.

Oribasius likewise recommends a combination of emollients with discutients; and Actuarius approves of the same practice.

Aëtius has a valuable chapter upon this subject. Besides the articles mentioned by our author, he recommends various rosins, turpentine, frankincense, and the like. He forbids the use of aluminous, sulphureous, and chalybeate baths. For indurations of tendons he recommends things possessed of attenuant and cutting properties combined with emollients, such as ammoniac dissolved in vinegar with melons.

The Arabians treat of scirrhus in much the same terms as the Greeks. Avicenna properly directs us to bleed when there is congestion of black blood in the part, and afterwards to use applications of a solvent and emollient nature. He and Serapion mention the same identical remedies as those of Paulus. For dissolving hard tumours he recommends an oil containing fenugreek, cyperus, and aromatic reed. Haly Abbas ascribes the formation of scirrhus to the same causes as our author, and recommends relaxant and emollient applications. Alsaharavius directs us to procure evacuations of black bile, and gives prescriptions for various emollient and discutient applications. When the usual remedies do not succeed, he advises recourse to be had to the operation. Rhases divides scirrhus into two varieties, that accompanied with sensibility, and that which is insensible. He mentions that Antyllus approved of extirpation and the actual cautery when the disease is of a corroding and cancerous nature.

XXXIII—ON STRUMA OR SCROFULA

Strumæ are indurated glands forming principally in the neck, armpits, and groins. Their gencral treatment therefore is the same as that for scirrhus, but in particular the flour of bitter lupines is to be boiled in oxymel and applied (this also answers with phyma;) or apply cows' dung boiled in vinegar. This discusses all indurated swellings. But strumæ may be properly discussed by means of quicklime mixed with honey, the sordes of baths, oil, or axunge; or, equal parts of quicklime and natron, and four times the quantity of cardamom and fenugreek may be boiled with honey for an emollient ointment and applied. This one discusses hard strumæ, and produces the rupture of suppurated swellings; the flour of darnel boiled with pigeon's dung, or linseed and wine: or, green olives, either wild or cultivated; or, the white cardamus triturated with liquid pitch and made into an emollient ointment may be applied; or, the ashes of the dried root of the wild cucumber, and the burnt dried leaves of the bay, may be mixed with turpentine and applied; or, equal parts of stavesacre and of natron, with double the quantity of rocket may be applied, with rosin; or, goats' or cows' dung boiled in vinegar; or, the flour of bitter vetches soaked in the urine of a young person not come to manhood, and added to melted pitch, wax and oil; or, a dead snake may be thrown into a pot, and being covered over with gypsum, it is to be put into a furnace, the ashes of it mixed with equal parts of fenugreek, and then added to honey and used. And the composition from asps is an admirable one, also that from fullers' herb, that from the wild cucumber and that from cedar rosin. The following one produces suppuration, or resolution of strumæ: Of myrrh, dr. x; of ammoniac perfume, dr. ij; of the mistletoe of oaks, dr. viij; of galbanum, dr. iv; of bee-glue, dr. j; pound in a mortar.

For strumæ and hardness of the breasts. Of wrought birdlime, of dry rosin, of wax, of each lb. j; of galbanum, oz. iij.

For strumæ ulcerated and not ulcerated. Of wax, of pine rosin, of axunge not salted, of horehound, of scraped birdlime, of each oz. vj.

An application for strumæ. Of old oil, lb. ij; of wax, lb. j; of colophonian rosin, oz. iv; of natron, oz. iv; the heads of garlic xij. Take away the cloves (nuclei) of the garlic, macerate in oil for three days, then having boiled until they are softened, throw them away, and melt in the oil those ingredients which are soluble, and after they are taken off the fire sprinkle on it levigated natron. It also breaks apostemes.—*Another*: Of the ashes of figs, oz. ij; of fissile alum, oz. j; of aphronitrum, oz. j; of liquid pitch, oz. vij.

A septic application for scrofula. Of fissile alum, of realgar, of each, dr. iv; of the flakes of copper, dr. j; of orpiment, dr. j; sprinkle the strumæ with it in a dry state; but if they are of a cancerous nature, mix with rose oil and use twice a day.

Commentary. See Hippocrates (De Glandulis); Galen (Meth. Med. xiv, 11); Oribasius (Synops. vii, 29); Aëtius (xv, 5); Actuarius (Meth. Med. iv, 16); Nonnus (Epit. 124); Celsus (v, 18); Scribonius Largus (153); Myrepsus (56); Marcellus (36); Serapion (v, 25); Avicenna (iv, 3, 2, 10); Albucasis (Chirurg. ii, 42); Alsaharavius (Pract. xxix, 1, 23); Haly Abbas (Pract. iii, 33); Rhases (ad Mansor. vii. 8; Cont. xxvii); Avenzoar (i, 10, 10.)

Hippocrates mentions struma as being one of the worst diseases of the neck, originating in inflammation, and being produced by a pituitous and indolent defluxion.

Galen directs us when scrofulous glands are not situated near large vessels to extract them with the knife, or consume them with septic applications. In another place he relates a case in which an imprudent surgeon, while removing a scrofulous gland of the neck, cut the recurrent nerves, and thereby occasioned loss of speech. (De Loc. Aff. i, 6.) For an account of the operation see the Sixth Book.

Part only of our author's applications are derived from Oribasius.

A very minute account of these complaints is given by Aëtius. He divides strumæ into the mild and the malignant. The mild are without inflammation or pain, and are attended with a moderate degree of hardness; the malignant are accompanied with inflammation, and a throbbing pain, feel unequal, have enlarged veins, and are exacerbated by handling or medicines. The latter are said to be incurable. He mentions, upon the authority of Leonidas, the accident related by Galen. He approves, however, of the operation in general. Incipient strumæ, he states, may be discussed like scirrhi, by a combination of emollients with discutients. He gives a long list of prescriptions for removing scrofulous tumours. One of them contains arsenic mixed with the fat of a goat or ox. With regard to the general treatment, he recommends laxatives, restricted diet, emetics, and the theriac.

Actuarius and Nonnus, as usual, borrow from our author.

Celsus remarks that strumæ occur most frequently in the neck, armpits, groins, sides, and the female breasts. He represents them as indolent affections of the glands, which come slowly to maturity and prove very troublesome to the physician. Some, he says, give white hellebore in these cases, and use applications for bringing them forward or for discussing them. Others have recourse to caustics, and when the eschar is removed, they heal the ulcer upon general principles. When the sore becomes clean he recommends exercise and a nourishing diet.

Scribonius Largus, Marcellus, and Myrepsus give nearly the same prescriptions as our author. Arsenic is an ingredient in the septic applications of Myrepsus.

Avicenna recommends emetics, phlegmagogues, bleeding in the arm, attenuant food, and avoiding all gross things and repletion. As a discutient he and Serapion commend the diachylon plaster. Haly Abbas likewise mentions this application, and also directs the swellings to be burnt with caustics. Alsaharavius briefly recommends excision or burning. Serapion evidently copies from our author. Avenzoar gives a very full account of scrofulous swellings, which, he says, are formed in general of a gross and viscid phlegm. Except in very particular cases he disapproves of bleeding. He approves in general of discutient applications; but when the swelling tends to suppuration, he directs us to promote it; and when pus is fairly formed he recommends us to let it out, but cautions the surgeon not to attempt this operation unless he has a practical acquaintance with anatomy, lest he wound any of the veins, arteries, or nerves.

Rhases forbids the knife when the scrofula is in the neck or deep seated. In certain cases he approves of destroying the tunic with septic applications.

Brunus, and the other surgical writers of that age, in imitation of the Arabian authorities, direct scrofulous tumours to be treated with discutients, excision, or septics. A discutient ointment recommended by Brunus consists of litharge, common oil, and the juice of melons and fenugreek. His septic medicine is a mixture of arsenic and quicklime, which is to be applied with honey. (Chirurg. Minor. 19.)

XXXIV—ON STEATOMA, ATHEROMA, AND MELICERIS

These things belong to the class of apostemes, as we said when treating of them, and each receives its peculiar appellation from the substance contained in the tumour. Thus one of them is like fat, another like honey, and the third like pap. The indication of cure in them all is to discuss the contents, produce the putrefaction of them, or to cut them out. Some tumours fall under all these three indications of cure, namely, those which contain a thin fluid, as the meliceris; others come under two of them only, as the atheroma, for it can only be cured by excision or putrefaction. But the steotoma admits of no cure except by a surgical operation, for it can neither be discussed nor made to putrefy. The diagnosis of each of these may be found in the Surgical part of the work, while the materials of which the discutients are formed are mentioned under the head of scrofula. This application is peculiarly adapted for discussing meliceris: Twenty raisins without their stones; of squama æris, dr. iij; having first fomented, apply.—*Another*: Of Cretan cistus, of bdellium, of galbanum, of ammoniæ perfume, of bee-glue, of turpentine, equal parts; to be pounded together in a mortar. It applies to scrofula, parotis, furunculus, and phyma. But Archigenes applies to meliceris aphronitrum, and double the quantity of hellebore, with hard cerate. But septics cannot be applied while the skin remains entire; we must therefore in the first place lay bare the meliceris, atheroma, or strumæ, with caustic medicines, of which the most simple is that consisting of quicklime (calx viva,) soap, and strained lye. The following one is more complex, and admits of being kept: Of calx viva, dr. iv; of red natron toasted, of burnt lees of wine, of each, dr. ij; of vermilion, dr. j; triturate in lye; and having made it of the consistence of liquid honey, boil three times, until it is of the proper thickness, and lay it up in a leaden vessel, pouring in some lye, so that it may not quickly become dry. It applies to acrochordon, myrmecia, pterygium, clavus, callus, and excrescences of the gums. The lees of wine should not be older than two months. Anoint the skin with this, and when it begins to dry clean it away with a sponge, and anoint again; and when the skin becomes black, wash away again, and use escharotics. When the eschars fall off, apply the septic medicines. A septic application which is not irritating: Of squama æris, dr. iv; of realgar, dr. ij; of black hellebore, dr. ij; use with rose oil.—*Another*: Of squama æris, of realgar, of nettle seeds toasted, equal parts; use with rose oil.—*Another*: Of burnt sea-urchins, of the shell of the cuttle fish, of arsenic, equal parts; use with rose oil, but rub all the parts around with cerate and oil. This also is a good application: Of quicklime, p. ij; of chalcitis, p. j; of arsenic, p. j.

Commentary. See most of the authorities referred to in the preceding section.

Our author's definitions seem to be taken from Galen. (De Tumoribus and Meth. Med. xiv.) Galen states that the steatoma is to be cured solely by a surgical operation; that the meliceris may be treated by discutients, septics, or excision with the knife; and that the atheroma admits only of excision, or the application of septics.

Aëtius may be referred to as an interesting authority upon this subject. The steatoma, he says, is a preternatural tumour, free from discoloration, and soft to the touch. He recommends excision for it. The contents of the atheroma consist of a pultaceous substance surrounded by a membranous tunic, within which are also sometimes found hairs; nay, Philoxenus affirms that he had found animals like gnats and flies. The meliceris also has a membranous coat, and its contents resemble honey. He approves also of the surgical operation for the meliceris and atheroma, but permits to attempt their reduction by means of discutients consisting of such ingredients as ammoniac, ceruse, turpentine, galbanum, vinegar, &c. He makes no mention of septics; indeed arsenic does not enter into any of his compositions.

Oribasius and Actuarius lay down the same rules of treatment as our author. Nonnus as usual epitomises him with some slight alterations. The active ingredients in one of his septic applications are sandarach and hellebore. Leo is brief and indistinct.

Celsus marks the differences of these tumours with his characteristic terseness and precision: "Atheromati subest quasi tenuis pulticula: meliceridi liquidior humor; ideoque pressus fluit: steatomati pingue quiddam." He recommends excision. (vii, 6.)

Avicenna's plan of treatment is so like our author's, that we need not give it in detail. The steatoma is to be removed solely by an operation. For the two others he permits the use of septic applications, such as arsenic, quicklime, hellebore, the lees of wine, &c. Haly's definitions are similar to those of our author, and he recommends either excision or the use of septics, such as vitriol. The treatment laid down by Alsaharavius is quite the same. In the barbarous translation of his works they are called by the names of *alsahamia, asalia,* and *accida.* (Pract. xxix, 1, 22.)

Vegetius, the veterinary surgeon, describes these tumours as they appear in cattle. He directs them to be treated by excision. (Mulom. ii, 30.)

It will be remarked from the text, that the ancients were well acquainted with the caustic powers of the *calx cum kali.* In fact, our author in this section has given a prescription for the paste now commonly used for forming issues.

It appears from the works of Fabricius of Aquapendente, that the practice of treating atheroma and meliceris by septic applications was sufficiently common in his time. Andreas Laurentius approves of removing *scrofulous tumours* in this way when they are deep-seated and have a broad base. He thus enumerates the septics used in his age: "Secundo extrahi potest struma caustico, nunc affixo in ejus medio candente ferro, nunc admotis erodentibus et putrefacientibus ut sandaraca, arsenico, argento liquido usto, oleo quod ex atramento sutorio igne elicitur, calce non extincta cum sapone, axungia porcina cum argenti sublimati portiuncula, pulvere mercurii, erinaceorum cumbustorum, testæ sæpiæ, auripigmenti." He also recommends us to tie the base of the tumour with a thread wet in a solution of arsenic (De strum. nat.) The treatment of atheroma by caustics is well described in the 'Bibliotheca Chirurgica' of Manget.

XXXV—OF FAVI

The favus is a swelling on the skin, having perforations through which a honey-like fluid is discharged. Wherefore dried grapes with rue are to be applied to it; or, the tender leaves of the fig tree with honey; or, cresses with linseed in honey; or, the root of the garden cucumber with honey; or, sulphur vivum with cerate or turpentine. You may vary the treatment of favi by transferring hither what is said in the Third Book regarding achores.

Commentary. Alexander states that the favus resembles the achores, differing from them solely in magnitude: for the openings of the pores by which the fluid escapes resemble the combs of bees, whence it takes it appellation; but in achores we cannot see the pores by which the fluid issues.

Aëtius gives a similar description of the complaint, which, he says, mostly attacks muscular parts, as the limbs, soles of the feet, over the sixth vertebra of the neck, and the sides. When it attacks the head, he says, it sometimes spreads to the skull. In this case he directs us to treat it with acrid applications, and even the actual cautery. For incipient favus he recommends an application consisting of sulphur, barley flour and meal.

Nonnus recommends the following application: of litharge, dr. ij; of alum, dr. iij; of the leaves of rue, dr. ij; of wine and rose-oil, q. s.

Celsus's description is so important, that we shall give a considerable part of it in his own language. He mentions two species of the favus, or κήϱιον. "Alterum est subalbidum, furunculo simile; sed majus, et cum dolore majore: quod ubi maturescit, habet foramina, per quæ fertur humor glutinosus et purulentus; nec tamen ad justam maturitatem pervenit. Si divisum est, multo plus intus corrupti, quam in furunculo, apparet, altiusque descendit. Raro fit nisi in capillis. Alterum est minus, super corpus eminens, durum, latum, subviride, subpallidum, magis exulceratum; siquidem ad singulorum pilorum radices foramina sunt, per quæ fertur humor glutinosus, subpallidus, crassitudinem mellis, aut visci referens, interdum olei: si inciditur, viridis intra caro apparet. Dolor autem, et inflammatio ingens est, adeo ut acutam quoque febrem movere consuerint." For the second species he recommends as external applications a dried fig, linseed boiled in mulse, and emollient plasters. To the other he also directs us to make applications containing figs, turpentine, rosin, &c. But when these have not the effect, he recommends us to cut the fungous excrescences down to the sound flesh, and then to dress the sore upon general principles. (v. 28.) The above account of an affection of the scalp, which we have often met with in practice, is the most accurate to be found in any author ancient or modern. We are even in doubt whether the complaint be at all noticed in modern works on surgery. It is not to be confounded with the Porrigo favosa, or Porrigo scutulata, of Dr. Bateman.

Avicenna's description of the achor and favus is far from distinct. (iv, 7, 3, 1.) The favi appear to be the pustulæ capitis quæ dicuntur *alsahafa* of Alsaharavius. (Pract. i, 11.) His description, however, is by no means distinct. He approves of general evacuants, and local applications of a stimulant nature, such as sulphur, mercury, birthwort, &c. Serapion has not described the favus very accurately, but he has given a full account of the treatment. He properly forbids strong applications at first. (i, 3.) Rhases recommends much the same applications as Serapion. (Ad Mansor. v, 16.)

XXXVI—ON THE SIMPLE ULCER

Since a simple ulcer is merely a division, if one will bring together the parts which are separated, and apply a circular bandage around, the divided parts will adhere together without more ado. It is necessary, however, when at one of its lips the ulcer is everted obliquely, to begin the bandaging there, and turn it to the opposite side. When it is deranged both ways, it will be proper to use a double-headed bandage, and thus to bring the lips together; for when nothing has fallen between the lips, such as a hair, or a sand, or oil, or filth, or the like, the ulcer will adhere completely. When the ulcer is large, so that the separated parts cannot be completely brought together by the aforesaid bandaging, they are to be first united with sutures, and then bandages are to be thus applied, and those remedies used which are called agglutinants, which have the power of drying and consuming the collected moisture, and prevent more from flowing to the part.

Commentary. On ulcers the following ancient authors may be consulted: Hippocrates (De Ulceribus); Galen (Meth. Med. iii, & iv); Oribasius (Synops. vii); Aëtius (xiv); Actuarius (Meth. Med. iv, 16); Nonnus (Epit. 259); Pliny (H. N. xxxii, 44); Celsus (v); Octavius Horatianus (i, 19, 20); Scribonius Largus (94); Avicenna (iv, 4, 1, 2, 3); Serapion (vii, 28); Averrhoes (Collig. vii, 32); Haly Abbas (Pract. iv, 18); Alsaharavius (Tract. xxix, 2, 2); Rhases (Ad Mansor. vii, 3; Divis. i, 138; Contin. xxviii.)

The author of the Hippocratic treatise quoted above particularly praises wine as a lotion for ulcers; and we may mention that Dr. Hosack, an intelligent American writer, states it as his opinion, that the surgeons of the present day might learn from him an important lesson upon its utility in such cases. He condemns the use of oils and fat.

Of all authors, ancient or modern, Galen has laid down the principles upon which ulcers ought to be treated with the greatest precision. He defines an ulcer to be, "a solution of continuity," a definition evidently very comprehensive, and including wounds as well as cases of spontaneous ulceration. His directions for the treatment of a simple ulcer or fresh wound are similar to those of our author; that is to say, he directs us to bring the lips of it together, and secure them with a bandage, or, if that is not sufficient, by sutures or clasps. Wine he pronounces to be the best of all applications to ulcers, in as far as they are ulcers.

Our author copies very closely from Oribasius.

In applying the bandage, Aëtius directs us to begin above the sore if only one simple bandage is to be used, but if two are necessary, as in fractures, he recommends us to begin at the ulcer and proceed upwards, and in like manner to begin again at the ulcer and roll downwards. He forbids us to loose the bandages oftener than every alternate day; and directs us not to apply water to the ulcer, but to remove the sanies with a soft, dry linen cloth.

Celsus describes very accurately the treatment of a recent wound or simple ulcer. He approves, according to circumstances, of bandages, clasps, or sutures, and his directions respecting the application of them are highly important, but too long for our limits. After the sore is dressed he directs us to apply over it a sponge soaked in vinegar, or, if that cannot be borne, in wine or cold water. This practice is deserving of imitation. He says afterwards: "Optimum etiam medicamentum quies est: moveri et ambulare nisi sanis alienum."

Octavius Horatianus directs us to avoid the bath, the fire, the sun, cold air, loud cries, intoxication, venery, and passion, lest these should occasion a rupture of the parts which had adhered.

Avicenna with his usual good sense gives judicious directions for the treatment of simple ulcers, but his principles are nearly the same as those laid down by Galen. He defines an ulcer to be "a solution of continuity, attended with a discharge of sanies or pus." This seems to be an unexceptionable definition. He forbids all oily and watery applications, and recommends us to observe that no body intervene between the lips of the wound when the bandage is applied. Rhases gives similar directions. He condemns the practice of those who put oil into a wound, and who allow the patient to take wine and heating food. Averrhoes lays down similar rules with considerable precision. Haly Abbas and Alsaharavius follow the practice of Galen without the slightest alteration.

Considerable difference of opinion has prevailed respecting the nature of the clasps (Fibulæ ἄγκτηρες) recommended by Celsus and other ancient authorities. Rhodius and Le Clerc maintain that no more was meant than a *simple interrupted suture,* but to this opinion we cannot subscribe. (See Le Clerc, Hist. de la Méd. iv, 2, 5, and Fabricius of Aquapendente Œuvres Chirurg. ii, 108.) They would appear to have been metallic clasps of a peculiar construction.

XXXVII—ON AGGLUTINANTS

Oak leaves applied, and those of the willow and cabbage; the fruit, leaves, and bark of the mezereon, and the juice of the more austere plantain, papyrus soaked in oxycrate or wine, and wrapped round in a circular manner. The following are agglutinants of fresh wounds: the leaves of the pine and spruce fir, and their fresh bark wrapped round like a bandage, with water, oxycrate, or wine; and new cheese pounded. But we must apply externally the leaves of dock, or of vine, or of beet, or of lettuce. But cheese made of acid milk cures even the larger sores; and the wild pears repress the discharge. The horse-tail (Hippuris) may be applied with advantage, even if the tendons are divided asunder; and the matured woad may be used to indurated bodies even when they occur in the heads of muscles. The leaves and shoots of cypress, and its recent and soft balls (pilulæ) may be applied to indurated parts, but we must mix with it some of the fine dust taken from a wall near a mill. Myrrh rubbed with water, or frankincense and earth worms, agglutinate even the divisions of tendons; also, cinquefoil leaves with honey, and garlic burnt and applied. Old ulcers again are remedied by barley burnt with cerate, and by ceruse with a quadruple quantity of myrtle cerate. For ulcers on the head sprinkle dried myrrh, and do not moisten it, for it will speedily produce adhesion. Or, having triturated dried aloes or birthwort, and having boiled it with honey in wine until it is of a proper consistence, spread upon a pledget and apply it. Of the compound agglutinants are those called the Barbarous, the Golden, that ascribed to Nicolaus, that from willows and dittany, and others of a similar nature, which can produce the adhesion even of very large sores.

Commentary. Celsus gives the following list: glutinant vulnus, myrrha, thus, gummi, præcipueque acanthinum, psyllium, tragacantha, cardamomum, bulbi, lini semen, nasturtium, ovi album, gluten, ichthyocolla, vitis alba, contusæ cum testis suis cochleæ, mel coctum, spongia, vel ex aquâ frigidâ, vel ex vino, vel ex aceto expressa, ex iisdem lana succida: si levis plaga est etiam aranea.

Our author's list is copied from Oribasius. Aëtius has a long chapter on the composition of applications for agglutinating fresh wounds. The ingredients of them are most various: sumach, litharge, wax, galbanum, bee-glue, turpentine, alum, chalcitis, &c. Actuarius merely extracts a few articles from our author's list.

Avicenna's list scarcely differs in any one particular from our author's, and nearly the same may be said of Haly's. Isaac (ap. Rhasis Contin. xxviii) particularly commends bdellium and myrrh, with honey and wine.

Galen has explained at considerable length the principles upon which these applications should be used. Agglutinants, he remarks, are austere and astringent medicines, being such as occasion a contraction and condensation of the fleshy fibres; and they must not possess detergent properties. They are principally applicable in the case of plane ulcers, that is to say, ulcers without loss of substance. (See Meth. Med. iii.)

XXXVIII—ON PAINFUL AND INFLAMMATORY SORES

To painful and inflamed wounds desiccant and anti-inflammatory remedies must be applied. Of liquid remedies the best is wine, but oxycrate is also a good remedy. But if the ulcer is foul as well as inflamed, much diluted hydromel may be used. Of dry medicines, those in general will apply which are mentioned for phlegmons, except such as are oily and acrid. This is a particularly excellent one: Having boiled the sweet pomegranate in wine and pounded, apply it. This is an admirable application and much used, for it applies to ulcers of the head, and those of the privy parts, and to very painful sores on all parts of the body, and to inflammations of the eyes. But if the erysipelas or the like attack an ulcer, we must have recourse to the remedies described for them.

Commentary. Hippocrates gives a long list of applications for inflamed sores. We have mentioned above that wine was one of his favorite remedies. If erysipelas come on, he directs us to purge either upwards or downwards.

Galen explains general principles. Our author copies closely from Oribasius.

Avicenna and Rhases agree with Paulus in approving of cooling or desiccative applications, such as a decoction of sweet pomegranate in Pontic wine. This application is recommended by Haly Abbas, who also mentions a cataplasm containing opium.

XXXIX—ON UNCONCOCTED ULCERS, AND SUCH AS HAVE NOT SUPPURATED

Recent ulcers, and such as being in an inflammatory state have not suppurated, may be digested and made to suppurate by these things: of simple things, tepid water poured on them, wheat flour, or chondrus, or bread, or glue for books, applied with turpentine, wax, saffron, frankincense, pitch, rose oil, axunge, or the fat of calves; but the compound application called tetrapharmacon may be applied upon a pledget mixed with rose oil. Old and callous ulcers are concocted by these simple medicines: the dried grape, storax, galbanum, myrrh, Cretan cistus, pitch, rosin, butter, Egyptian mastich and unwashed wool; and by these compound ones: Galen's plaster without wax, dissolved in oil of ricinus, and applied upon a pledget with old oil, or oleum ricini; and in like manner those called dichromos and basilicon, and the like.

Commentary. Celsus's list is not very different from our author's: Concoquunt et movent pus, nardum, myrrha, costum, balsamum, galbanum, propolis, styrax, thuris et fuligo et cortex, bitumen, pix, sulphur, resina, sevum, adeps, oleum. These articles furnish the ingredients of most of our modern applications. For further information respecting each article, the reader is referred to Dioscorides, Galen, and Serapion.

XL—ON HOLLOW ULCERS

The hollow ulcer requires the filling up of the deficient flesh, the *materiel* of which is a moderate quantity of good blood. Wherefore we procure a moderate supply of it by a sufficiency of food, and produce a proper temperament of the sore by food of wholesome juices, and a suitable temperament of the part in which the sore is seated. With regard to the discharge, that which is thin renders the sore more humid, and that which is thicker makes the sordes adhere to it; on that account it requires applications that are moderately desiccant and detergent; such as frankincense, the flour of barley, that of beans and tares, iris, birthwort, calamine, panax, and pompholyx. When one incarnative remedy does not answer another must be tried. But if the sordes of the ulcer appear greater, and the ulcer more humid, it is to be understood that the medicine has not dried properly, and its powers are to be increased by a mixture of honey. If it is clean, but with less moisture than natural, the medicine has dried more than was proper, and we must apply a cerate mixed with more oil. It sometimes happens when the application is too strong, that the flesh is melted down, so that the ulcer appears foul and moist, like those which have been imperfectly dried; but that from the melting of the flesh becomes more hollow, its lips are callous, and it is red and inflamed; and sometimes the patient has very acute pain. But the other, which arises from the applications being less desiccant than proper, is attended with none of these characters. Wherefore the caries of wood, more especially of such as is possessed of a moderate degree of astringent and detergent qualities, as that of the elm, purges and incarnates clean ulcers; or anemone may be applied for the same purpose. Having shaven down the bark of the pine and pounded it with cerate, and rubbed it upon pledgets, apply it to hollow ulcers, more especially to such as are recent, for it will fill them. The compound medicines for ulcers which are clean, are, that from snails, that ascribed to Manetho from the lees of wine, that from aloes, the dry powder called meletera, that containing equal parts of starch, of manna, of halica, and of tares; and in like manner, the composition from frankincense and that called aphroditarium. But when the ulcers are fouler the powders called cephalic are to be applied, and of those applications that are made upon pledgets, that called trophos, the isis and the athena, and that from distaff-thistle (atractylis,) and moreover that called Italicum, and any others of tried efficacy.

Commentary. The resemblance here pointed out between an ulcer too strongly stimulated and one too little is highly deserving of attention. Our author appears to have borrowed his description from Oribasius, who however abridges it from Galen. Galen and Aëtius give a somewhat fuller account than our author, but their principles of treatment are the same. They remark that frankincense in humid intemperaments engenders flesh, but in dry ones only pus. Pompholyx burnt and washed; calamine and the shells of oysters are said to be incarnant and dissiccant without pungency. Galen inculcates that the greatest difficulty in treating these ulcers, is to find out the nature of the intemperament of the part, and correct it.

Celsus gives the following list of incarnants: Carnem alit et ulcus implet resina pinea, ochra attice, vel asterace, cera, butyrum. He recommends the use of hot water; an application consisting of butter, roses, and a small portion of honey; or the tetrapharmacum with roses. He approves of giving wholesome and nutritious food, such as fowls, venison, pork, and even wine. The list of the Pseudo-Dioscorides contains nearly the same articles as that of Celsus. (Euporist. i, 186.)

Octavius Horatianus recommends a composition of equal parts of honey, turpentine, rosin, and wax, melted in a vessel; or a mixture of powdered rosin, wax, and fat.

Scribonius Largus recommends basilicon, and a composition consisting of calf's marrow, the fat of geese, butter, stag's marrow, wax, turpentine, honey, and roses.

Avicenna remarks, that in treating hollow ulcers we must not use very desiccative applications, as they dry up the fluids which are necessary for forming flesh; nor for the same reason, very astringent applications, nor abstergents of any greater strength than to remove the sordes. Rhases recommends a mixture of equal parts of olibanum, aloes, sarcocolla, and dragon's blood. Camphor is an ingredient in one of his incarnative applications. Alsaharavius makes mention of an application from olibanum, like that of Rhases.

All the ancient authors say that round ulcers are more difficult to heal than those of any other shape; and Cassius Medicus and Alexander Aphrodisiensis assign various reasons for this, the most probable of which seems to be, that in this case the sound parts are further removed than in any other.

Apollonius Dyscolus states that ulcers are prevented from healing by pregnancy, by disease of the spleen, and by varicose veins. (Histor. Mirab. 42.)

XLI—MEDICINES FOR CLEANSING FOUL ULCERS

Foul ulcers, whether hollow or level with the surface, may be properly cleansed by birthwort in honey, turpentine with an equal portion of rose oil and honey, or instead of rose oil butter may be substituted, with Illyrian iris and honey; and by pickled olives applied. To nervous parts, turpentine melted with butter may be applied. When the sores are very foul and spreading, horehound with honey is a good application, which removes the eschars. The following are compound applications: Of boiled lees of oil, of scummed honey, of the species of alum called phormion, equal parts.—*Another*: Of the dried serapias, called also triorchis, of Illyrian iris, of dried horehound, of birthwort, of each, dr. viij; of the flour of tares, dr. x; use in a powder and with honey. And for foul ulcers the Egyptian cerate is useful, also those from salts when melted, the Indian, that called athena, the green plasters diluted, the powder of dried pumice stone, those from tares, the trochisk called melanchlorus, and in like manner that called criogenes.

Commentary. The following are the most important articles in Celsus's long list of substances for cleansing ulcers: Purgant, ærugo, auripigmentum, quod ἀρσένικον a Græcis nominatur; (huic autem et sandarachæ in omnia eadem vis, sed validior est) squama æris, thus, resina, et pinea, et terebinthina liquida, misy, chalcitis, galla, sulphur, pix, oleum, ruta, ammoniacum, &c. Hippocrates makes mention of many of these, namely, arsenic, verdigris, flowers of copper, frankincense, myrrh, hellebore, &c.

Scribonius Largus recommends honey, Illyrian iris, and a compound application containing arsenic, scales of copper, elaterium, and burnt paper.

One may find in Galen and Aëtius many compound applications, but as they are all formed from much the same ingredients as those of our author, it will be unnecessary to take further notice of them. Aëtius commends a combination of turpentine and honey.

Avicenna and Haly Abbas recommend the same applications as our author. They make no mention of arsenic. Alsaharavius gives very particular directions for treating these ulcers; when the edges are hard, he directs us to rub them until they become red, or to cut them off and apply to the sore the green ointment; and when the ulcer is covered with much sordes, he recommends us to dress it with the Egyptian ointment. Rhases mentions antimony as an excellent application for cleansing foul ulcers. He properly recommends us to consider whether the foulness of the ulcer be the effect of too much or too little stimulation. He relates a case of the former description, in which the sore got worse under the application of the green ointment. (Cont. xxviii.)

XLII—FOR WORMS IN ULCERS

For worms which form in ulcers, the first thing to be done is to stop the humidity and the putrefaction which occasion them. Worms may be killed by all the things in general which are described for those in the ear. But for those which form in ulcers Archigenes says, mix equal parts of ceruse and poley with liquid pitch, and anoint with it.

Commentary. Aëtius recommends dried plantain, the ashes of the wood of figs, and the juice of calamint. Galen and Avicenna also mention calamint.

Pliny mentions the gall of frogs.

XLIII—ON FUNGOUS ULCERS

The fungous flesh of ulcers is to be removed by medicines which are powerfully desiccant, such as diphryges sprinkled upon it, the squama æris, all the testacea burnt, both the echini (the hedgehog and sea-urchin,) burnt entire. But the following things are moderately cleansing, and repress the fungous flesh: the flower of the Asian stone, and still more powerful than it, the sori and chrysocolla, chalcitis and misy (when burnt they are less caustic,) and the flos æris in like manner; but verdigris is the most powerful of all. Salts, when burnt, consume the foul flesh, and in like manner charpie that has been soaked in strong brine and dried, consumes fungous flesh that is moderately large. But verdigris with the squama æris is powerfully repressing. Of the compound applications the powder called rhodium, and the psarum, and that named yellow, repress fungous growth without being pungent. But the trochisks called phaustiani, when levigated and sprinkled on the sore, and the dry medicine (or powder) called heliocaes, make fungous flesh slough off to the bottom. But the application consisting of equal parts of calx viva, squama æris and manna, answers with fungous flesh; with honey it cleanses such as resemble a mushroom, and with cerate it proves incarnating.

A powder for keeping down fungous flesh: Of litharge, of chalcitis, of verdigris, of plumbago, equal parts.—*Another*, which represses strongly without being pungent, and applies also to spreading ulcers, and more especially the epulis of the gums, and whitens the teeth: Of quicklime, lb. j; of arsenic, oz. vj; having triturated the dried arsenic with water, add the lime washed like calamine, and, having rubbed them together dry and use. And of the trochisks, that called pantolmios, and those described for polypus, are excellent for repressing fungus in ulcers. But the green plasters, more especially the one from Cappadocian salts, and in like manner the isis, are most effectual in preventing fungous flesh in ulcers.

Commentary. The powerful applications mentioned by our author will be found amply sufficient to fulfil every intention in conducting the treatment of these ulcers. Many of them are mentioned by Hippocrates.

Galen lays it down as a rule that these fungous excrescences are to be repressed by powerfully desiccative substances, such as misy, chalcitis, or more especially verdigris; when burnt and washed they become mild detergents. (Meth. Med. iii.)

Aëtius gives many useful prescriptions for such preparations, but they are entirely formed of the ingredients which enter into those of our author.

Celsus gives a long list of caustics highly applicable in such cases: Adurunt, auripigmentum, atramentum sutorium, chalcitis, misy, ærugo, calx, charta combusta, sal, squama æris, veratrum et album et nigrum, cantharides, sandaracha, alumen scissile, &c. Pliny speaks of a composition of unwashed wool, with barley flour, and verdigris.

Octavius Horatianus recommends the Phrygian stone pulverized, and a powder consisting of the recrementum plumbi, verdigris, aloe, and quicklime.

Rhases and Avicenna copy from our author. Haly Abbas speaks of removing the superfluous flesh with an instrument.

XLIV—ON SPREADING ULCERS, PUTRID ULCERS, AND PHAGEDÆNA

Spreading and putrid ulcers are to be bathed with vinegar and oxycrate, an astringent wine, cold water, sea-water, or the decoction of lentil, of pomegranate rind, of the flowers of the wild pomegranate, of lentisk, of myrtles, of Egyptian thorn, or some other astringent and desiccant medicine. Cataplasms are to be applied to them of the flower of tares and liquid alum, the inner part of bread made of similago, an old goby fish, or some other old pickle, unwashed flesh, and liquid turpentine; these things are to be all pounded together in equal proportions. Or the parts may be anointed with equal proportions of birthwort, and the juice of the leaves of the Palma Christi, and half the quantity of verdigris, made with water to the thickness of honey; but if the eschar is not removed an equal proportion of elaterium is to be mixed with the verdigris. For putrid ulcers sori levigated and sprinkled on them is an effectual remedy, and above is to be put dried charpie; or the round birthwort and galls in equal quantities may be rubbed in with oil; or the root of the wild cucumber, or of cabbage, or of beet, or the leaves of dock are to be bound in a piece of linen, and put into ashes; when they are softened triturate with salt and apply; they will cleanse powerfully.

Or apply green olive leaves boiled in wine with honey; or apply chalcitis, or parsley seed levigated, or apply linseed triturated with copperas, or use an application of thyme, dried grapes and boiled figs, or of fig leaves triturated with honey; or of nitre, cumin, and fine flour with honey; or of the root of the wild cucumber, or of squill boiled with honey; or of sori, dr. xij; of chalcitis, dr. x; of misy, dr. iv; triturate with half an hemina of the strongest vinegar until it is dried, and taking it off use by dipping a specillum in it, and rubbing it over the ulcer, and placing above it a double pledget out of wine and oil. But if it is inflamed apply henbane with polenta, or cabbage with honey.

For putrid and spreading ulcers on all parts of the body.—Of quicklime, of chalcitis, of each dr. ij; of arsenic, dr. j. This may be used for pterygia of the fingers, for phagedæna and carbuncle, with honey if on the genital organs, but dry if on any other part of the body. Above apply an oblong pledget with rosin.

An universally applicable powder for all spreading sores, and those of the mouth, for hemorrhages, and for repressing fungous flesh. Of chalcitis, of misy, of both in a crude state, dr. xx; of squama ferri, dr. vj; of immature galls, dr. viij.

For spreading and putrid sores. Of salts, dr. ij; of any species of alum which has been burnt, dr. j; of squama æris, of burnt pumice stone, equal quantities. Scraped verdigris, with burnt misy mixed with liquid pitch; and the flakes of iron with oil also answer well.

For spreading ulcers of the pudendum. These things will apply to them, and also the composition called meliterium, the powder of the wild myrtle, and that from paper; also the composition from oxymel called coracion, the trochisk of Andron and the like, will answer with all spreading ulcers. The same things also apply with phagedæna; for phagedæna is an ulcer that spreads by eating.

For foul and fetid ulcers. The Lemnium sigillum (Lemnian earth) mixed with vinegar, oxymel, oxycrate, or wine, until it is of the consistence of clay, may be rubbed on them with advantage; or the leaves of cypress, its shoots, and tender balls (pilulæ), or the ashes of dried gourd burnt, or of the burnt bark of the plane tree, or of burnt dill in like manner, or of foul wool burnt, or of plaintain; also woad by itself or with polenta, or the dried root of hog's fennel.

Commentary. It will be remarked that the milder applications mentioned in this section are all powerful desiccants and astringents. Most of them are mentioned by Dioscorides as possessing these properties.

Galen recommends the compound applications mentioned by our author, containing verdigris, squama æris, &c.

For these spreading and putrid sores Aëtius, among other prescriptions, gives one which would no doubt be applicable in the worst cases: "Of crude misy, of crude chalcitis, ā dr. viij; of ochre, dr. iij; of sandarach, dr. iv; of quicklime, dr. ij; of the scales of copper, of alum, ā dr. ij; of diphryges dr. iij; m." These caustic and escharotic medicines enter into the composition of many of his applications. Some of them contain astringents and desiccants, such as sumach, galls, alum, fossil salts, frankincense, calamine, birthwort, pomegranate rind, &c. In short the ingredients in his applications correspond with Celsus's list of corrosive substances: Rodunt, alumen liquidum, sed magis rotundum, ærugo, chalcitis, misy, squama æris, sed magis rubri, æs combustum, sandaracha, galla, thus, auripigmentum, calx, nitrum et spuma ejus, alcyonium, resina, squama ferri, atrumentum sutorium, veratrum, &c.

The other authorities give only combinations of these substances; for a full account of which preparations we refer the reader to Galen. (Med. sec. gen. iv.)

Octavius Horatianus recommends lentils boiled and mixed with honey; the leaves of cabbage, coriander, or ivy, all mixed with honey.

The Arabians, although they supply nothing new, add their authority in confirmation of the remedial virtues which the Greeks assigned to the substances mentioned above. Avicenna and Rhases recommend arsenic, copperas, misy, sori, chalcitis, flos æris, quicklime, alum, galls, ammoniac, the trochisk of Andron, &c. When a part becomes black and putrid, Haly Abbas directs us to open a vein leading to it, if the age and state of the patient permit, and afterwards to apply odoriferous things, such as camphor, &c.

XLV—ON ULCERS REQUIRING CICATRIZATION

By drying and constringing the flesh of ulcers requiring cicatrization to such a degree as not only to dissipate the preternatural superfluity, but also to touch upon that which is in its natural state, we may render the surface of the sore like skin, and make the ulcer cicatrize. This is promoted by immature galls, the moderately desiccant bark of pomegranate, and whatever else is desiccant without being possessed of pungent astringency. And such things as these promote cicatrization: myrrh, litharge, and oysters if burnt, for they must be sprinkled on the sore dry. And these things often produce cicatrization: pine bark with myrtle cerate, ivy flowers with cerate, the root of the lily with rose-oil, dried pine-rosin, burnt pumice stone, the flakes of copper; they are to be used in equal proportions dry. The following also repress: mix a small quantity of manna and of diphryges with levigated pumice, and use; or of litharge p. j; of diphryges p. ss, apply on a pledget with cerate. Birdlime with frankincense cicatrizes old ulcers, also verdigris with an equal portion of diphryges and with myrtle cerate, or the small centaury applied fresh. To the more humid apply the root of cypress. To those about the anus and pudendum, more particularly if inflamed, use levigated aloes, either in a dry state or with water, or squama æris; or soften chrysocolla in the sun with wax, and apply.

A dry application for producing cicatrization. Of oysters, dr. xij; of manna, dr. vj; of calamine, dr. iv. It applies also to spreading sores.—*Another*: Of birthwort, dr. vj; of pine bark, dr. vj; of manna, dr. vj; of pumice, dr. iv; of Colophonian rosin, dr. iv; of iris, dr. iv.—*Another*: Of hart's horn burnt, dr. iv; of pine-bark, oz. vj: of ceruse, oz. iv; of scraped verdigris, oz. ix; of calamine, dr. xviij.—*Another*: Of the flowers of pomegranate, of copperas, of each, dr. xvj; of squama æris, of fissile alum, of each dr. viij; of galls, dr. j.—*Another*: Of ceruse, of litharge, of each, oz. viij; of the dross of lead, of galls, of dried myrrh, of each, dr. iv.

A cicatrizing application. Take of fissile alum, oz. j; and having levigated it, macerate in a sextarius of water: when dissolved in the water soak pledgets in it, and having dried them apply.

A plaster for cicatrizing the more simple ulcers. Of wax, dr. xl; of litharge, dr. xxxv; of diphryges, dr. viij; of myrtle-oil, half a hemina. The plaster called phœnicinum, that from calamine, the myrsinatum, and the like, are also applicable in such cases. For ulcers of difficult cicatrization: Of wax, of myrtle-oil, of each, dr. vj; of calamine, oz. vj; of lead, of frankincense, of each, dr. ij; of fissile alum, of burnt copper, of each, oz. j; of scraped verdigris, dr. ij; dissolve them singly. For chronic ulcers, and such as are of difficult cicatrization: Of calamine, dr. viij; of chrysocolla, dr. viij; of fissile alum, dr. viij; of verdigris, of the flakes of copper, of each, dr. j; of pine-rosin, dr. xl; of wax, dr. c; of myrtle-oil, q. s.—*Another*: Of wax, of pine-rosin, of each, oz. vj; of calamine, oz. vj; of crude chalcitis, oz. iij; of myrtle-oil, q. s. The calamine and the chalcitis are to be triturated with wine during the season of the dog-star; use it upon a broad compress, and apply above it a pledget and sponge out of wine.—*Another*: Of burnt copper, oz. ij; of fissile alum, oz. ij; of sal ammoniac, dr. ij; of wax, oz. vj; of Colophonian rosin, oz. vj; of myrtle-oil, oz. ij; the dry things are to be triturated in the vinegar in the sun for twenty days, and when it becomes of the consistence of honey, having melted the wax, mix it and soften. The medicine from pumice-stone, the isis, and the like, are also applicable in such cases.

Commentary. Celsus gives the following list of the more active articles of this class: Crustas ulceribus tanquam igne adustis inducunt, præcipue, chalcitis, utique si cocta est, flos æris, ærugo, auripigmentum, misy, et id quoque magis coctum.

For a variety of applications suitable to this class of ulcers, we refer the reader to Galen's 4th book of 'De Med. sec. gen.' The ingredients of them are powerfully desiccative, astringent, and escharotic. Many of our author's prescriptions will be recognized in it. For an account of the isis, and the other compound medicines mentioned towards the end of this section, we refer the reader to Galen (l. c.) and to the Seventh Book of this work. Galen, in another place, and after him Aëtius, give the following important directions for the use of these applications. The ulcers to which this mode of treatment is applicable, being very foul and filled with a vitiated discharge, are first to be wiped clean with a soft linen cloth, and then the cavity of them is to be filled with the medicine, and a splenium (oblong compress) applied externally. Then having put a piece of linen above the splenium and bound it on, we are to place over it a sponge squeezed out of cold water or wine, endeavouring to keep the sponge cold during the whole time of the treatment, which may easily be done by pouring cold water upon it without loosing the bandages. They are not be removed until the third day. Galen states that the articles which answer best in such applications are galls, pomegranate-rind, alum, chalcitis, misy, and the like.

A similar mode of treatment, without any material alteration, is described by the Arabians. Haly Abbas remarks, that cicatrizing medicines are powerfully desiccative with some astringency, such as galls, alum, and the like.

XLVI—ON THE MALIGNANT ULCERS CALLED CHIRONIAN AND TELEPHIAN

Old ulcers which are difficult to get cicatrized are called chironian, as if requiring Chiron himself to cure them; and telephian, from Telephus having long laboured under such a sore. We must attend then whether the whole body being in a state of cacochymy, sends such defluxions to the ulcer, and the prevailing humour is to be evacuated by appropriate remedies. Or if it is a varix which sends these humours to the legs, the ulcer being in it, it is to be cured as will be described in the Surgical part of this work; or the humours are to be evacuated by venesection, taking away blood frequently, and then using topical applications which have the property of extirpating the disease without being pungent. These therefore are simple applications; those from pumice and diphryges, and flakes of copper, verdigris, and lime moderately washed; sprinkle fissile alum levigated, or of unwashed wool, dr. iv; of dried grapes, dr. iv; of natron, dr. ij; having previously anointed with honey, sprinkle of flakes of copper, dr. x; of alum, dr. ij; and having softened in the sun with dr. x of wax, apply.

These are compound medicines. *A plaster for chironia.* Of ceruse, oz. viij; of fissile alum, oz. ij; of the flakes of copper, dr. ij; of sal ammoniac, of frankincense, of scraped verdigris, of pomegranate rind, of each, oz. ij; of quicklime, oz. j; of wax, lb. j; of myrtle-oil, lb. j. ss; triturate the dry things with wine. At first it removes callus; and it is laid by and kept, and at last when used, being softened with myrtle-oil, it cicatrizes.—*Another*: Of litharge, lb. j; of oil, lb. ij; of black chamæleon, of the roots of birthwort, of immature galls, of each, oz. j; of galbanum, of ammoniac perfume, of frankincense, of each, oz. ij; prepare, stirring with the roots of green reeds.

From Archigenes, for chironia, and malignant ulcers in the legs and breast, for struma, and parotis. Of the fat of an ox lb. iij; of turpentine, oz. v; of manna, oz. vij: of the earth called sarda which painters use, oz. v: having put the soluble and dry articles together and melted, use.—*Another*, of Archigenes: Of wax, oz. iv; of oil of unripe olives, of manna of frankincense, of diphryges, of the flakes of copper, of each, dr. iv; having triturated the powder with vinegar, and made of the thickness of honey, mix with the cerate, and use upon a pledget.—*Another*, for the malignant ulcers of women, and of other persons having a soft skin: Of Tuscan wax, dr. viij; of bulls' fat, of turpentine, of burnt lead, and of pepper, of each, dr. j; use on a pledget with rose-oil or myrtle-oil.

Commentary. Celsus describes the chironian ulcer as being large, and having hard, callous, and swelled edges, with a copious discharge of thin sanies. It is attended with no inflammation, the pain is moderate, it does not spread, and therefore it is not dangerous, although not readily cured. Sometimes, he says, it becomes covered with a thin cicatrix, and then again the ulcer breaks out. It occurs mostly in the feet and legs. From this description it is evident that by the chironian ulcer Celsus meant merely an ill-conditioned ulcer, and that he distinguished between it and the *cacoethes*, or malignant ulcer, which last he held to be nearly allied to the carcinoma. However, most of the Greek authors apply the term malignant to the chironian ulcer. For the cure of it Celsus recommends an application consisting of squama æris, lead burnt and washed, calamine, wax, and a small quantity of roses.

Galen furnishes us with an account of the manner in which Thessalus the Methodist proposed to cure all chironian and malignant ulcers. Thessalus lays it down as a rule for the treatment of all sores which are difficult to cure, or which break out again when healed, to remove the exciting cause, whether local or constitutional, by means of proper alteratives. He adds:

"In cases of chronic ulcers which cannot be got healed, we must remove the parts which prevent adhesion, and convert the sore into the state of a recent ulcer; and then having allayed the inflammation proceed accordingly. Those sores which heal up and break out again during their exacerbations, and when ulcerated, are to be cured like recent inflammations by soothing applications until the irritation subside, after which cicatrizing applications are to be used, and then the surrounding parts are to be covered with a malagma of mustard, or some other rubefacient and alterative, to remove the indolence. If this is not sufficient, we must attend to the general health, attempting to effect a change of the system by repeated exercise, gestation, a diet increased or diminished according to circumstances, and at the commencement by administering an emetic of radishes, or even the white hellebore." (Galen, Meth. Med. iv.) Although Galen, who all along displays a strong hostility to the *Thessalian asses*, (so he calls the Methodists,) has animadverted in severe terms upon the rules here laid down, they would appear to be highly proper and ingenious. Galen in another place (Med. sec. gen. iv) gives from Asclepiades, Andromachus, and others, a great collection of applications for chironian, malignant, and indolent ulcers. One by Asclepiades consists of the scales of copper, scraped verdigris, wax, and larch rosin. Others by Andromachus contain sori, misy, chalcitis, verdigris, alum, turpentine-rosin, and the like, mixed with wax. Hippocrates directs us to treat a callous ulcer by applying to it septic medicines to make the hard parts slough off, after which the edges are to be brought together. (De locis in homine.)

The directions of Aëtius, more especially respecting the constitutional treatment, are highly important. In cases where there is a redundance of blood he recommends venesection, in others both purging and bleeding; and in certain cases he directs us to pay attention to the state of the liver and spleen. He relates a case of an ulcer on the hand, which he cured by opening a vein leading to it. He also directs us to scarify or cut off the callous edges of the ulcer. He gives various prescriptions for sores of this description, containing verdigris, sori, chalcitis, burnt copper, alum, &c.

Octavius Horatianus recommends a plaster consisting of equal parts of chalcitis, wax, and alum. For phagedænæ Pliny mentions an old shad-fish triturated with sandarach. (H. N. xxxii, 44.)

The Arabians treat of these ulcers very fully. Avicenna in particular gives very proper directions for the constitutional treatment. When the state of the ulcer is occasioned by an intemperament, it is to be corrected, and if the blood is deficient in quantity or quality, this is to be remedied by a proper diet; and when on the contrary it is connected with plethora, venesection is to be had recourse to, and if the veins leading to it are varicose, it may be proper to open them. When the sore is kept from healing by a spiculum of bone, we are to cut down and remove it. His applications consist of the same ingredients as those used by the Greeks, namely, the flower of copper, copperas, alum, ceruse, lime, arsenic, &c., mixed with wax and oil. The directions given by Rhases are less circumstantial, but to the same purpose. He particularly directs us to remove the callous edges by friction, scarifications, and septics. He speaks of turpentine as an excellent addition to other ointment. (Contin. xxviii.) He mentions that in case of malignant ulcer on the leg connected with varix, Galen opened the enlarged vein.

The *cacoethes* of Celsus was evidently the disease called *noli me tangere* by Theodoricus; a very absurd appellation, which however has been retained to the present day. Celsus has pointed out its resemblance to carcinoma, and recommended the only mode of treatment which ever does any good in these cases, namely, the application of septics, such as arsenic, quicklime, &c., or the actual cautery. As our limits will not permit us to enlarge further on this subject at present, we must be content with referring to No. 108 of the 'Edinburgh Medical and Surgical Journal,' where we have given a full exposition of the ancient principles of treatment. (See also the Commentary on s. xxvi of this Book.)

XLVII—FOR BLACK CICATRICES

Let the root of the white and black bryony be boiled in oil until they are reduced to the state of juice, and the oil applied will take away black scars; and so in like manner calamint boiled in wine, and litharge washed with white rose-oil. But the scars from lichen, and all other kinds are made like the other skin by anointing them with the fat of asses; or the seed of rocket triturated with the gall of a goat, of an ox, and of a sheep may be rubbed in with litharge; or a lamb's foot burnt may be triturated with austere wine for the same purpose; or, ammoniac perfume may be rubbed in with swines' gall. These are compound applications: Of litharge, of mint, of frankincense, equal parts with honey.—*Another*: of natron, of ammoniac perfume, of sulphur vivum, of myrrh, equal parts; having triturated with vinegar, white wine, or water, rub in but a very little, so as not to produce an ulcer.—*Another*: Of Cimolian earth, of pigeons' dung, of soap, of frankincense, equal parts with vinegar. A detergent ointment for black scars: Of Cimolian earth, dr. xiij; of aphronitrum, dr. v; of white hellebore, dr. v; of the greasy dregs of nut-ben, dr. iv; scrub with it while in the bath.

Commentary. Avicenna condenses all the information contained in the authors who preceded him. He sets out with stating that the class of medicines which are applicable in such cases are the abstergents; of which he enumerates verdigris, stavesacre, the scales of copper, and even arsenic.

Among the less active ingredients he mentions, like our author, the fat of asses. We need not give extracts from the other authorities, as no one has treated of this case so fully as Avicenna.

XLVIII—ON SINUOUS ULCERS

When the skin adjacent to an ulcer is not united with the parts below, we call such a complaint a sinus. When, therefore, the sinus extends upwards, the ichor readily flows out from the sore, and adhesion easily takes place; but when it extends downwards the ichor by remaining within corrodes the continuous parts, and unless you first make an incision for its discharge, you will be able to effect nothing; for the sores can neither be incarnated nor the parts made to unite. But if the sinus is in any of the limbs, as the arms or legs, one may produce adhesion without a counter-division by putting the limb in a declining position. Thus when the sinus is in the arm, and the mouth of the sore is near the elbow, by placing the hand in an elevated position, you will render the discharge from the ulcer below easy. And when the sinus is in the thigh, and has its outlet near the knee, you must make the position declining by putting a soft pillow below the back part of the knee, so that the groin may be in a lower position than the knee; and if the sinus does not require incarnation, forthwith by means of a straight and hollow pipe having a bladder attached to it, syringe it with honey so diluted with water that one could drink it, in order to clear away the ichor from the sinus. For promoting adhesion when about to take place, do it with wine, or wine and honey, and then proceed to the agglutinating medicine. But if the sinus being hollow requires incarnation, first inject a little of the composition from dried paper with much rose-oil, then plug up the mouth of it with charpie, and afterwards the plaster of iris, or of Machærion, or of some such, may be melted with liquid rose-cerate, and injected in like manner. If the sinus is moderately incarnated you may apply some of the agglutinating medicines, as if you were curing a case of recent bloody wound. Such are those called the barbarous, dichromos, and gilvus; and more especially that prepared from the oil of palma Christi and the metals without wax which is called the dun plaster of Galen, is applicable. After the application of the medicine, a recent sponge out of wine and honey, or wine alone, is to be put on particularly in a soft manner, and the bandaging is to commence at the bottom of the sinus and end at its orifice. The folds of the bandage should bind the bottom of the sinus firmly, yet so as not to occasion pain, but ought to be gradually relaxed towards its orifice; and the plaster which is put on should be so cut as to leave an opening at the orifice for the escape of the matter, but another small plaster of the same materials should be applied to it in a loose state, so as to favour the discharge. This is to be left on till the bandages are loosed, which is to be done on the third day, when they are to be taken off and changed, but the application along the sinus is to be left. You may judge whether the bottom of the sinus has adhered, from observing if the matter be small and well concocted, or if there be no discharge at all; and moreover if there be no sensible pain along the sinus nor swelling, but the whole part is contracted, dry, and free from pain. But if you see a little well concocted pus at the orifice, you may still more confidently entertain good hopes. If on the second or third day a thin ichor be discharged from the sinus, you need not despair that adhesion has taken place, for often the strength of the medicine squeezes out from the parts below a thin fluid, which being discharged the parts become dry and adhere. But if on the third or fourth day from the commencement the matter appear unconcocted as it runs from the opening, you may be sure that the sinus has not adhered, and you must persevere with the same application. When owing to the moisture of the part it falls off, as is not unlikely, it will not be improper to make some change in the medicine itself.

On sinuous ulcers with a thin covering of skin. When the abscess is too long opened, owing either to the unskilfulness of the surgeon, or the timidity of the patient, the skin which lies over it becomes thin and ragged, and it cannot be removed, then after the syringing which has been described, we must have recourse to an agglutinating application of a humid consistence, but of desiccative properties, such as that from chalcitis called phœnicinum, diluted with old oil, so as neither to be very hard nor of such a consistence as not to stain the finger; and afterwards it is to be mixed with moderately old wine, and applied in a circular form with corresponding bandaging. To skin in this ragged state honey, as was said, is not one of the least proper applications when boiled to the consistence of a plaster and applied. It will be better, however, if after spreading it on the rag you sprinkle over it from a sieve some myrrh finely pulverized, or aloes, or frankincense, or all of these together. I have also found the lesser centaury a wonderful application for the same purpose; next to it is comfrey, after which is the root of the Illyrian iris, and after these is the flour of tares. Sometimes during the process of boiling we sprinkle these upon the honey when the vessel is about to be taken off from the fire. It is better, however, to do so after it is taken off, and then it is to be stirred about, and when it becomes tepid applied to the sinus, and bandaged as aforesaid.

Commentary. Similar directions are given by Galen and Aëtius, but upon the whole those of our author are superior; and as those of the other two supply no additional information, it will be unnecessary to multiply extracts from them. (See Galen, Therap. ad Glauc. ii.)

Actuarius, in like manner, briefly directs that unless the sinus open downwards, it shall be cut open and dressed with an agglutinative application. You may think well of the case, he adds, when the part is dry and free from pain, or when only a little well-concocted pus is discharged from it.

In the translations of the Arabians, the sinus is described by the names of *absconsio* and *caverna*. Avicenna states that the sinus differs from the fistula in having a larger cavity, and its edges not being indurated. He lays down very correct rules of treatment, but they are all copied from Galen. Thus he directs, when the orifice of the sore is above the cavity of the sinus, that it should be cut open; or, if this cannot be conveniently accomplished, he recommends us to introduce a tent smeared with some incarnant or detergent application. Upon the authority of Dioscorides he recommends the lesser centaury in such cases. His directions for the application of the bandages are similar to those of our author.

Celsus, and other of the ancient authorities, do not treat of the sinus separately from the fistula.

XLIX—ON FISTULA

Fistula is a callous sinus formed for the most part from abscesses, and deriving its appellation from the pipes of reeds (fistulæ). If, therefore, it terminate with a bone, it cannot be cured without a surgical operation, unless in process of time a scale of the bone come off spontaneously. But if it does not terminate with a bone, it is to be cured by the applications for removing callosities, and the agglutinative medicines. The applications for removing callosities are such as these: the root of spondylium scraped around and applied removes the callus of fistulæ. And in like manner black hellebore applied removes the callus in two or three days; also lees of oil boiled and injected; sori in a crude state, or burnt and injected with some diluted wine, or sori and crocomagma with hydromel. Or make collyria by mixing elaterium with turpentine, and apply. Or syringe with the juice of the root of laserwort. This melts down the callus: of verdigris, dr. xij; of ammoniac, dr. ij; mix with vinegar, and form into an oblong collyrium.

A collyrium which I use for removing the callosities of fistulæ. Mix with vinegar equal parts of ammoniac perfume, of copperas, of verdigris, of misy, of chalcitis, and of gum.—*Another*, from the surgical works of Heliodorus: Of calamine, of misy, of copperas, of burnt copper, of gum, of each, dr. iv; of crude chalcitis, dr. iij; mix with the urine of a young person not come to manhood, and form collyria. Put this collyrium into the fistula, and apply externally the inner part of bread soaked in water, changing it until the inflammation subside, and the eschar fall off.—*Another*, which I received in Alexandria: Of the roots of alkanet, of toasted misy, of chalcitis, of verdigris, of fissile alum, of copperas, of aloes, of each, oz. j; triturate along with fine cantharides in vinegar, and make collyria.—*Another*: Of copperas, dr. ij; of chalcitis, of verdigris, of each, dr. j; mix with ammoniac and use, and when the callus is thrown off, cleanse with verdigris and eight times the quantity of the purest honied water; but after the discharge of the callus, incarnants must be used. An incarnative collyrium: of aloes, of myrrh, of ammoniac, of the cinders of egg shells, equal parts; having triturated with water form collyria, and apply.—*Another*: Of myrrh, of aloes, of frankincense, of pomegranate rind, equal parts, mix with water; but some use bull's gall. The oil of unripe olives is incarnative when injected. I knew a person who injected cedar-rosin into fistulæ, and succeeded surprisingly. After it is incarnated we must have recourse to the agglutinative medicine, according to the plan described for other sinuses. "When the fistula is narrow and long," says Galen, "and does not appear to me to contain callus internally, but only sordes, I first inject lye into it, and then allowing it to remain in the fistula until I expect that the sordes has fallen completely off, I afterwards apply the medicine." It was the one from the oil of palma Christi, mentioned above.

Commentary. We shall have occasion to refer to the Hippocratic treatise 'De Fistulis,' in the Sixth Book.

Celsus treats of fistulæ with more than his wonted minuteness. This is his definition: "Id nomen est ulceri alto, angusto, calloso." He has described all the complications of it with great accuracy. He directs us to commence by making an inspection with a probe or sound, so as to ascertain the state of the parts and of the discharge. If a soft body is felt at the bottom, we conclude that the fistula terminates in the flesh, but if a hard one is felt, we know that it ends with a bone. If the probe slide readily over the bone, it is free from caries, but if it does not so, and yet no inequalities are felt on it, caries has taken place, but it is still smooth: if it feel unequal and rough, the bone is eaten with caries. For a simple and recent fistula, not deep-seated or in a joint, the plaster for recent wounds will be sufficient, provided salt, or alum, or the scales of copper, or verdigris, or any of the other metals, be added to it. The application is to be made upon a piece of linen, and a sponge soaked in vinegar is to be put over it, and is to be removed on the fifth day. The patient must live upon nutritious food. If the fistula is at a distance from the præcordia, emetics with radishes are said by him to be proper. When the fistula is old it becomes callous, and requires stronger applications, containing such ingredients as calamine, atramentum sutorium, verdigris, galls, lime, orpiment, or realgur. He mentions as a very ready application a solution of ammoniac in vinegar, with some verdigris added to it. However, he remarks, any other caustic will accomplish the same purpose. If the fistula is long and transverse, an incision is to be made at its commencement, after which the collyrium may be applied. When the fistula is double, or consists of still more passages, he recommends us to blow in with a writing pen the medicines in the form of powder, or to apply them dissolved in wine, mulse, or vinegar. But whatever the internal dressing be, he recommends us to apply on the outside of it something of a refrigerant and repressing nature, as the parts around are generally affected with inflammation. When the dressings are removed the fistula is to be syringed with wine if the discharge of the pus is copious, with vinegar if its edges are callous, but with mulse, or a decoction of tares, if the passage be clean. By the means we have been describing it will generally happen, he says, that the inner coat of the fistula will slough off, and leave the ulcer in a clean state. Agglutinants are then to be applied, especially a sponge smeared with boiled honey. When the sides of the fistula are clean there need be no apprehension lest they do not adhere, since, he remarks, we often see in ulcerations of the fingers that without great care one finger is apt to adhere to another.

In the 'Euporista' of the Pseudo-Dioscorides, it is recommended first to dilate the fistula with a piece of sponge, and then to use a stimulant application containing verdigris, ammoniac, &c.

Aëtius gives an excellent account of fistula, but it is mostly borrowed from Galen. We can afford room only for a few extracts. When a fistula extends obliquely, nothing can be done without making a free incision, for which purpose he directs us to introduce a sound and cut along it. His directions for examining into the nature of a fistula are such as ample experience alone could have dictated. He seems to be decidedly of opinion that, except in cases of a recent fistula, or when it is not deep-seated, an incision ought always to be made at first; after which applications for removing the callus may be used. When, however, the patient refuses to submit to an operation, and the case is recent, the cure may be attempted by means of escharotics and incarnants, such as verdigris, misy, alum, &c., mixed with frankincense, aloes, and myrrh.

Oribasius briefly recommends white hellebore, a mixture of equal parts of verdigris and ammoniac, and a few other such articles, as applications for fistulæ.

Scribonius Largus mentions several compound applications containing misy, chalcitis, verdigris, alum, &c.

Marcellus gives one consisting of ceruse, ammoniac, and oil.

Actuarius gives a brief but distinct account of the nature and treatment of fistula, but it is taken almost entire from our author.

Avicenna inculcates that a fistula is only to be cured by a free incision, or by removing the callous sides of it by burning with fire or caustic medicines, such as arsenic, ammoniac, sulphur, the flour of copper, or mercury. This in fact is the sum of the medical practice in such cases. There is nothing particularly interesting in Haly Abbas. Alsaharavius truly states that a diseased bone is the common cause of fistulous ulcers not healing, and inculcates that in this case there can be no hope of recovery until the carious portion be removed. Rhases, upon the authority of the celebrated Antyllus, directs us to use corrosive applications when a fistula cannot be operated upon with the scalpel. He intimates that this is particularly the case when the disease is seated in the groins.

The earlier modern surgeons, such as Gulielmus de Saliceto, Arnoldus, Rogerius, Rolandus, and Guy of Cauliac, in imitation of the Arabians, direct fistula to be treated by the application of septics, the actual cautery, or incision. Rogerius recommends a tent spread with quicklime and soap, or with arsenic. Guy of Cauliac, like Avicenna, speaks favorably of sublimed quicksilver or corrosive sublimate.

L—FOR SORES WHICH BREAK OUT AGAIN

Some sores which have become cicatrized, often after no long time become inflamed and break out again; for a bone being diseased, sometimes the flesh which covers it heals up readily and appears sound, but in a short time a strong defluxion taking place from the corrupted bone below, inflammation supervenes, and pus is formed which corrodes the cicatrix. What then is the cure of such ulcers? Dry the diseased bone to such a degree that it may exfoliate. But the diseased part of the bone may easily be brought up if you apply a cataplasm, consisting of fig leaves triturated with fine dried barley flour and wine. Or you may apply equal parts of the reed of henbane and of copperas triturated together. The root of hog's-fennel speedily removes the laminæ of bones.

Commentary. This chapter is copied from Aëtius, who gives some additional prescriptions, such as one consisting of the scales of copper, frankincense, alum, sal ammoniac, pomegranate rind, and ceruse, with or without cerate; and another consisting of red arsenic finely triturated with bear's fat.

Avicenna recommends strong attractive applications, such as a plaster of the leaves of the black poppy with fig leaves; and another containing the atramentum sutorium (sulphate of copper.)

LI—ON ULCERS IN THE JOINTS

The joints being drier than the fleshy parts, they therefore require when ulcerated more desiccative applications. Wherefore the trochisk of Polyides, when rubbed with wine until of the consistence of the sordes of baths, is an excellent application; and in like manner all equally desiccative medicines. And we have seen them benefited by bathing with sea-water and brine frequently. Wherefore we must use the most desiccative applications to the joints.

Commentary. This is copied from Oribasius. (Synops. vii, 19.)

LII—THOSE THINGS WHICH EXTRACT SHAFTS, JAVELINS, THORNS, AND THE LIKE

Javelins, reeds, and shafts, and thorns, are extracted by the two pimpernels, the round birthwort, ammoniac with honey, the fruit of henbane triturated and sprinkled upon the part. Mix the pounded root of calamus with honey, put it into a piece of linen, and use in great quantity; it will speedily extract them.

Commentary. This subject will be more fully treated of in the Sixth Book.

Our author copies from Oribasius. (Synops. vii, 17.)

Most of the articles here enumerated are mentioned by Dioscorides as possessing strongly attractive properties. Avicenna, Rhases, and Haly Abbas, speak of similar articles, without any new remedies of consequence. See in particular Haly. (Pract. iv, 24.)

The applications mentioned by Pliny are ridiculous. (H. N. xxx, 42, and xxxii, 43.)

LIII—ON HEMORRHAGE FROM VEINS AND ARTERIES

In cases of hemorrhage from parts, the contrary position to that for sinuses will be the proper one, that is to say, the upright, but that must not be in too great a degree, for there is danger of pain being excited, and of the blood bursting forth from the vessel again; for nothing produces hemorrhage and increases inflammation more than pain. Wherefore apply your finger immediately to the part from which the blood flows, putting it gently upon the orifice of the opening in the vessel, and pressing it so as not to excite pain, for by this means you will restrain the bleeding, and block up the opening with a thrombus, and should the bleeding vessel be deep-seated you will thereby ascertain most correctly its situation and magnitude, and whether it be an artery or a vein. After this, if the vessel be small we must use some of the styptics. The best of these are the obstruents, composed of roasted rosin, of fine flour of wheat, and of gypsum, and such like, mixed up with the white of an egg and applied upon the down of a hare. When the vessel is large seize it with a hook, stretch and twist it moderately. When the bleeding is stopped, endeavour if it is a vein to restrain the blood without a ligature, by the same medicines. But if it is an artery, one of two things must be done, either apply a ligature around it, or cut the vessel asunder, by which means you will restrain the blood. Sometimes, too, we are obliged to apply a ligature to large veins, and also occasionally to cut them asunder transversely. We are sometimes driven to this necessity with regard to veins which arise from a deep-seated place, more especially when they run through a narrow passage or important parts, for thus the portions will be retracted on either side, and the wound will be blocked up and covered by the parts above it. But the safer practice is to do both these things, applying a ligature to the root of the vessel and then dividing it. Having done these things, the wound is to be incarnated as quickly as possible, before the ligature slip from the vessel. For if it is not speedily incarnated, but the emptied portion is dilated, the disease called aneurism is formed. You may know whether it is a vein or an artery that pours forth the blood, from this, that the blood of an artery is brighter and thinner, and is evacuated by pulsations, whereas that of the vein is blacker and without pulsation.

The most excellent of all the incarnative medicines which we know, is that used with safety for hemorrhages from the meninges of the brain, and which may be used in wounds of the neck, even for those of the jugular veins; for it will restrain the bleeding from them without a ligature. It contains of the fattest frankincense, p. j; and of aloes, when applied to soft bodies, p. ss; but when too hard, an equal quantity, and instead of the frankincense manna is to be substituted. These are to be mixed with the white of an egg until they become of the consistence of honey, when it is to be applied upon the soft down of a hare to the vessel and the whole wound; and a bandage is to be put on externally, the first four or five turns of which we are to make upon the bleeding vessel, and from thence extend to the root of it. Then having loosed it on the third day, if the medicine should still be properly applied to the wound, we are to put on another one all around, soaking it, as it were, and then bandaging. But if the first pledget come away of itself, the finger is to be pressed gently upon the root of the vessel, so as to prevent all discharge, and it is to be removed softly and another pledget applied.

Thus it is to be treated until the vessel heal up, the upright posture being still preserved, but so as not to excite pain. Those things which form sloughs render the part more exposed than it was naturally, owing to the falling off of the sloughs; for in many cases a hemorrhage which can hardly be restrained supervenes upon the falling off of the sloughs. And yet we must have recourse to them when a great necessity compels us. A great necessity for using escharotics, or cauteries with fire, occurs when the bleeding proceeds from the vessels being corroded by mortification; and indeed, when in such affections we cut off the whole mortified part, it is safer to burn, as it were, its root, or to use escharotic medicines. This happens more especially upon the pudendum and fundament. The object of escharotics is to produce heat with astringency, as in chalcitis, misy, and copperas. Those from quicklime are stronger indeed, but owing to the want of astringency in the lime, the eschars from them fall sooner away; but it is better that they should remain longer, for thus will flesh have time to form previously at their root, and become as it were a cover to the vessels. In such cases of hemorrhage matured woad (isatis sativa) when sprinkled upon the part is excellent for restraining the bleeding, or burnt galls, but they must first be heated in the fire, and extinguished in vinegar or wine. The following Simples stop hemorrhages: Aloes, frankincense, manna, Samian earth, the rust of iron, the ashes of burnt wool finely powdered, the dung of an ass or of a horse, a small quantity of bitumen, pomegranate-rind, diphryges, galls, dried myrtle, all kinds of alum whether crude or burnt, roasted rosin, the bark or green leaves of the vine, and the down of the peels of the plane tree, more especially when the vessels throw off their crusts. In particular, hemorrhage from the nostril is to be restrained by the application of the fruit of the sharp rush, the juice of nettle leaves, chalcitis, burnt anthyllis, the down of a hare, the middle part of a ferule when burnt with vinegar, an ass's dung dry or moist, the juice of leeks with frankincense applied upon lamp-wick. The following are compositions for restraining all kinds of hemorrhage: Having soaked a fresh sponge in liquid pitch, and smeared it with bitumen, burn it in a new pot. Mix together of the ashes of it, p. ij; of lead, p. j; of antimony, p. j.—*Another*: Sprinkle on the part equal quantities of the manna of frankincense, and sulphur vivum.—*Another*: Of chalcitis, dr. viij; of frankincense, or of its manna, dr. xvj; of roasted rosin, dr. viij; of burnt gypsum, dr. viij.—*Another*, an escharotic styptic: Of chalcitis, of burnt copper, of copperas, of roasted misy, equal parts. And the medicine called the Rhodian, and that called the yellow, are excellent styptics.

Commentary. See Celsus (v, 26); Galen (Meth. Med. v, *et alibi*); Oribasius (Med. Collect. x, 22; Morb. Curat. iii, 36; Synops. vii, 20); Aëtius (xiv, 51); Actuarius (Meth. Med. vi, 4); Palladius (Comment. in Hippocr. Epidem. ed

Dietz, ii, 189); Albucasis (Chirurg. i, 58); Avicenna (iv, 4, 2,16); Averrhoes (in Avicennæ Cantic. ii, 2, and Collig. vii, 23); Serapion (v, 16); Haly Abbas (Pract. iv, 21); Rhases (Divis. i, 139; Contin. xxviii.)

Contrary to what is often stated in modern works on surgery, the ancients appear to have been very well acquainted with the proper treatment of hemorrhage. Celsus directs us when a dangerous hemorrhage is apprehended from a wound, to fill it up with dry pledgets, then to apply a sponge squeezed out of cold water, and to make pressure with the hand. If the bleeding does not stop, he directs us to change the pledgets often, and if dry ones do not answer to soak them in vinegar. For fear of inflammation he recommends us not to use caustics and escharotics except in urgent cases. When all other means fail, he directs us to seize upon the vessels (venæ) which pour forth the blood, and having tied them in two places about the wound, to cut them asunder, so that they may contract and still have their mouths shut up. If circumstances prevent this from being done, they are to be burnt with a red-hot iron. He also speaks of stopping bleeding by revulsion, as for example, by applying a cupping-instrument to the hindhead for bleeding in the forehead.

Galen has treated of this subject at great length in the Fifth Book of the 'Meth. Med.' When blood is discharged from a wounded artery, he directs us to apply a finger to the orifice of the vessel firmly, yet so as not to occasion pain, and thus a thrombus will be formed that will stop the flow of blood. When the vessel is deep-seated he advises us to examine accurately into its situation and size, and to ascertain whether it be an artery or vein; after which it is to be seized with a hook and twisted moderately. If the flow of blood is not stopped thereby, he recommends us, if the vessel is a vein, to endeavour to restrain it without a ligature by means of styptics, or things of an obstruent nature, such as roasted rosin, the fine down of wheaten flour, gypsum, and the like. But if the vessel is an artery, he says, one of two things must be done,—either a ligature must be applied to it, or it must be cut across. He adds, we are even obliged sometimes to apply a ligature to large veins and cut them across. From this extract of Galen's practice, it will be readily perceived how much our author is indebted to him. He makes mention of the ligature in many other parts of his works. He also recommends the actual cautery.

To stop bleeding, Oribasius directs, in the first place, cooling and astringent applications to be used, and if these do not succeed, caustics, such as misy, chalcitis, copperas, or the actual cautery. Upon the whole, his account of hemorrhage is nearly the same as our author's, only he says nothing of the ligature.

Aëtius treats of this subject in the same terms as Galen, recommending the ligature under the circumstances mentioned by him. Some of his styptics are powerful escharotics and astringents, such as copperas, chalcitis, alum, galls, quicklime, rosin, and frankincense. He informs us that Ammonius, the famous Alexandrian lithomist, used a composition of arsenic, sandarach, chalcitis, and quicklime.

Actuarius recommends a composition containing burnt copper, chalcitis, galls, frankincense, &c.

Palladius, in his Commentary on the 'Epidemics' of Hippocrates, treating of hemorrhage says, we often stop the bleeding by applying a ligature to the divided vessel.

Albucasis mentions four methods of stopping the discharge of blood from an artery: 1, by the cautery; 2, by dividing the artery across; 3, by using the ligature; 4, by styptics applied upon a bolster or compress, and tightly bandaged.

Averrhoes recommends to stop bleeding by styptics, the cautery, or the ligature. He says distinctly, that when the bleeding cannot be stopped, the artery or vein is to be secured with a thread.

Avicenna treats of all the modes of stopping hemorrhage with singular accuracy, but at so great length that we can only afford room for a few remarks. He recommends stupefying things, cold water, exposure to cold, escharotics, and the actual cautery. He also directs in extreme cases the vessel to be cut across, or a ligature to be applied, namely, a flaxen thread. His description of the process of taking up and tying an artery has quite a modern complexion. He also recommends the application of a compress with tight bandaging when the ligature cannot be applied.

Rhases makes mention of the cautery, of the application of snow, of the ligature, of styptics, and of cutting the vessel across. He mentions that Galen in certain cases approved of two ligatures, as it sometimes happens that the inferior portion will pour forth blood. He further speaks of his having occasionally used two or three ligatures for the sake of greater security. He also mentions torsion of the artery.

Haly Abbas gives an interesting account of hemorrhage, and makes mention of bandages and the ligature. He and Serapion agree in recommending strongly as a styptic a mixture of one part of frankincense, with a half part of aloes, applied upon the down of a hare. This is the application called the plaster of Galen, and is much recommended by Zacutus Lusitanus (Pract. Admin. i, 85), by Scultet (Arsinal de Chirurg. Tab. 33), by Brunus (Chirurg. Maj. i, 12), and Lanfrancus (Chir. parva. 5.)

The early modern writers on surgery make mention of all the ancient methods of stopping hemorrhage. Guy of Cauliac recommends the ligature upon the authority of Galen and Avicenna (iii, 1, 3.) It is also recommended by Brunus (i, 12), Theodoricus (i, 13), Rolandus (ii, 1), and Lanfrancus (iii, 1, 9.) It appears, therefore, that the use of the ligature for stopping hemorrhages was well understood by the ancients, and had never been lost sight of even in the darkest ages.

LIV—ON WOUNDS OF THE NERVES

When the nerves are wounded or pricked, they experience great inflammation and pain owing to their great sensibility; and therefore fever and convulsions supervene upon them, and in some cases delirium, owing to the continuity of the nerves with the brain. And sometimes phlegmons and abscesses form in the other parts adjacent to the wound, arising from the wounded nerve, owing to their continuity with it. Wherefore we must preserve the wound of the skin from adhering, that the ichor may escape by it. And in punctures, if they appear blind, the part must be divided by two incisions intersecting one another. With regard to the treatment, if the body is plethoric, and the inflammation strong, it will be proper to begin with venesection; and when the body appears to be in a state of cacochymy, purging must also be had recourse to. We must apply to the wound medicines for allaying pain, and for increasing the discharge, more especially if the cross incisions have not been practised. It is necessary to know that warm water, which is most applicable to other inflammations, is inimical in these cases, and it is better to bathe the part with a thin oil which has no astringency and is warm to the feeling; for nothing either very cold or very hot can be applied without detriment. Of medicines turpentine-rosin is beneficial by itself in the case of children, women, and persons of tender flesh, but softened with euphorbium for those of a firmer fibre; and if it become too hard it is to be mixed with some of the thinner oils. To nerves in a state of inflammation and mortifications, we may use cataplasms consisting of the flour of barley or of beans, or by boiling that of tares in trained lye with oxymel. But without boiling we may use the following cerate for punctures: of wax, oz. iij; of euphorbium, oz. j; or of pigeon's dung; for harder parts, of oil, oz. ij; and sometimes of turpentine, oz. j. When you wish to give the medicine the form of a plaster, you may add to the preparation from euphorbium, of wax, of boiled rosin, of oil, and of fat pitch, of each, oz. vj; but you will make it better by substituting the fattest bee-glue instead of the rosin. The following is a good remedy for punctured nerves, applying also to persons bitten by mad animals: Of vinegar one sextarius, of fat pitch, lb. j; of opoponax, oz. iij; having dissolved the opoponax in the vinegar triturate it more, and having melted the pitch, boil. This medicine is applicable to punctures of the nerves not allowing the mouth of the puncture to close up, as in the case of persons bitten by rabid animals it does not permit the wound to cicatrize. But it answers only with hard bodies, and when you wish to apply it to the punctures of children, or of persons of soft skin, you must melt it in some discutient article such as the oil of marjoram, of opobalsam, or old oil.—*Another* suitable application is basilicon with the addition of natron, or quicklime, or euphorbium, or sulphur vivum, or wild pigeon's dung, or opoponax, or sagapene, or Cyrenaic juice, or castor, adding to a pound of the ointment an ounce of one of these medicines. It answers well for wounds of nerves, and more especially punctures. And in the country when one is not supplied with any other medicines, one may apply fresh and fat bee-glue to the wound, or leaven more especially if old, by itself or mixed with bee-glue, or with the juice of tithymal. But cataplasms may be applied made of oxymel, or of strained lye, with the flour of beans, or of tares, or of chick-peas, or of bitter lupines, or of barley, or of the flour of polenta, not only when in a state of inflammation, but they may be used from the commencement. But relaxing cataplasms are to be entirely rejected for wounds of nerves. If the nerve is not cut, but laid bare by a wound, the surrounding skin being divided so that the nerve appears naked, and is wounded longitudingly and not transversely, we must use none of the afore-mentioned from euphorbium, nor any thus acrid, for the nerve being bare will not bear their power which is strong, but one may use lime that has been washed often in the warm season mixed with much honey. The preparation from pompholyx, and that from honey melted with much rose-oil, are also excellent ones. But these things must not touch the wound, for the nerve is sensitive, of a cold temperament, and continuous with the most important part. And neither is it proper to bathe such an ulcer with oil, for it will make it become foul, and we must only wipe away the ichor with soft wool wrapped about a probe. When all things succeed agreeably to our wish, there will be no danger in fomenting with must. For stronger persons the trochisk of Polyides with sodden must may be used upon a warm pledget. After the exposed nerve has been covered over, we must apply externally pledgets, with some of those things which are fitting for narrow wounds, such as that from euphorbium, or that from pigeon's dung, taking in also much of the sound parts. When the wound is transverse there is greater danger of convulsions, but everything relating to the cure is in this case the same, except that while the wound is recent some have used sutures and certain of the agglutinative applications; but the sutures must not be applied very superficially lest the part below remain ununited, but more deeply, taking care however that the nerve be not punctured by the needle. It is to be known once for all, that in wounds of the nerves the medicine which cures punctures being of a bitter nature, it is not possible to cure with it the division of the nerve, as the parts cannot endure pungency and inflammation. And neither does the medicine which cures incisions answer with punctures. For its strength does not reach the bottom of it, the incision of the skin being narrow. A spare diet is to be allowed, and a soft couch; and warm oil is to be applied to the armpits, head, and neck; but when the wound is in the leg, the medicine is to be applied to the groins, pubes, and the parts there. Baths, until the inflammation is on the decline, are to be abstained from, water not agreeing with these wounds, as we have said. But since some from habit cannot bear to want the bath, if the wounded art be the hand it must not, if possible, be wet in hot water, and still less in cold; but when the wound is in the foot, since it is impossible to preserve it from being wet, when about to go into the bath apply to the wounded part some of the plasters, and externally a compress consisting of many folds and moistened with oil; and again external to that a linen bandage; and after having done these things when the person affected is about to take his seat in the bath pour oil once more upon the bandage. When he comes out of the bath take away all those applications, and have recourse to the treatment described above. When there is only contusion of the nerve, if along with it there be contusion of the skin and ulceration, the cataplasm of the flour of beans and of oxymel will be a fit one, but you may add sometimes the flour of tares, and some iris; and when the contusion is attended with pain, you may mix a little liquid pitch with it. If there be no contusion of the skin, it will be more discutient to bathe frequently with an oil of a heating nature, I mean that of dill, of rue, of iris, or of marjoram. When the whole nerve is cut asunder no danger will result from it, but the part will be mutilated; and the treatment is to be conducted as in the case of other ulcers. The treatment of the wounds of nerves by simples is sufficient for accomplishing the whole cure, but some are in the practice of using compound applications in such cases, as the plaster from metals, those called barbarous, and the cissinum, that from groundsel, the melanchlorum, the indicum, harmonica, and athena, the composition of which, and the manner of using them you will find described in the Seventh Book. And since some very wealthy people are fond of using expensive applications to wounds of the nerves, Galen has described the following for punctures of the nerves: Of cinnamon, oz. j; of dittany, oz. j; of marum, oz. j; of amaracus, dr. ij; of wax, oz. viij; of opobalsam, oz. x; of turpentine, oz. x.—*Another*: of cyrenaic juice, oz. j; of wax, oz. iij; of opobalsam, oz. xij. This is an application for exposed nerves: Of wax used for ointments, oz. iij; of the ointment called spicatum, or foliatum, or that of nard, oz. xij; of washed pompholyx, oz. j; of spikenard, oz. j; of amomum, oz. j; of the leaf (malabathrum), oz. j. And these, Galen says, are superlatively excellent.

Commentary. Galen has devoted a whole book of his work 'De Med. sec. genera' to the consideration of wounds of tendons, membranes, ligaments, and nerves properly called, and he also treats of them more generally in the sixth book of his work 'Meth. Med.' He professes to have had ample experience in the treatment of these cases while attending wounded gladiators. As our author has given a very comprehensive abstract of Galen's principles of cure, it will be unnecessary for us to enter into any minute detail of them. He states very decidedly that cold applications, especially cold water, are highly dangerous, and inculcates that calefacient oils are the most proper applications. He particularly praises oils medicated with spurge, or sagapene, or turpentine-rosin. They are to be applied upon soft wool. In certain cases, he says, I have mixed the powerfully desiccant substances, such as quicklime, misy, chalcitis, pompholyx, arsenic, and sandarach, with the oils or cerates. When tendons are cut across he directs us to unite the ends together by sutures. Wounds of membranes and ligaments are said to be less dangerous than those of tendons. In general he further recommends either bloodletting or purging.

Oribasius, Aëtius, and, in short, all the subsequent authorities, like our author, copy everything from Galen. As a specimen we shall give an abstract of the method of treatment recommended by Octavius Horatianus, who, it is probable, belonged to the Methodical sect. He commences with stating that wounds of nervous parts are in general very dangerous, and recommends applications of a digestive nature to avert the violent symptoms and pains. In such cases he directs us to bleed and purge, forbids all fomentations of warm water, but approves of those made with tepid oil, after which dressings composed of turpentine-rosin, either by itself or with some sponge, are to be applied. But for women and children of a delicate frame he recommends turpentine alone; for others, however, he recommends turpentine with spurge and oil, to which occasionally may be added bee-glue, sagapene, assafœtida, and opoponax. He also from personal experience speaks favorably of an application prepared from lime washed in water, spurge, sulphur, turpentine, wax, and pitch. He mentions other preparations from rosin, spurge, with oil and sea water.

The Arabians copy from Galen very closely. Thus Avicenna condemns cold applications, and recommends calefacient ones. He approves of sutures when the tendons are cut asunder. Haly Abbas cautions against cold water, and particularly commends wool dipped in hot oil of violets. When spasm (tetanus) supervenes owing to the wound of a nerve, he directs us to divide it asunder lest the affection of it spread to the brain and prove fatal. Rhases also forbids all relaxing applications. He commends hot stimulant oils, and basilicon mixed with spurge, natron, lime, assafœtida, castor, &c.

Gulielmus de Saliceto, Guido de Cauliaco, Severinus, and Lanfrancus in laying down the treatment of wounded nerves and tendons, follow closely the principles delivered by their Arabian masters. They approved of sutures when the tendon is cut across.

LV—ON ANCYLOSIS

Contractions of joints arising from impacted humours, or some nervous tension, we are accustomed to call ancylæ and ancylosis, which cases require emollient and relaxing applications. Wherefore, in general, those things recommended for scirrhous parts, but still more particularly the applications to paralysed members will be proper, and more especially pouring upon the part water and oil, in which linseed, fenugreek, marshmallows, bay, the root of the wild cucumber, and the Sicyonian oil itself, have been boiled. After bathing we may apply first the more simple acopa, such as that from poplar, that from fir, the one called bromium, that ascribed to Basilius, and the pyxis; and after these the Aristophanian, and that ascribed to Azanites. But the strongest are those called lysoponium and varium. Of plasters, that ascribed to Amathaon, and the anicetum. This is a most excellent one: Of bdellium, of calves' fat, of ammoniac perfume, of Illyrian iris, of each, dr. xvj; of opoponax, of galbanum, of the seeds of rosemary, of storax, of frankincense, of each, dr. viij; of pepper, clx grains; of wax, lb. ss.; of turpentine-rosin, lb. ss.; of the lees of the oil of iris, q. s.; of wine, q. s.; the medicine is pounded. It forms a good acopum when diluted with oil of iris, of privet, or of bay. Intermediate between the acopa and plasters is the preparation from bacon called polymigmaton. The acopa are to be used with soft and continued friction, along with gentle attempts to bend and stretch the affected joint.

Commentary. The principles of treatment here laid down are the same as those inculcated by all the other authorities. For a complete account of the formation of malagmata, we refer the reader to Galen (Med. sec. gen. vii), and to Aëtius (xii, 42.)

Actuarius recommends an acopum composed of old oil, the oils of bay, iris, and storax, with turpentine, spurge, castor, ammoniac, pepper, opoponax, galbanum, and stag's marrow. He remarks that emollient and relaxing medicines are indicated. (iv, 16.)

Celsus recommends, "ad recenti vulnere contractos articulos, quas ἀγκυλας Græci nominant," a malagma consisting of frankincense, rosin, galbanum, ammoniac, and bdellium, with wax. (v, 18.) Avicenna makes mention of a similar one. Scribonius Largus gives a prescription for ancylosis consisting of bdellium, opoponax, ammoniac, galbanum, calves' fat, &c. (civ.)

LVI—ON RELAXATION OF THE JOINTS

The joints often become relaxed from protracted febrile complaints, and from colic, and paralytic affections, especially when a hot and humid intemperament seizes them; and hence the motion of the joint is impeded. In these cases the juice of acacia mixed with water may be poured upon the part; or a decoction of bramble, of myrtle, of lentisk, or of the bark of elm roots will answer well; or the rind of pomegranate may be formed into a cataplasm, or myrtle leaves with myrtle ointment may be applied. For the ligaments require to be strengthened by astringent and desiccative powers; and such applications are therefore to be made to the joints, as that from willows, that called oxyrum, and the phœnicinum, with the addition of an astringent wine or vinegar. Some imagining that the weakness of the joints proceeds from cold, and having had recourse to more heating remedies, have only increased the mischief.

Commentary. Our author has correctly stated that relaxation of the joints is to be cured by astringent desiccant applications. Aëtius makes mention of the simple articles enumerated here (xiv, 72), and Oribasius recommends a few of the same. (Synops. vii, 23.) Our author is much fuller than Oribasius on this head. (Ibid.)

LVII—ON WORMS

There are three different sorts of worms, the round, the broad, and thirdly, those called ascarides. They are all the offspring of crude and thick pituitous matters with a suitable putrefaction, such matters collect in children, and others who take too much food. But they do not grow from hot, acrid, or melancholic humours; for these being too strong for nutrition, are inapt for the generation of worms; and, on the contrary, bilious superfluities are particularly destructive of them. Or if at any time yellow bile be discharged along with worms, either downwards or by vomiting, you may be sure that they have been formed in the intestines, whereas the bilious humour had been collected at the mouth of the stomach, or in some other part. We shall now describe the form, generation, situation, diagnosis, and cure of each variety, beginning with the round.

Of the round worms. The form of the round worms must be known to everybody, because they are more common than any of the others. They are generated principally in the small intestines, and are very prevalent in the stomach; wherefore they are often discharged by the mouth, and sometimes by the nose. They are most common in children, more especially in fever. For they are formed about the commencement of fevers from a corruption of the matters; at their acme from the malignant nature of the disease; and during the decline from a change of the whole system to a better state. Wherefore Hippocrates says, "it is a good symptom when round worms are evacuated at the crisis of the disease, and these speedily die." Those who have round worms experience pain of the intestines and stomach, small dry tickling cough, and in some cases hiccough, sleep with palpitations and irregular startings; and some start from their sleep with a scream, and again fall over asleep. The pulse is unequal, and the fever has irregular exacerbations, making its attacks with coldness of the joints, and coming on three and sometimes four times in the day or night without any stated form. Children have mastication and projection of the tongue without cause, and grinding of the teeth; they shut their eyes and wish to remain silent, and are offended when disturbed. Their eyes appear bloody, their cheeks red, and again change to pale. But these things occur at intervals in a short time. Sometimes the worms crawling up to the stomach occasion nausea, gnawing pain, and anorexia to the patients. When forced to take food they can scarcely swallow for nausea, or they vomit what they have taken, or their bowels are loose with corruption of the food, or are inflated like a bladder; but the rest of the body is wasted in an unaccountable manner, there being neither famine nor any extraordinary evacuation. But one must not expect to find all these symptoms in all cases, but certain ones, according to prevailing circumstances, and occasionally the most of them. These symptoms occur from the animals turning themselves about in the intestines and biting them, and the febrile heat raising noxious vapours to the brain from putrid humours collected in the belly, in which case we must sometimes pay attention alike both to the fever and the worms, and sometimes we must bestow little attention to the fever, and direct our efforts to remove the worms from the body. Many having neglected them have been eaten through by them, and have died convulsed. And others say that they have seen them come out from the groins of the patient. You may remove them from the body by killing them, and you may kill them principally by using bitter remedies. When both the treatment of the fever and of the worms is common, the simple remedies will be proper. Wherefore the patients must first drink a decoction of camomile, and of the fruit of the sebesten plum, or these medicines themselves may be given boiled. We may also give the juice of endive, or coriander seed, triturated with hot water or with oxycrate; or a decoction of the herb mouse-ear, or the shavings of hart's horn, or sinopic vermilion finely levigated. And they may swallow by degrees two spoonfuls of the oil of bitter unripe olives, for by its bitterness it kills them, and by its lubricity it drags them along and evacuates them with the fæces. When inflammation and distension of the intestines are present, we must have recourse to a cataplasm of linseed and of the flower of lupines, and of wormwood, and of the roots of bryony in hydromel, or pour upon the hypochondria the oil of camomile, wine, and the infusions of the fruit of wormwood and aloes. When the fevers are not very troublesome we may mix with the sebesten plums some mint, and give them: and when there is no fever we may administer the more drastic medicines, such as the decoction of seriphum, or of calamint, or of fern, or the seed of cardamon, or a decoction of the root of acid pomegranate reduced to one third, or of toasted cumin, and of tawny-coloured natron, of each, scr. iij; or wormseed, or southernwood, or both made into pills with honey, or scr. iij of bitter lupines, or the levigated seed of cabbage or of rocket, or wormwood which is often sufficient alone. We may give of washed aloes to the amount of scr. iij; which is one of our most celebrated remedies; but to stronger persons we may give them unwashed. And since children will not take the aloes from a cup, they are to be secured upon their back, and their mouth being forced open by a spoon, we are to inject in spite of them the aloes by means of a syringe having a strong pipe, throwing it in as far as possible. This is an admirable method with children who can hardly be prevailed upon to take medicines, and in this way we may often inject soup in cases of anorexia. And cyphi and masuaphium may be properly administered, and burnt hart's horn with pepper in honey or oxymel; and we may also endeavour to give the other medicines in oxymel. But the vinegar of squills will be still better, especially when given to adults. Or mustard with oil and vinegar may be given to the amount of a spoonful. Those whose bowels are troubled with a flux owing to worms may take a potion of the juice of plantain, or the plaintain itself may be given in a dry state, for it is of use both for the flux and the worms. We may apply to them cataplasms of crude barley flour, of fern, of wormwood, of the flower of lupines, of wormseed, and of southernwood, and likewise pomegranate rind, acacia, galls, and the flowers of the wild pomegranate are to be mixed with them. And since many people often loathe bitter draughts, we may give of those we have mentioned, such as are not decidedly bitter, and in addition, ground pine and horehound, elecampane, bay berries, cassia, thyme, pennyroyal, carpesium, cyperus, polypody, iris, bastard-saffron, madder, Egyptian thorn, with an equal quantity of pepper, to the amount of scr. vj, to a decoction of mint, the juice of the root of mulberry, or the decoction of stone parsley, or of other aromatic seeds. Externally we may use aloes with the oil of apples and wine. This also whets the appetite, which is a thing to be much attended to. With the aloes we may often mix wormwood; or the navel may be filled with bull's gall along with some of the bitters formerly mentioned; or the oil of rose-bay may be constantly rubbed in, or cedar-pitch may be applied alone and along with cerate to the whole belly; or dried pitch may be levigated and sprinkled on it; or it may be anointed with mint and gith in rose-oil; or we may mix with them the decoction of seriphum; or we may triturate peach leaves and apply. We may use stag's marrow in the form of an ointment to the navel, pubes, and loins; and, if necessary, we may apply the cerate of aloes, of wormwood, of the flour of lupines, of seriphum, of gith, of each, scr. vj; of wax, oz. jss; of oil of camomile q. s.; triturate the powders with bull's gall. We may give them frequent injections of honied water, that the worms may be attracted downwards by the sweetness of the honey. But if they putrefy in the deep-seated parts, and are not discharged, but on the contrary raise effluvia, we must evacuate them by giving aloes, or the medicine called picra, prepared from it. In certain cases a moderate evacuation, by means of a suppository, is not unuseful to them.

Of the broad worm (tænia). The broad worm is (if I may say so) a conversion of the membrane which lines the inside of the intestine into a living body, which is often either discharged whole, when its size appears incredible to be seen; or it is evacuated in parts; but when loosed from its attachment it does not form again. It occurs most frequently without fever, but sometimes in fever after a protracted disease, when it brings on constant gnawing pains of the stomach, and an insatiable desire of food; for the animal which is formed in the intestines seize the food lying there, so that another supply is straightway required, and, if not furnished with it, the worm will bite the bowels. It is accompanied with emaciation of the body and loss of strength, with anomalous symptoms: but the most unerring symptom is when certain substances, like the seed of gourd, are discharged with the fæces. The cure resembles that of the former kind; taking the bitter draughts, eating garlic, drinking or injecting a decoction of fern, or of centaury, or of calamint, of dittany, or of pennyroyal. And we may also inject brine. The patient may also drink this potion, which is not unserviceable to those who are troubled with other worms, if they happen to have fever: Of red natron, of pepper, of cardamom, equal parts: the dose is gr. iij, with wine or hot water.—*Another*, a linctus: Of pepper, of pure bay berries, of Ethiopian cumin, of mastich, equal parts; of honey, q. s.; the dose is a spoonful taken in the morning and at bedtime. But if you wish to make it stronger, add an equal part of red natron.—*Another*: Of elecampane, of ammoniac perfume, of pepper, (in another formula, of fern,) of each, dr. v, with hot oxymel; and after an interval give adults one or two drachms of euphorbium in a draught.—*Another*: Of fern, an acetabulum; of natron, dr. ij; give it in a hemina of water, but it will be better if a little scammony be added to it.—*Another*: Of the bark of the roots of sour pomegranate stripped of its rind above, dr. iv; of pepper, dr. iv; of cardamom, dr. vj; of horehound, dr. ij; give it in honey to the patient after he has previously eaten of garlic, until the affection is completely removed. Give also of theriac, when not prevented by strong fever.

LVIII—ON ASCARIDES

Ascarides, as we formerly mentioned, are a kind of intestinal worms resembling earth-worms, being formed about the extremity of the rectum and the beginning of the sphincter ani, and occasioning a great itching of the parts. This species is formed by bad diet, cold, and indigestion of the food. Wherefore they are to be discharged, in children, by suppositories of honey with a moderate quantity of salts or natron; but in adults by acrid brine, or a decoction of centaury with natron and honey, or of colocynth, or of wormwood, or of chamæleon, or of alkanet, or of bastard saffron, or of hyssop, or of pennyroyal, or of calamint, or of lupines. After the injections we may anoint the rectum with these simples: Acacia, or hypocistis with natron, or Syriac sumach with liquid alum; and in those which are bound, with Lemnian earth in wine, and with these compound medicines, the trochisk of Andron and the like. And we may give them an injection of cedar-rosin with a syringe having many perforations, such as those used for the uterus; or salted flesh is to be adapted to the part and secured with a bandage, as long as it can be allowed to remain, and changed often. In general all those infested with worms derive benefit from fumigations with the hairs of ichneumon. The food should contain wholesome juices, and such as are easily distributed over the system, neither increasing the cause which engenders the worms, nor allowing the strength to sink; and on that account we may give some diluted wine. And we must give food frequently on that account, and in order that the worms may not bite the intestines for want of their food. The best time for taking food is when the worms are full. If there be a defluxion of the belly you may be sure that the worms are on the increase, the food not being properly distributed, and we are to give soups with a mixture of astringents, such as pears, apples, and pomegranates, more especially such as are acid; and we may apply to the belly, externally, astringent remedies as mentioned above.

Commentary. On this curious subject consult Hippocrates (Aphor. iii, 26; De Morbis, iv, 27); Aristotle (H. A. v, 9); Celsus (iv, 17); Cælius Aurelianus (Pass. Tard. iv, 8); Scribonius Largus (36); Serenus Samonicus; Marcellus (31); Octavius Horatianus (ii, 30); Dioscorides (pluries); Galen (Meth. Med. xiv; Isagoge;) Aëtius (ix, 39); Oribasius (Morb. Curat. iv, 90); Actuarius (Meth. Med. i, 21); Nonnus (172); Myrepsus (8); Avicenna (iii, 16, 5); Serapion (iii, 30); Averrhoes (Collig. vii, 37); Avenzoar (ii, 7, 22); Haly Abbas (Theor. viii, 28; Pract. vii, 29); Alsaharavius (Pract. xvii, 2, 9); Rhases

(Divis. 169; Contin. xxvi); Alexandri Tralliani Epistola ap. Alb. Fabricii Bibl. Græc. xii, 602, and ed. Ideler, 1842.

Hippocrates states that the round and broad lumbrici are often passed with the first discharges from the bowels of children. This is a fact very difficult to account for. When, and how did the *seed* of the worm get access to the belly of the child? He rejects the opinion that the rings of the broad lumbricus (tænia) which are passed from the bowels are its offspring. He says it does not occasion death, but continues to live as long as the man lives.

Aristotle divides intestinal worms into the lumbrici teretes, the l. lati, and ascarides. He remarks that the broad produce something resembling the seeds of the gourd. He believed in spontaneous generation.

The pomegranate seems to have been a popular remedy for intestinal worms. Cato the Censor gives directions for medicating wine by the addition of pomegranate and fennel, of which, he says, "Id vinum tinias perpurgat et lumbricos, si sic concinnes." (De re rust. 127.)

Celsus treats of the lumbrici lati and teretes. For the cure of the former he recommends a draught containing lupine and the bark of mulberry, with the addition of hyssop, pepper, or scammony. He also recommends emetics with garlic, or pomegranate rind with some nitre. For the teretes he recommends the same, and also the seed of nettle, or of cabbage, or mint, or wormwood, or hyssop with mead, or the seed of cresses with vinegar. He advises, likewise, to eat garlic, and use clysters of oil.

Scribonius Largus directs first garlic and old soft cheese to be eaten, and then Macedonian fern to be taken with honey. After four hours a mixture of aloes and scammony with honied water is to be given, and a clyster of warm water administered. He also recommends wormseed and the shavings of hart's horn. Marcellus mentions the same remedies.

Serenus Samonicus recommends hartshorn, calamint, garlic, southernwood, coriander, pennyroyal, horehound, &c.

The beginning of the chapter of Cælius Aurelianus on lumbici unfortunately is lost. He mentions the usual symptoms which accompany them, namely, occasional deliquium, agitation, grinding of the teeth, change of colour, convulsions, &c. Worms are discharged by the mouth or anus, sometimes single, and at other times in great numbers rolled up in a ball; sometimes dead, and at other times alive; and they are of various colours. For ascarides he recommends when there is inflammation of the rectum an injection of oil, to which may sometimes be joined a decoction of wormwood and centaury. But if bloody scrapings of the bowels are discharged, he directs us to give a decoction of pomegranate-rind, and, if the complaint continue, equal parts of burnt paper and of arsenic, to the amount of six drs., with the infusion of plantain. Surely there must be some mistake as to the amount of the dose, for so great a quantity could not be injected with safety. When there is putrefaction he recommends an injection of salt water, with other suitable remedies. When complicated with any other disorder he properly directs us to pay attention to it; after which the animals may readily be discharged by drinking oil, or a decoction of sebesten plums (myxæ), or of liquorice: these things, he says, will obviate constriction and swelling, while by lubricating the bowels they will promote the discharge of the worms. When complicated with relaxation he recommends astringents externally and internally, such as vinegar with honey, lupine, the shavings of hart's horn, &c. Sometimes, he says, in order to expel them we must have recourse to acrid substances, such as onions, garlic, mustard, cresses, cardamus, assafœtida dissolved in vinegar, wormwood, &c. In stating the detail of the treatment he mentions various other anthelmintics, such as the hiera of aloes, gentian, mulberries, squills, spurge, alkanet, colocynth, and scammony. All these things may be given by the mouth or in injections, with a considerable admixture of oil. For the lumbricus latus he directs, first, an emetic of oil, and next day a clyster with nitre or salt. Saltish things are also to be given in drink, with liquorice, or scammony, or polypody, &c. When the animals are discharged, to prevent a renewal of the complaint, he recommends friction, vomiting, acrid food, calefacient plasters, sinapisms, paroptesis, and the like.

Pliny recommends the ashes of hart's horn for tænia. (H. N. xxviii, 59.)

Dioscorides ascribes anthelminthic properties to various acrid and bitter substances, such as garlic, cresses, fern, gith, mulberry, pomegranate rind, lupine, cabbage, nettle, hyssop, mint, calamint, wormwood, wormseed, rue, coriander, thyme, &c. Similar remedies are recommended in the 'Euporista,' which is falsely ascribed to him.

Galen mentions that bitters in general are destructive of intestinal worms. The teres, he adds, is killed by the absinthium; but the latus and ascaris require stronger medicines, such as the filix. The author of the 'Isagoge,' a work generally ascribed to Galen, divides intestinal worms into the broad, the round, and the ascarides. The round are about the length of a span or somewhat more, especially such as are formed about the stomach. The ascarides are short, and form in the rectum. The broad, called also fasciæ or tæniæ, from their resemblance to tape, are said to be sometimes the length of the intestines. The round are most common in children, the ascarides before manhood; and these are difficult to remove except by bitters, elecampane, and acrid food.

Oribasius treats briefly of lumbrici, recommending for the l. rotundus, southernwood, wormwood, calamint, gith, &c., taken internally or applied outwardly; for ascarides, the juice of calamint, and cedar rosin, in like manner; and for the tænia the bark of the root of mulberry, and the roots of fern in honied water, and also the root of the white chamæleon and costus.

Aëtius gives a full and accurate detail of the symptoms and treatment of lumbrici, but as his remedies are much the same as our author's, it will be unnecessary to deliver any account of them. He remarks, that anthelminthics either kill worms by their acrimony, or remove them by their bitterness, or irritate them so as to expel them, or by lubricating the parts facilitate the expulsion of them.

Actuarius gives a sensible account of the formation of worms, which he ascribes to putrefaction or indigestion. White worms, he says, are the product of indigestion, but the red, and those of any other colour, arise from putrefaction.

Nonnus merely abridges our author's account of this subject.

The ingredients in the compositions recommended by Myrepsus, are such as aloes, scammony, southernwood, and bitter almonds.

Octavius Horatianus gives a good account of worms, but it contains scarcely anything that is not to be found in our author's. He says, that from long experience he had great confidence in a purgative draught consisting of scammony, the ashes of burnt peas, euphorbium, and nitre, given in sweet wine. But garlic, and other acrid things, are to be first eaten.

The Epistle of Alexander Trallian on worms, first published by Hieronymus Mercurialis, and afterwards by Albertus Fabricius, and again lately by Ideler, contains an interesting exposition of the ancient views on this subject. He divides intestinal worms into three genera: the ascaris, the strongylus or round, and the latus or broad. He remarks that the small worms (ascarides) are generally found in the large intestines, the round in the small intestines, and hence they are often vomited up; while the broad worms (tænia) are sometimes as long as the intestines, some having been discharged sixteen feet in length. He states that they are engendered by corruption of the food, and putrefaction of crude humours. He lays down at great length the plan of treatment, which he varies according as they are with or without fever. His remedies consist of cathartic, acrid, oily, acid, and bitter substances. Of purgatives he mentions aloes, scammony, and hellebore; of acrid articles, garlic, cresses, and the like; of oily medicines, the oil of roses, castor oil (oleum ricini), and common oil boiled with rue; of acids, salt and nitre (soda); and of bitters, southernwood, wormwood, hyssop, fennel, and the like. For the expulsion of the strongylus he speaks favorably of a decoction of gagate stone (jet). For ascarides and lumbrici he recommends a lavement prepared from juniper. He concludes his treatise by stating that "ten thousand" other things had been recommended as anthelminthics by the ancients.

Avicenna in his account of worms condenses all the information contained in the Greek authors, but we do not find that he supplies anything new. He in particular copies freely from Aëtius and our author. The same may be said of Serapion, who recommends wormwood, bitter lupines, calamint, peach leaves, cabbage, onions, thyme, colocynth, &c. Averrhoes says that the lumbrici in general are removed by bitters, such as wormwood or wormseed, but that the cucurbitini (tæniæ) require strong medicines. Of the pineæ nuces he says, "Occidunt vermes qui sunt in ventre." (Collig. v, 42.) Probably this hint may have led to the use of turpentines for the cure of tænia. Avenzoar attributes the formation of worms to ill-digested food in the stomach, and recommends much the same remedies as the Greeks. Haly Abbas describes the three species of worms, and details the symptoms of them. He remarks that these animals are to be killed by medicines of a hot and dry nature, such as bitters. He recommends wormwood, fern, and the like, pounded with honey, vinegar, &c. The remedies mentioned by Alsaharavius are oils, bitters, and drastic purgatives. He treats of lumbrici very fully. Rhases recommends in general terms bitters; for the round, wormwood, for the broad, (tæniæ, called by him semina cucurbita) seriphium, bitter lupines, narcissus, &c. And for the ascarides he directs us to apply a suppository of wool dipped in the gall of a bull. He remarks that they occur most frequently in autumn, being engendered by fruit. He states correctly that they often bring on epilepsy, and looseness of the bowels. He much commends the oil of unripe olives.

Vegetius recommends nearly the same medicines for removing the vermes of cattle as those already mentioned, namely, wormwood, cresses, coriander, fenugreek, and the like, boiled in oil, and administered by the mouth and in clysters. (Mulom. i, 44; see also Columella vi, 25.)

According to Michaelis and Sprengel the ancient Brahmins were acquainted with the anthelminthic properties of the dolichos pruriens.

We have stated above that the most celebrated of the ancient *savans* believed in the *spontaneous generation* of animals. This doctrine, although generally rejected at the present time, has been advocated by many modern naturalists of great eminence, such as Baron Buffon and Professor Rudolphi. Virey gives a very impartial statement of the arguments for and against this physiological doctrine. (See Hist. des Mœurs et de l'Instinct des Animaux, ii, 121.) Mr. Madden, the traveller, relates that the bark of the pomegranate is still considered in the east as a specific, not only for ascarides, but also for the tape-worm. He says, "I have rarely seen it fail in the cure of tænia. They make a decoction of two oz. of the fresh bark in a pint of water, this they drink daily till the worm is expelled, which it generally is the third day." (Travels in Egypt, ii, 371.)

LIX—ON DRACUNCULUS, OR THE GUINEA-WORM

In India and the upper parts of Egypt a class of worms called dracunculi, resembling the intestinal, are formed in the muscular parts of the body, such as the anus, thighs, legs, and in the sides of children, under the skin; and they move in a perceptible manner. Then in process of time at the extremity of the dracunculus matter is formed in the part, and the skin being opened the head of the dracunculus comes forth. But if the worm be dragged it occasions pains, and particularly when it breaks. Wherefore some say that it is proper to fix a piece of lead to the worm in order that its discharge may not take place at once, but gradually with the weight of the lead. Some disapproving of this practice, inasmuch as the worm is apt to break with the weight of the lead and occasion violent pains, direct the part to be put into hot water, in order that the dracunculus being warmed may come forward, when it is to be seized with the fingers and dragged forth by degrees. But Soranus is of opinion that the dracunculus is not an animal originally, but a nervous concretion, which has only the appearance of moving. Whether this or the former be the true account of the matter, it appears to Soranus, Leonides, and others, that they are to be treated with the affusion of warm water, and digestive cataplasms made of honied water and the flour of wheat or barley; and they approve of sometimes using a plaster possessed of similar properties. Wherefore that from bay-berries, and the one from honey are proper. For by the use of these the dracunculus or concretion dies and falls out. But when suppuration takes place, if it does not fall out, the skin is to be divided, and the part being laid open, that which is contained in it is to be taken out, when a tent is to be put into the skin, and then the treatment for suppurations is to be applied.

Commentary. The following authors treat of the vena medinensis, or dracunculus, now generally called the Guinea worm: Galen (De Loc. Affect. vi, 3; Isagoge;) Aëtius (xiv, 85); Pollux (Onomast. iv); Plutarch (Symp. viii, 9); Theophrastus (H. P. ix); Actuarius (Meth. Med. vi, 8; iv, 16); Avicenna (iv, 3, 2, 21); Avenzoar (ii, 3, 20); Haly Abbas (Theor. viii, 18); Alsaharavius (Pr. xxviii, 12); Rhases (ad Mansor. vii, 24; Cont. xxvi.)

Galen admits that he had never seen the dracunculus, and that therefore he could not be positive respecting its origin and nature. He had known many persons, however, who had seen it, and was inclined to believe that it is of a nervous nature, and resembles lumbrici only in colour and thickness. The author of the Isagoge states that dracunculi resemble varices, and that when they project or move about they occasion great pain, and are to be removed by making an incision of the skin as for varices.

Plutarch briefly mentions the dracunculus as being a disease which had newly attacked the inhabitants of the country adjoining the Red Sea.

Aëtius professes to derive his account of the dracunculus from Leonides. He says, like our author, that it is formed most commonly in the legs and muscular parts of the arms in India and Ethiopia, and that the generation of it is not dissimilar to that of intestinal worms. He adds, that in process of time suppuration takes place at the end of the worm, when an opening is made in the flesh, and the head of the dracunculus protrudes. If dragged out considerable disturbance is produced, especially if the worm should be broken, for what remains occasions the most excruciating pains. He directs us, therefore, to put a ligature round the arm, and to tighten it every day so that the dracunculus may come forth by degrees without breaking. The part is to be washed with honied water, with oil in which wormwood or southernwood has been boiled, or with some such anthelminthic decoction; but all acrid things are to be avoided for fear of inflammation. He recommends us to forward suppuration by means of maturative cataplasms, and the other means mentioned by our author.

Pollux calls the dracunculus a piece of *corrupted nerve* which sometimes comes from the sores of Ethiopians, but seldom troubles other people.

Actuarius, like our author, mentions that the dracunculi occur most commonly in the region above Egypt, being generally formed in the muscular parts, and that in process of time the part becomes livid and suppurates. They are killed, he adds, by bitter and acrid things.

Avicenna comprehends in his account whatever information could be gleaned from preceding writers. He says the dracunculus is called *vena medine*, from Medine, the name of the country where it is most prevalent. It occasions a blister in the part which bursts, when a red and somewhat blackish substance protrudes and gradually increases in length. He directs us to correct the habit which gives rise to it by baths, humid food, and the like. His treatment is similar to that of Aëtius and our author, namely, binding a ligature round the arm, fastening a piece of lead to the worm, using fomentations of warm water, and the like.

Haly Abbas mentions the vena as being a worm which forms principally in the legs of the inhabitants of warm countries, such as India, Egypt, Ethiopia, and Lybia.

Avenzoar says that the complaint most commonly attacks negroes, being formed by gross humours, for dispelling which he recommends internally various sharp and acrid medicines, such as squills, nettles, colocynth, &c. He further directs a piece of lead to be bound firmly over the worm so that it may be made to crawl out gradually, which, however, he says, will not be accomplished in less time than a year.

Alsaharavius states the danger of breaking the worm (vena). He recommends the same treatment as Avicenna. The conclusion of his chapter on the dracunculus decides him to be the same person as Albucasis.

Albucasis recommends us to fasten to the end of the animal a piece of lead from one to two drs. in weight, and thereby to extract it gradually. He says that in some cases the animal is as long as fifteen palms, nay, that he had seen one twenty palms long.

Rhases says that the dracunculus takes place in hot and squalid bodies, and is formed by the use of potherbs and fruits. He recommends gradually increased doses of aloes, and when the animal protrudes it is to be wrapped round a leaden reed one dr. in weight, so that it may be dragged out gradually. He cautions us not to leave any part of it in the body. He also approves of incision as described by our author. In his 'Continens' he collects the opinions of Galen, Paulus, and others. He says that it forms most commonly in the bodies of persons who bathe frequently, and drink much wine. He says that he had seen it extracted by making free incisions.

See an interesting account of the guinea-worm in No. 66 of the 'Edinburgh Medical and Surgical Journal,' by Mr. Scott, surgeon, Madras.

Bertapalia, Guy of Cauliac, and all the early modern writers on medicine, repeat the ancient accounts of the vena civilis vel medine. They direct us to extract it by attaching a small piece of lead to its extremity. Ambrose Paré adopted Galen's notion, that it is corrupted animal matter; but Andry held that it is a real animal. It appears, however, from some statements which we have seen in the periodicals of the day, that some of our English surgeons in the East Indies still advocate the doctrine of Galen; but we are inclined to think that the other opinion is the more correct one.

BOOK V

SECT

I—ON THE PRESERVATIVES FROM VENOMOUS ANIMALS IN GENERAL

In giving an account of animals which emit poisons we shall begin with some general remarks upon them, treating of the preservatives from them in the first place. If therefore a person be compelled to sleep in places infested by venomous animals, especially in such as salamanders, phalangia, or reptiles abound, it will be proper to shut up their holes under ground with garlic pounded in water, or some of the herbs about to be mentioned; and to fumigate with hartshorn, the hoofs or hairs of goats, gagate stone, bitumen, bdellium, galbanum, the shavings of the cypress or cedar, gith, hog's fennel, the leaves of the chaste tree, calamint, sagapene, castor, the root of rosemary, fleabane, or some of the strong-scented things. Gnats in particular are driven away by fumigations with copperas, the seed of wild gith, and of cumin in equal proportions, and by cows' dung. In addition to these, frequent fires should be lighted, for reptiles commonly flee from the light. A couch should be prepared by strewing asphodel, calamint, chaste tree, pennyroyal, poley, fleabane, and southernwood; or if it is not possible to make a couch entirely of these, they should at least be laid around the bed. Attention should be paid to such things as are to be boiled, to the water, and wine vessels that they be properly covered up. Fires for the purpose of cooking should not be lighted under particular trees, more especially pitch trees or pines, for salamanders and deadly caterpillars abound on them, which being warmed by the heat of the fire fall upon the victuals, or any other vessels which happen to be uncovered. Those who wish to be particularly guarded, anoint their bodies with a liquid cerate composed of wax, rose-oil, and a little galbanum, and with a little of the shavings of hart's horn, or Ethiopian cumin. The leaves of mallows triturated with oil when rubbed on the skin protect in an especial manner from bees and wasps.

Commentary. The following is a list of the ancient authorities on Toxicology:

Nicander (Theriaca et Alexipharmaca); Dioscorides (Liber de Venenis); Celsus (v); Scribonius Largus (47, et seq.); Galen (Ther. ad Pison.; Meth. Med., De Antid.); Aëtius (xiii); Pliny (Hist. Nat. pluries); Oribasius (de Morb. Curat. iii); Solinus (Polyhist. 40); Serenus Samonicus; Nonnus; Simeon Seth (de Alimentis pluries); Actuarius (Meth. Med. v); Vegetius (de Mulo-medicina, iii, 77); Avicenna (iv, 6); Rhases (ad Mansor. viii, and Cont. xxxv); Haly Abbas (Pract. iv, Theor. viii); Alsaharavius (Pract. xxx); Serapion (pluries); Anonymi (Fragmentum apud Bernardi Reliq.) The work of Ælius Promotus on Venomous Animals and Poisonous substances, which exists in MS. in the Bibliotheca Vaticana, has never been published as far as we know. It is quoted by Hieronymus Mercurialis (Var. lect), and is noticed by Albertus Fabricius (Bibl. Græc. xiii, 780.) Fabricius supposes it to be the production of Æschrion Empiricus. It is proper to state that whenever we quote the work, it is from the extracts given in Schneider's Annotations on Nicander.

It is to be borne in mind that the work on Poisons, usually published as the production of Dioscorides, is not held to be genuine by his latest editor, Sprengel; still, however, it is acknowledged by all to be a work of considerable antiquity and of great authority on the subject of ancient Toxicology. The work 'Euporistôn,' which is also published with the works of Dioscorides, is generally admitted not to be genuine. It contains, however, some valuable matter on Toxicology and other medical subjects.

These directions of our author for driving away reptiles are mostly taken from Nicander, who recommends fumigations with hartshorn, gagate-stones, sulphur, bitumen, galbanum, juniper, and other such articles. (Ther. 35.) See also Dioscorides (M. M.); Orpheus (de Lapidibus); Geopon. (xiii, 8); and Nonnus (Epit. 261); also Aristot. (H. N. iv, 8); and Pliny (H. N. x, 90).

Virgil makes mention of this practice:

"Disce et odoratam stabulis accendere cedrum,

Galbaneoque agitare graves nidore chelydros."

Georg. iii, 314.

See a long list of substances used in fumigations for driving away serpents in Lucan. (Pharsal. ix, 916.) It is different from that of Nicander and our author. For example: it contains tamarix, costus, thapsos, &c. Arsenic occurs among the articles mentioned by Rhases. (Cont. xxxv.) It is also mentioned in the Geoponics (l. c.)

Nicander affirms, and it has been generally believed, that human saliva proves destructive to serpents. Galen says that it will kill the scorpion. Aristotle states, that it is destructive to most venomous reptiles. (H. A. viii, 28.) Redi maintains that this is an ancient error; but Andreas Laurentius declares that he knew from experience that the human saliva is destructive to serpents.

Nicander recommends a composition containing cedar-berries, fleabane, sage, and other such articles for preserving the body from venomous reptiles. Paxamus directs us to smear the face with a composition made of the roasted flour of fenugreek, with the juice of the wild mallows and oil. (Geopon. xv, 6.) He says it preserves the face from the stings of bees in particular.

The κώνωψ, here translated *gnat*, as it is in the English version of the scriptures, (Matt. xxiii, 24,) is proved by Bochart (Hierozoon. iii, 442); and by Harris (Nat. Hist. of the Bible), from Aristotle, Plutarch, and others, to mean properly a kind of insect that is bred in the lees of wine.

II—THE GENERAL TREATMENT OF ALL PERSONS BITTEN OR STUNG BY ANY VENOMOUS ANIMAL

If a person happen to be bitten or stung by any venomous animal he ought immediately to get the part sucked. The person who sucks it should not be fasting, and he ought first to rinse his mouth with wine and retain oil in it; and then, if the part admits, it should be cupped with much heat, scarifying also the surrounding parts; for the poison is forced back out of the body along with the spirits and blood which are drawn out. The part in which the wound is situated ought also to be burnt and eschars formed on it, and amputation of the extremities may then be seasonably practised if the animal that inflicted the bite be of a deadly nature, such as the asp, the cerastes, the viper, and the like: as Galen relates that a certain vine-dresser being bitten by a viper, and knowing the animal, immediately cut off the finger that was bitten with his pruning hook, and was entirely freed from the danger. But if the poison be already distributed over the body, venesection ought to be had recourse to immediately, especially if the person bitten be plethoric; and pepper and garlic given to eat with the food, and strong wine to drink, whereby the system will be filled with fresh vapours and a suitable heat. Afterwards cataplasms are to be applied that can warm and stimulate the bite, such as a mixture of the ashes of cabbage or of fig with vinegar, or with the strained lye, or with the sauce of pickle. Likewise onions may be mixed with polenta or bread, and strong leeks with salts, or warm liquid pitch with salts, or cedar-rosin, or goat's dung. It will also be proper to pour upon the parts hot vinegar in which calamint has been boiled, or with vinegar and sea water, or with brine. We are to apply to the part fowls, more especially hens, cut up and still warm, or other such animals, for they absorb the poison and soothe the pains. And we must have recourse to plasters, such as that formed from salts, that from rosemary and adarce, and on the whole such things as are of an acrid nature. And in general all persons bitten or stung by any venomous animal ought, unless the deep-seated parts are wholly unhurt, to take in the first place potions containing endive, heath, or astragalus with vinegar, or bitumen and Christ's thorn in like manner, or a decoction of Christ's thorn; or two drachms of dried weasel with wine, which is a cried-up remedy; or the blood of the sea-tortoise, or a drachm of castor with diluted wine, or a drachm of frankincense, or of Sicyonian root, or the juice of leeks, or ground pine, or alsander, or cinnamon, or birthwort, or the seed of the chaste tree, or cypress balls, or seseli, or pepper, or the seed of trefoil, or bay berries, or river crabs roasted or boiled. Use the following compound theriac.

A theriac for venomous animals, and deleterious substances, and for persons bitten by vipers and scorpions. Of bryony, of opoponax, of Illyrian iris, of the root of rosemary, of ginger, of each, dr. iv; of birthwort, dr. v; of frankincense, of wild rue, of each, dr. iij; of the flour of tares, dr. ij; form trochisks with wine, and give three oboli with wine. Purging will also be proper for them, with sudorifics, and taking the theriac of vipers.

Commentary. These general directions are mostly taken from Dioscorides, who is greatly indebted to Nicander. Neither of them, however, makes mention of venesection among his remedies.

The remedial means recommended by Dioscorides are scarification, cupping, sucking, excision; and in extreme cases, amputation; clysters, and acrid applications to the part in order to clear out the venom; pure wine, must, or acrid substances to extinguish it and counteract its effects; and finally as adjuvants of these means, purging of the bowels, sweating, and some other particular remedies as stated under their proper heads.

The general remedies mentioned by Nicander are, sucking the wound, applying cupping instruments to it, and afterwards strong stimulants, hot irons, and leeches. He directs that the person who sucks it should not be fasting; from which it may be inferred that he had a correct idea that the vessels absorb most readily when in an empty state. This physiological doctrine was lately announced as a new discovery; but frequent allusions to it are to be met with in the works of Galen, our author, Avicenna, Avenzoar, Averrhoes, and Haly Abbas. The dangers resulting from an empty state of the vessels, whether produced by fasting or venesection, is well expressed by Gorræus in his Preliminary Dissertation on the Alexipharmics of

Nicander: "Nec vero id tantum incommodi habet fames, sed in multo majus periculum adducit hominem, quando et venæ plurimum exinanitæ et cibum vehementer appetentes, venenum avidius ad se pertrahunt et in intima viscera, cordisque arcem immittunt." "Quod si quis etiam abundare videatur, et nihil eorum repugnet quæ sunt in venæsectione observanda, sanguinem audacter mittamus, non quidem per initia (sic enim in venas deleteria traherentur, a quibus omni studio atque industriâ excludi debent) sed post vomitus alvique dejectiones," &c.

Serapion, contrary to most of the authorities, recommends that the person who sucks a poisoned wound, should be in a fasting state; but as he is a servile copyist from his predecessors, it might be suspected that the text is in fault, if the same directions were not given by Rabbi Moyses, with this explanation: that a fasting person will perform this office with more risk to himself, but with greater advantage to the patient, than one who had taken food immediately beforehand. (De Venenis, i, 1.) All this shows how well the ancient savans were acquainted with the physiological fact, that the absorbent powers of the vessels is in the inverse ratio of their state of repletion.

Celsus recommends nearly the same general remedies as Nicander. Thus he directs us in the first place to apply a ligature round the limb, but not too tightly, for fear of occasioning torpor; and then to extract the poison by sucking, or by a cupping instrument along with scarifications. His local applications are of a hot stimulant nature. As internal remedies he recommends emetics, which may be supposed to expel the poison from the system by the concussion which they produce, and various articles of a calefacient nature, such as wine and pepper; because, says he, "maxima pars venenorum frigore interimit."

Isidorus states in still more general terms that the poisons act by oppressing the vital heat. He says, "Omne autem venenum frigidum est, et ideo anima quæ ignea est, fugit venenum frigidum." He states, likewise, that poisons do not act upon the system unless mixed with the blood: "Venenum autem dictum eo quod per venas vadit. Infusa enim pestis ejus per venas vegetatione aucta discurrit et animam extinguit. Unde non potest venenum nocere nisi hominis tetigerit sanguinem." Lucanus: "Noxia serpentum est admixto sanguine pestis."

This, however, is an imperfect account of the action of poisons, whether such as act by being introduced into the stomach, or those that prove deleterious when applied to a wound. Perhaps the classification given by Avicenna may be mentioned as the most complete of any proposed by the ancient authorities. He states that poisons act either by some certain quality, or by their whole substance. Of the former class some are corrosive and putrefactive, like the lepus marinus; some inflammatory and calefacient, like euphorbium; some frigorific and stupefying, like opium; some prove obstruent of the respiratory passages, like litharge; some act with their whole substance, as the wolf's bane, and these are the most deleterious of all. Of these some act upon one member in particular, as cantharides upon the bladder, or the lepus marinus upon the lungs, and some upon the whole body as opium. (iv, 6, 1.) Schulze, in his 'Toxicologia Veterum,' has stated the ancient arrangement somewhat differently, and we are at a loss to think what authors he has followed. He says, the ancients arranged poisons according to their properties into the frigorific (ψυκτικὰ), corrosive (διαβιβρώσκυντα), and septic (σηπεδονώδη). The frigorific, he properly remarks, are those substances now called narcotics; to which class, as Galen mentions, the conium, poppy, henbane, and mandrake belong. On the action of narcotics, see section xliii. Galen remarks that the human frame becomes habituated to bear the action of these medicines without injury. He mentions the case of an old Attic woman, who by little and little had accustomed herself to take hemlock in any quantity. (De Simpl. iii.)

Avicenna states that the great indications of cure in all cases of poisoning are to comfort and rouse the vital heat, and to resolve (neutralize?) or expel the poison. When the poison is distributed over the system, his remedies are venesection, purging, and the like. He states decidedly that the proper time for venesection is either when the poison is distributed over the body, more especially when it is in a plethoric state, or when the poison is a substance not likely to be absorbed. His other remedies are such as expel the poison from the body, namely, emetics and sudorifics, or such as prevent it from entering the system, namely, ligatures to the extremities, prohibiting sleep, applying cupping instruments, or leeches, sucking the wound, amputation of the limb, using actual and potential cauteries, and keeping the wound long open. Upon the whole the general remedies recommended by him and the other Arabians are little different from those of the Greeks, especially of Dioscorides, who is the great authority upon theriacs.

Haly Abbas allows bleeding when the poison is distributed over the body, and like the others also, makes mention of cupping with heat and of amputation. He also joins in the general praise of the theriac.

Alsaharavius recommends strong ligatures, cupping, and, in urgent cases, amputation. He also approves of applying the bodies of hens still warm. Serapion approves of bleeding under the same circumstances as the others, and of the same general treatment that they recommend. Rhases recommends sucking and cupping the wound, and the application of stimulant dressings, such as a plaster consisting of mustard, lime, and pitch. He, and most of the ancient authorities on toxicology, recommend salt as an application to the wound. Most of them also join Dioscorides in recommending the application of caustic leys. They also in general direct us to prevent sleep. The ligature to prevent absorption is recommended by Rhases, as it is in fact by most of the ancient authorities. As a matter of course all of them speak highly of the theriac, and acquiesce in Galen's celebrated eulogy upon its virtues. (Ad Pison. ii, 457, ed. Basil.)

The Arabian authorities notice cursorily the treatment of poisoned weapons of war, more especially of the Armenian arrows. Galbanum and assafœtida administered internally, and applied to the wounds in various forms, are the two articles which are most generally approved of by them. They also recommend sucking the wound, as in other cases of poisoning by a wound. (See further, B. vi, 88.)

III—ON PERSONS BITTEN BY MAD DOGS, AND ON HYDROPHOBIA

We have placed the account of persons bitten by mad dogs before all the others because these animals are numerous and domestic, and are frequently seized with madness; because the complaint is difficult to guard against, and the danger inevitable, unless one have recourse to many and suitable remedies. Dogs for the most part become mad during violent heat, but also, as Lycus says, sometimes in extreme cold. When mad they shun drink and food, for they are thirsty but do not drink, and for the most part they pant, hang their ears, and emit much frothy saliva. Generally they utter no sounds, and are as it were delirious, so that they do not recognize persons with whom they are familiar. Wherefore they attack equally without barking all animals, whether wild beasts or men, and bite them. Their bite at first occasions nothing disagreeable except the pain of the wound; but afterwards it brings on the affection called hydrophobia, which makes its attack with convulsions, redness of the whole body, but especially of the countenance, sweating, and anxiety; and those affected shun water when they see it, and some every fluid that is presented to them. Some bark like dogs and bite those who approach them, and so doing they occasion the same affection. The cause of the other symptoms is obvious, being occasioned by the poison affecting all the parts, but as to the dread of water some have said that it is occasioned by inordinate dryness, as if the whole fluids of the body had undergone a change. But Ruffus has pronounced it to be a species of melancholy which affects them, the poison putting on the nature of that humour in like manner as we know other melancholic persons dreading some one thing and some another; which reason accords also with those who say that they think they see the image of the dog that bit them in the water. Of persons falling into this affection we know none who has been saved, except that we have learned the histories of one or two cases, and these were of persons who had been bitten, not by a mad dog, but by some person who had been bitten and imparted the disease to them. But before the affection has made its attack many, even of those who have been bitten by a dog, have been saved. Wherefore we must begin the treatment from thence. And since often from the attack of hydrophobia having not yet come on (for most commonly it comes on about the fortieth day, and in some cases after six months, nay, instances are related of its coming on after seven years,) some supposing that the dog who inflicted the bite was not mad, and making haste to heal up the wound have thereby given rise to the complaint. By the following experiment you may ascertain whether the bite was inflicted by a mad dog or not: Pound walnuts carefully and apply them to the wound, and next day take and present them for food to a cock or hen. At first indeed he will not touch them, but if he is compelled by hunger to eat of them, observe, for if the dog that inflicted the bite was not mad, then the fowl will live, but if mad he will die next day; and then you must hasten to open the wound, and after a few days repeat the same experiment; and when the fowl does not die you may bring the wound to cicatrization, inasmuch as the patient is then freed from danger. Oribasius recommends this experiment: If from the symptoms which we have mentioned we know for certain that the dog is mad, we must have recourse to medicines for laying open the sore, the principal of which is that from pitch, very acrid vinegar, and opoponax, which is described accurately in the section on the wounds of nervous parts. But if the person who has been bitten has a tender skin, it is to be diluted with oil of iris, of balsam, or the like; or having first fomented the sores, apply a cataplasm of garlic. This also forms eschars. A dry escharotic for persons bitten by mad dogs: Of fossile salts, dr. viij; of chalcitis, dr. xvj; of squills, dr. xvj; of green rue, dr. iv; of scraped verdigris, dr. iv; of the seed of horehound, dr. j; use it at first dry that it may form an eschar, and then with rose-oil that the eschars may fall off. Keep the parts from cicatrizing for forty-two days at least. A cataplasm for persons bitten by mad dogs, which keeps the mouth of the wound open: Apply a cataplasm of onions with salts and rue, or of laserwort with salts, or of old pickle, or of the cinders of burnt wood with oil, or of garlic, or apply the leaves of the elder tree, or mint, or baum, each with salts, or walnuts with onions, salts and honey, or the ashes of figs mixed with cerate. Wash the sore with a decoction of camomile in water, and the root of the wild dock. But some burn the sore with heated irons. They ought in the first place to get draughts of simple things, such as buckthorn, wormwood, the juice of laserwort, germander, the water germander, and poley. These are compound applications: Of river crabs, of the shoots of the white vine burnt in a vessel of copper or bronze two spoonfuls, of gentian root triturated one spoonful, give to drink for forty days, with two cyathi of old undiluted wine. Some add two spoonfuls of the blood of the partridge. The crabs are to be taken when the moon is on the increase before sun-rising. But to those who do not drink it every day give a double doze, and sometimes a triple. And the theriac from vipers may be given with advantage. The patient is to be purged with the preparation from the wild cucumber, which is to be given every day with the decoction of sage, or with the Heraclean ironwort, which is also called alysson. Some also give the liver of the dog that inflicted the bite to eat. Such a diet is to be given as blunts and extinguishes the power of the poison, and at the same time prevents it from being carried deeper into the system. Both these ends may be accomplished by drinking old sweet wine that is both undiluted and strong, or milk, and in like manner by eating garlic, onions, and leeks. But if from some hinderance at the commencement the remedies which we have described have been neglected, scarification, cupping, or burning the wound, must not be had recourse to, because the poison has already been carried to the deep-seated parts; but we must use the remedies called metasyncritica, that is to say, when the attack of hydrophobia has not come on. Purging with hiera and divided milk is also to be had recourse to, with sudorifics; and calefacient plasters, and sinapisms are to be applied to every part of the body. But the most effectual of all remedies is a course of hellebore frequently repeated.

Commentary. Aristotle is the first author who mentions hydrophobia, but his account of it is remarkably incorrect, if the text be not corrupted. He says, all animals that are bitten by a rabid dog are affected with the disease *except man*; and that the disease proves fatal to all animals *but man*. (H. A. viii, 22.) But see the Annotations of Schneider. (l. c.) Ovid ranks inveterate gout and hydrophobia among the incurable diseases:

> "Tollere nodosam nescit medicina podagram,
>
> Nec formidatis auxiliatur aquis."

Ex Ponto, i, 3, 24.

Celsus, also, was well aware of the fatal nature of the disease, for which he says the only remedy is to plunge the patient unexpectedly into the cold bath, after which, to prevent convulsions, he is to be put into warm oil. He also approves of giving undiluted wine. As a preventive of the disease he directs the wound to be cauterized. (v, 27.)

Pliny in like manner reckons the disease dangerous, and mentions hellebore as a remedy for it. (H. N. viii, 63; xxix, 32.)

But without doubt the best account of hydrophobia contained in any ancient author is that given by Cælius Aurelianus. We shall now give a short abstract of it. He says the disease may be produced not only by the bite, but likewise by the breath of a rabid dog. This fact is mentioned by other authorities, such as Aretæus (Morb. Acut. vii), and Vegetius (Mulo. Med. iii, 84); and it is confirmed by modern writers, as Gokel, Lister, Rhazouz, and others. He also relates the case of a sempstress who fell into the disease from having sewed a robe which had been torn by a mad dog. Similar cases are related by Hildanus and Heister. He likewise states, what is confirmed by the Arabian authorities, and also by modern experience, that the disease may be brought on by the bite of wolves, bears, leopards, horses, and asses. He mentions the case of a person in whom it was occasioned by a wound inflicted with the spurs of a cock while fighting. Sometimes, too, he adds, it arises in the human subject without any manifest cause, which also is confirmed by modern experience. We once saw *the horror of water* in a case of Phrenitis. He mentions a singular case of hydrophobia in a child which was affected with a horror of its mother's breast. His description of the symptoms, if compared with modern descriptions (for example that given by Dr. Goden in Hufeland's 'Journal,' Jan. 1816), will be found in every respect complete and accurate. Thus Cælius says that the pulse is *densus, parvus, inordinatus,* and Goden found it intermittent and irregular. Cælius says there is a frequent desire of making water, which Goden found to be a constant attendant of the disease. Cælius thought that the stomach is more deranged than any other part, and Goden is of opinion that the splanchnic nerves are particularly affected. In short, Cælius maintained that it is an *incendium nervorum*; and it appears from him that some of the ancient authorities believed it an inflammatory affection, and treated it by bleeding. He treats it upon much the same principles as Tetanus, that is to say, his great object seems to have been to remove constriction, and with this view he recommends friction with tepid oil, venesection, and all remedies of a relaxant nature. He also directs us to administer clysters of tepid water and oil; and proposes to quench the thirst by forcing a cooling injection up to the stomach; for which purpose pressure with the hands is to be applied externally. He makes mention of the internal administration of hellebore, but disapproves of it. The use of white hellebore, however, is favorably mentioned by Aëtius (vi, 24), by Actuarius (Meth. Med. vi, 11), by Theomnestus (Geopon. xix, 3), by Dioscorides (ii, 3), by Alexander Trallian (i, 15), and by Avicenna (iv, 6, 9.)

Galen, in his work on 'Antidotes,' gives prescriptions for several compositions of this sort for the prevention and cure of hydrophobia; and mentions the disease incidentally in several parts of his works, but has nowhere given any description of it. Dioscorides' account of the symptoms, and his plan of treatment are nearly the same as our author's. He strongly recommends the cautery.

The external application of the cautery is also commended by Celsus, Galen, Pliny, Scribonius Largus, Aëtius, Actuarius, Nonnus, Avicenna, Rhases, and Alsaharavius.

See a good account of hydrophobia in Haly Abbas (Theor. viii, 20); and in Alsaharavius (Pract. xxx, 2, 30.) None of the ancient authorities insists with so much earnestness as Haly Abbas on the necessity of applying strong stimulants to the wound, namely, the most acrid vinegar, copperas, and the like, so as to keep up a discharge from it for a considerable time. Rhases is a strong advocate for bleeding when the poison is distributed over the system. (Cont. xxxv.)

Perhaps Alexander Aphrodisiensis is correct in stating that the disease in the dog is a species of fever. (Problem.)

There is a sensible account of hydrophobia in a 'Fragment' of an anonymous Greek author, published in Bernard's 'Reliquiæ.' The complaint is said to arise either from the bite of a dog, or from humours engendered in the body. It is correctly stated that persons affected with it dread all liquids, so that at the bare mention of them they start up with a scream, trembling, cold sweats, and chattering of the teeth. Among other things cold applications over the stomach and chest are recommended.

IV—FOR THE BITES OF DOGS THAT ARE NOT MAD

On the bites of dogs that are not rabid, as even in this case they possess some poisonous quality, immediately sprinkle some vinegar, and strike the bite with your hand spread out, and then having rubbed nitre with vinegar, pour it from above upon the part. Afterwards, having soaked a new piece of sponge in vinegar or in the vinegar and nitre, apply it for three days, and moisten it; for it will effect a complete cure. Or apply the flour of tares mixed with oil, or new sponge, or unwashed wool soaked in vinegar and oil may be applied; or triturate the leaves of bramble with vinegar, and apply; or onions triturated with honey, or equal parts of the hair of marjoram, of salt, and of onions with honey; or black horehound, which they also call ballotes, with salts. When the bites have already suppurated, apply the flour of tares mixed with honey, for it is particularly applicable. When they are inflamed anoint with litharge triturated with water.

Commentary. See Rhases (ad Mansor. viii, 9; Cont. xxxv); Haly Abbas (Pract. iv, 28); Alsaharavius (Pract. xxx, 2, 31). Haly adopts the treatment laid down by our author. Alsaharavius recommends a composition of fat, wax, pitch, and galbanum.

V—ON WASPS AND BEES

Those who have been stung by bees experience pain, redness, and swelling in the wound, the surrounding parts become tumefied, and the sting remains in the wound; and those stung by wasps experience all the other symptoms, and that in an aggravated degree, only the sting does not remain. Both cases are remedied by rubbing the parts with clay, or cow's dung, or with the juice of figs, or with the triturated leaves of sycamore, or of mallows; or by applying a cataplasm of barley flour mixed with vinegar. Foment also with brine or sea-water.

Commentary. See a similar plan of treatment recommended by Aëtius, Dioscorides, Nonnus, and Rhases. Simeon Seth recommends the decoction of mallows, which appears to have been a domestic remedy generally used in such cases. See also Geopon. (xii, 12); and Pliny (H. N. xx). Virgil alludes to this practice in a passage which has been often misunderstood. (Georg. iv, 230.) Haly Abbas recommends cold water or snow, also Armenian earth with vinegar, and other applications of the same nature. (Pract. iv, 34.) Alsaharavius mentions the same remedies as Haly, but expresses himself sceptical as to their efficacy. (Pract. xxx, 2, 29.) Rhases, among other applications, mentions a composition of camphor and vinegar; and another containing opium, henbane, and camphor, to be used along with a cloth moistened in snow-water. The Arabian writers on husbandry also recommend the composition from mallows and oil, as a preservative of the face and hands from the stings of bees and wasps. (Casiri, Bibl. Arab. Hisp. 335.)

VI—ON THE PHALANGIA, OR VENOMOUS SPIDERS

When a person has been bitten by a phalangion the part itself appears red, and as if pricked by a sharp-pointed instrument, but it does not swell, nor is it very warm, but it is moderately red, cold, and itchy. Those who have been stung experience a great sense of cold, trembling, heaviness of the body, a cold sweat, constant pain, paleness, and a perpetual desire to make water; in some cases there are dysuria, erection of the genital member, humid eyes, and spasmodic distension about the groins and thighs, a violent gnawing pain of the stomach, loss of taste in the tongue, vomiting of water, or of substances resembling webs, and sometimes these substances are discharged by the urine or bowels. By going into hot water they are freed from pain, but the pain returns again with violence. They are relieved by the application of the ashes of figs mixed with salts triturated in wine, or of the pounded root of the wild pomegranate, or of birthwort with barley flour mixed with vinegar. Bathe the ulcers with hot sea-water, or with the decoction of baum, the leaves of which may also be applied. Recourse must also be had frequently to baths, and potions composed of these things, the seed of southernwood, dill, birthwort, wild chick-peas, Ethiopian cumin, pounded cedar-berries, the bark of the plane tree, the seed of the herb trefoil, the fruit of tamarisk; give two drachms of each of these with one hemina of wine, or a decoction of the green parts of cypress, or of its balls mixed with wine. Some say that the river crab when reduced to juice, with milk, and the seed of parsley, and given, removes the mischief.

Commentary. Nicander describes several species of phalangia, whose bites occasion a variety of symptoms, such as a cold horror, tremblings of the limbs, and in some instances tension of the genital members. On the phalangia, see Aristotle (Hist. Anim. ix, 39); Xenophon (Memorab. i, 3); Pliny (H. N. xix, 9, and xxix, 27); Ælian (H. A. xvii, 11); Solinus (Polyhist. xvii); Phile. (66). The distinction between the phalangia and common spiders is thus stated by Humelbergius: "Araneorum primâ divisione duo genera sunt, unum eorum qui innoxii sunt quos Græci arachnas, Latini araneos dicunt, quorum etiam a Dioscoride duo genera recensentur, unum quod holcon et lycon vocat, alterum vero dicit esse quod candidas, tenues et densas telas operetur. Alterum genus est eorum qui noxii sunt, quos et Græci et Latini phalangia vocant." (Apud Apuleium.)

Similar modes of treatment to that of our author are recommended by Dioscorides (vi, 42); Celsus (v, 27); Nonnus (270); Aëtius (xiii, 16); Actuarius (Meth. Med. vi, 10); Haly Abbas (Theor. viii, 22); and Alsaharavius (Pract. xxx, 2, 26).

Sprengel allows that there is considerable difficulty in determining the nature of the ancient phalangia. He attempts, however, to refer the different species described by Nicander to their proper names in the Linnæan classification. (Comment. in Dioscoridem.)

Many modern authorities, for example, Gesner, Baglivi, and Andreas Laurentius, have held that the Tarantula, so famous in the annals of the Dancing Mania, was a species of the phalangium. See further Hecker's Epidem. 113. This seems to be confirmed by Rhases calling a species of the phalangium by the name of tarantula (Contin. xx and xxii); and, indeed, Ardyen seems to settle the question that the tarantula is a species of the phalangia. (De Venen. viii, 5.)

VII—ON THE BITE OF THE SPIDER

There is also a kind of spider, the sting of which occasions intense pains about the middle of the hypochondrium, difficulty of making water, erythema, and sometimes convulsions. Those who are stung by such animals, are relieved by the Theban wild cumin, the seed of the chaste-tree, and by draughts from the leaves of the white poplar, or by applying garlic alone, and taking full draughts of undiluted wine.

Commentary. For the sting of the spider, Celsus recommends garlic mixed with rue and pounded in oil. (vi, 27.) See also Pliny (H. N. xxix, 27); Haly Abbas (Pract. iv, 35); Alsaharavius (Pract. xxx, 2, 24).

VIII—ON THE STING OF THE SCORPION

When one has been stung by a scorpion, the part immediately begins to inflame, becoming hard, red, tense, and painful, being seized at one time with heat, and at another with cold; and when pain is an attendant symptom, it has remissions and exacerbations. These symptoms are followed by sweating, a sense of shivering, trembling, coldness of the extremities, tumour of the groins, and erection of the genital member: sometimes there is a discharge of flatus by the anus with a loud noise, and horripilation, and a painful discoloration on the skin, the pain resembling the prick of a needle. These are immediately relieved by having the juice of the fig poured into the wounds, and the scorpion which stung the person may be pounded and applied to the bite; afterwards salts triturated with linseed and the seed of marshmallows may be applied. Native sulphur, mixed with rosin or turpentine, is also of service; and in like manner, galbanum, spread out into the shape of an oblong pledget and applied, or calamint pounded and applied; and crude barley-flour prepared in wine and the decoction of rue; and in like manner the pounded seed of the herb trefoil may be applied with advantage. They may also take propomata containing two drachms of birthwort, more particularly of its bark with wine; or gentian pounded, or pennyroyal properly boiled, and ten bay-berries bruised, and calamint long boiled with oxycrate, and cyperus with wine; and in like manner, rue, the juice of the fig, and laserwort, if at hand; but otherwise we must use the Parthian juice. The fruit of trefoil and the seed of basil-royal may be taken in a draught with advantage. Silver immediately applied to the wound has a wonderful effect. The benefit of all these may be increased by the frequent use of the bath, copious perspirations, and drinking strong or diluted wine. The following compound propomata may be taken: Of sulphur vivum to the size of an Egyptian bean, with eight grains of pepper in half a hemina of wine, or the juice of laserwort triturated with crabs in wine, or equal parts of gith, Ethiopian cumin, and the seeds of the chaste-tree in wine.

For severe stings of scorpions and phalangia. Of the lees of wine, dr. xvi; of pellitory, dr. iv; of the seed of wild rue, dr. iij; of castor, of the seeds of rocket, of each, dr. ij; let them be mixed with the blood of the sea-tortoise. The dose is four oboli with wine, or three cyathi of unmixed vinegar.—*Another*: Of pellitory, of birthwort, of each, oz. iv; of pepper, dr. ij; of the juice of the laserwort, dr. j. The dose is the size of an Egyptian bean.

Commentary. Nicander describes several species of the scorpion. The white, he says, is innoxious. The red occasions a fiery heat with restlessness and great thirst. The black brings on inquietude, delirium, and laughter. The green occasions chilliness with horror. The symptoms superinduced by the other species are also detailed. (See Theriac. 775.) Ælius Promotus gives a very circumstantial description of the effects produced by the sting of the different species of scorpions, but it would appear to be mostly taken from Galen and other Greek authorities. On the nature of the scorpion, see further, Pliny (H. N. xi, 25); and Ælian (vi, 20.)

On the medical treatment, see in particular Dioscorides (vi, 44); Aëtius (xiii, 19); Nonnus (269); Actuarius (Meth. Med. vi, 10); Celsus (v, 27); Rhases (ad Mansor. viii, 3); Haly Abbas (Theor. viii, 22, and Pract. iv, 33); Alsaharavius (Pract. xxx, 2, 20); Avicenna (iv, vi, 5.)

Galen gives a variety of prescriptions for the composition of antidotes for the cure of persons stung by scorpions. The following one may be taken as a specimen of them: Of birthwort, dr. iv; of pepper, dr. ij; of opium, dr. j; of pellitory, dr. iv; form into trochisks of the size of an Egyptian bean, and give to swallow along with two cyathi of undiluted wine. (De Antidot. ii.) Rhases gives another receipt of Galen's for the sting of the scorpion, viz. equal parts of opium and of the seed of henbane given with honey. (Contin. xx, 24.)

On the use of venesection for the cure of the sting of the scorpion, Celsus says, "Cognovi tamen medicos qui ab scorpione ictis nihil aliud quam ex brachis sanguinem miserunt." Rhases has pointed out the proper time and circumstances which require venesection: "When you have administered the theriac, and the pain has subsided, if fever supervene, bleed the patient on the following day in the morning, and give him barley-water and diluent food." The symptoms as detailed by Haly Abbas are pain, swelling, hardness, and inflammation, which occasionally superinduce asphyxy and epilepsy. He directs a ligature to be put immediately around the member, and a bruised scorpion to be applied to the wound. He also mentions cataplasms with olive oil, and recommends the internal use of wine either alone or with garlic. The treatment as given by Alsaharavius is very similar. Dioscorides, Aëtius, Haly Abbas, Alsaharavius, Actuarius, and Nonnus, omit to mention venesection.

The veterinary surgeons recommend bleeding, scarifications, and burning with red-hot irons. See Vegetius (Mulom. iii, 77, and Geopon. xvi, 20.)

Sprengel remarks that Nicander's division of scorpions is adopted by modern naturalists. (Hist. de la Méd.) Conrad Gesner gives a very elaborate dissertation on them. The *scorpio Europæus, L.*, is not venomous. The African, however, is a very dangerous reptile. The inhabitants of Morocco, at the present day, treat its bite with the ligature, the cautery, and by applying the body of a dead scorpion to the wound. See Jackson's Morocco (108). The Arabian authorities describe a highly venomous species of scorpion, which they call *scorpius rastellans, carrareti,* and *algreta.* See in particular Rhases, Haly Abbas, and Alsaharavius.

IX—ON THE LAND AND SEA SCOLOPENDRA

When one is bitten by a scolopendra the general symptoms are lividity of the parts around the bite, and swelling; sometimes it is of a feculent appearance, and sometimes, though rarely, red; and a painful and ill-conditioned ulcer takes place, beginning with the part that is bitten; and in addition to these, there is a sensation of pruritus over the whole body. Those bitten by the sea scolopendra in particular have a watery and transparent swelling, whereas that occasioned by the land scolopendra is red. It is proper therefore to apply to the wound pounded salts, or levigated rue, or ashes mixed with vinegar, or squills. Bathe the part with vinegar and brine; but Archigenes directs it to be done with much hot oil, and thus to apply the things formerly mentioned; and to administer potions containing birthwort with wine, or wild thyme, or calamint, or wild rue, or trefoil, or the juice of the root of asphodel to the amount of half a hemina with wine.

Commentary. Nicander says, that the scolopendra has two heads, and walks in both directions upon its many feet. Avicenna admits that he was wholly unacquainted with it. See in particular Ælian (H. A. iv, 22; and vii, 35.) Our author and Actuarius copy almost every word from Dioscorides. See also Aëtius (xiii, 15); Nonnus (272); Alsaharavius (Pract. xxx, 2, 23); Avicenna (iv, vi, 3.) Avicenna calls them, *saculufudurni*; and Alsaharavius, *alhatrabay*. Alsaharavius approves of wine with birthwort, rue, mint, &c., internally; and of salt, with honey, vinegar, &c., externally. The Pseudo-Dioscorides recommends salt with vernix, pitch, and honey. (Euporist. ii, 121.) We need have no hesitation in deciding with Sprengel and the other authorities on this subject, that the land scolopendra is the *scolopendra morsitans*, and the sea, the *aphrodite oculeata, L.*

X—ON THE STELLIO OR SPOTTED LIZARD

Those bitten by the spotted lizard experience intense pain and lividity of the part, but are relieved by the immediate application of cataplasms consisting of onions and garlic to the wound; and some by eating these things and drinking undiluted wine have been cured.

Commentary. That the galeotes and ascalabotes are but different names for the same animal is evident from Aristophanes (Nubes, 170, et seq.); and from the Scholiast's note on Nicander (Ther. 484.) Pliny says of the stellio: "Hunc Græci coloten vocant et ascalaboten." (H. N. xxix, 28.) On the stellio, see further Bochart (Hieroz. ii, 510); Harris (Nat. Hist. of the Bible, in the word spider); and Dr. Martyn on Virgil (Georg. iv, 244.) All agree that it was a kind of lizard. In short it is the *lacerta stellio, L.* A learned modern authority says it is venomous in Greece, but innocuous in Sicily. He describes it as resembling the lizard in shape, and the chamæleon in nature. (Agricola de Anim. Subterran.)

Dioscorides does not treat of the stellio. Aëtius recommends very nearly the same treatment as our author. (xiii, 12.) Avicenna and Rhases direct us to get the wound sucked, to put the patient into a warm bath and administer the theriac. The harbæ of Avicenna is probably only a species of the stellio.

Alsahaya and alvesghe of Alsaharavius seem to have been two species of stellio. (Pract. xxx, 2, 27.) He approves of the same treatment as that recommended by Avicenna and Rhases.

XI—ON THE MUS ARANEUS OR SHREW-MOUSE

When persons are bitten by the shrew-mouse, throbbing pains supervene, erythema of every part pierced by a tooth, blisters along the skin filled with an ichorous fluid, and all the surrounding parts are livid; and if the skin be stripped off from the blister, the ulcer appears white, owing to the skin being torn into nervous membranes. In addition to these symptoms, the mortified parts drop off, the disease extending like a spreading ulcer; and besides tormina supervene, with dysuria and the discharge of a cold fluid. They are relieved by the application of galbanum in the form of an oblong pledget, by itself, or triturated with vinegar, or of barley-flour mixed up with oxymel. And the shrew-mouse itself which inflicted the bite may be torn in pieces and applied, and pellitory may be applied, or the boiled rind of the sweet pomegranate, or wild mallows, or pounded garlic, or mustard triturated with vinegar; and the parts may be bathed with warm brine, and then a cataplasm of burnt barley with vinegar may be applied. They may take propomata of southernwood boiled in wine, or sisymbrium, or wild thyme, or rocket, or galbanum, or sage, or the tender balls of cypress with oxymel, or pellitory with wine, or the root of chameleon, or the rennet of a kid or of a lamb, or gentian root, or vervain. These things may also be administered in the form of a cataplasm. But some give in a potion the shrew-mouse itself that inflicted the bite, having triturated it with wine. This one also is effectual: Of myrrh, dr. vj; of the bark of birthwort, dr. iv. To the bites of the shrew-mouse and of the scolopendra apply salts with liquid pitch, or cedar-rosin with honey, or garlic with the leaves of the fig-tree and cumin, or the leaves of calamint, or barley with vinegar.

Commentary. Nicander says that the bite of the blind Mus araneus is mortal. Our author's plan of treatment is taken from Dioscorides. Oribasius recommends garlic and cumin, mixed with oil. (De Morb. Curat. iii, 70.) Aëtius says that the Mus araneus is an animal resembling the weasel. His plan of treatment is similar to our author's. (xiii, 14.)

Isodorus says of it: "Mus araneus, cujus morsu aranea moritur, est in Sardiniâ animal perexiguum, araneæ formâ, quæ solifuga dicitur, eo quod diem fugiat." (Orig. xii, 3.)

Vegetius, the veterinary surgeon, recommends garlic pounded with nitre, or with salt and cumin. (Mulom. iii, 82.) See also Columella (vi, 17); and Ælian (H. A. ii, 37.)

Most of the Arabians treat of this case in the same terms as the Greeks.

Without doubt it is the *sorix araneus, L.* The accounts which the ancients give of its venomous qualities are said by Buffon and Sprengel to be exaggerated. Probably Agricola states the matter correctly when he says, that the mus araneus is venomous in warm climates, but innocent in cold. In size, he says, it is nearly equal to a small weasel. (De Anim. Subter.)

XII—ON VIPERS AND ECHIDNÆ

When persons have been bitten by the viper or echidna, or some such venomous animal, pain supervenes, at first of the part which has been bitten, but afterwards of the whole body. In the bite there appear two perforations at a little distance from one another, from which there is a discharge of blood and ichorous fluid, and afterwards of an oily one, but in all cases of a poisonous fluid, which they affirm to be the poison of the reptiles. Swelling comes on around the wound, which is reddish and livid; there is paleness of the whole body, vertigo, and resolution of the stomach, deliquium animi, and in some cases bilious vomitings and dysuria. Around the bite blisters arise, as from burning with fire, the disease spreads by extending to the surrounding parts, and the gums discharge blood. Trembling, heavy sleep, and a cold perspiration succeed these symptoms. Those bitten by the echidna appear to escape with less danger than those by the viper; and of these they run the least risk who have previously taken food. In treating them the most effectual remedy is eating garlic and drinking wine, so that if one can endure this course he will not stand in need of any other remedy.

And let them eat also leeks, onions, and acrid pickle. Some likewise give frogs prepared with sauce to eat. The following things are effectual, each of which may be taken with wine: the dried blood of the sea tortoise with wild cumin, the rennet of a hare or a hind to the amount of three oboli, a drachm of the dried testicle of a stag, a whole alkanet with the slender leaves, which also some apply as an amulet. In like manner the juice of leeks, to the amount of half a hemina, in honied water, the juice of baum leaves, wild rue, the brains of domestic fowls, the root of panacea boiled in wine, one drachm of agaric, juniper berries, the root of asphodel, pounded pistachia, the seed of the chaste tree, two drachms of dried weasel, the root and juice of vipers' bugloss, river and sea crabs alone or with stavesacre, salts and poley, the root of birthwort with equal parts of myrrh, gentian, and bay-berries mixed with honey. The following is an admirable remedy of Oribasius for persons bitten by vipers: Of anise, an acetabulum; of pepper, dr. iv; of the bark of birthwort, of opium, of castor, and of myrrh, of each, dr. j; triturate with must, and form to the size of a Grecian bean, and give according to the patient's strength in three cyathi of diluted wine.—*Another*, from the works of Lycus, a medicine for the bites of vipers: Of myrrh, of castor, of pepper, of purslain, of each, dr. j; of the seed of dill, an acetabulum; triturate in must, and give.—*Another*, from the works of Archigenes: Pound carefully twenty crabs with a sufficient quantity of wheaten flour in a mortar, and having mixed some calamint and salt with it, form trochisks of it, and dry. Use in a cataplasm with milk, and give one in a draught with honied water. But, says he, if you have not river-crabs, use sea-crabs. Goat's dung applied externally to the wound with wine is a powerful remedy; or bay-leaves boiled with oil, or bay-berries, or calamint, heath, rue, parsley, southernwood, galbanum on a pledget, green marjoram pounded; also young fowls torn in pieces, and applied warm and frequently changed, the flour of tares mixed with wine, the pounded bark of radish, boiled squills, raw barley-flour in oxymel, the leaves of the wild cucumber with fine polenta, the lees of wine in like manner with fine polenta, rue with salts and honey, bran boiled in vinegar, ashes with vinegar, cedar-pitch with salts, liquid pitch with salts. Bathe also with the decoction of trefoil, or of pennyroyal, or with vinegar and brine. When the blisters become bloody let out their contents without taking off the skin, then bathe with much water, and apply a cataplasm of boiled lentils with honey till the cure is completed. The antidote of vipers is particularly efficacious, both when taken in a draught and applied externally.

Commentary. Most of the ancient authorities appear to have considered the echidna the female viper; but, as will be seen below, there is reason to suppose that it was a different species altogether. It is the colubra of Celsus. (v, 27, 3.)

Our author's description of the symptoms is closely copied from Nicander, who also recommends similar treatment. Dioscorides in like manner directs us to give wine, and various articles of an acrid and calefacient nature, such as garlic, onions, pepper, squills, &c. Archigenes (ap. Aëtium, xiii, 21) affirms that eating garlic and drinking undiluted wine, constitute the most effectual part of the treatment. Of course these things were given upon general principles with the view of supporting the strength and vital heat. Hence it may be understood why the ancients reposed so much confidence in the theriac of Andromachus, most of the ingredients of which were stimulant, acrid, and calefacient substances. The body of the viper, which entered into this famous composition, is said by a modern authority on the Materia Medica, Moses Charras, to contain a certain volatile oil. (See Book VII, sec. ii, of this work.)

Avicenna delivers his plan of treatment at great length, enumerating many Arabic substances, the nature of which cannot now be easily determined. His general principles, however, seem to have been much the same as those of our author. He recommends in the first place the ligature, and cupping with scarifications. Wine and the theriac are to be given unless inflammatory symptoms come on, in which case the patient is to be bled. (iv, 6.) In another place he praises the juice of the citron as a remedy against the sting of the viper. Haly Abbas recommends immediate amputation of the part when this is practicable, and otherwise directs us to apply a ligature around it, to make scarifications, and use stimulant applications, such as onions, leeks, &c. Like most of the other authorities, he recommends the theriac, and wine, with other stimulants, such as pepper, birthwort, bay-berries, &c. In certain cases he also approves of bleeding. (Pract. iv, 32.) Alsaharavius recommends cupping, the ligature, and in short nearly the same plan of treatment as Haly. (Pract. xxx, 2, 18.)

Garlic was used in common cases as a substitute for the theriac, both internally and in cataplasms. (See, in particular, Geopon. xii, 30.)

On the viper, see Ælian (H. A. x, 9); Phile (70); Galen (Ther. ad Pison.) The ancient stories of the fatal copulation of the male viper with the female, and of the loves of the muræna and viper, are probably fabulous. (See De Pauw, apud Phile.) The latter story is told by Aristotle (H. A. v, 10); Ælian (i, 50); Oppian (Hal. i, 554); Pliny (ix, 23); Athenæus (vii); Achilles Tatius (i.) One of Athenæus's authorities, however, questions the truth of it. (Deipn. l. c.)

According to Sprengel, the Asiatic ἐχίδνα is the *coluber Ægyptius*; the ἔχις, probably the *C. ammodytes*; and the European ἐχίδνα, the *C. berus*. (Comment. in Dioscor.)

It is clear, however, from Nicander's description of the viper, that the term ἔχις was applied to a considerable variety of venomous snakes. It must not then be supposed to apply in all cases to the coluber ammodytes. It is also certain, as will be seen under their proper heads, that other serpents, to which specific names were given, such as the cerastes, the hæmorrhus, and the asp, were merely varieties of the *vipera*.

The seps is not treated of by the Greek authorities on Toxicology, except Nicander, but is briefly noticed by the Arabian under the name of *famusus*. Avicenna states that the treatment of the viper applies to it. (iv. 6, 3, 48.) From the description of it given by Nicander, it would appear to have been a variety of the hæmorrhus. (See Theriac, 320, with the Commentary of Eutecnius.)

XIII—ON THE AMPHISBÆNA AND SCYTALA

The same symptoms follow their bites, and the same remedies are applicable to them; therefore it is unnecessary to treat of them particularly.

Commentary. Nicander says that the amphisbæna is a small serpent with two heads, and small eyes. The scytala, he says, is like the amphisbæna, but thicker and larger towards the tail. Avicenna doubts whether the amphisbæna moves both ways. He says it is a serpent of equal thickness at both extremities, which probably gave rise to the supposition that it had two heads. He calls it a snake of the fragile nature, which description evidently points to the blind-worm. (See further, Matthiolus, Comment. in Dioscor.) We suppose the altahban and alhuidia of Alsaharavius are the amphisbæna and scytala. (Pract. xxx, 2, 19.) He recommends general treatment, namely, the ligature, cupping, scarifications, with cold water to drink.

Sprengel inclines to think that the scytala was the *anguis eryx*. He makes the amphisbæna to be the *anguis fragilis*, L.; he questions, however, the accuracy of the ancient accounts respecting its venomous qualities. (Notæ in Dioscor.) But, indeed, Aëtius states distinctly that these serpents are not venomous, and that their sting merely occasions inflammation like that of wasps and bees. (l. c.) Nicander also merely describes these serpents, and says nothing about their being venomous.

XIV—ON THE DRYINUS THE INTRODUCTION FROM GALEN

The dryinus, that lives at the roots of oaks, is so pernicious and destructive an animal, that if one tread on him he will excoriate one's foot, and great swelling will seize upon the whole limbs; and, what is more wonderful, they say that if one attempt to dress the wound, one's hands will be excoriated; and that if any person attempts in defence to kill the animal, he emits such a stench as overpowers all other smells. When one has been stung by the dryinus, tumefaction of the part takes place with redness, and blisters on the surrounding parts, along with a discharge of a watery ichor. These symptoms are followed by cardialgia and tormina. Birthwort given as a draught with wine is serviceable in these cases, and the herb trefoil, and the root of asphodel, taken in like manner, and the fruit of all kinds of oak triturated and taken in a draught. In like manner the roots of the ilex pounded and applied to the part are of use.

Commentary. Nicander says it is also called chelydros and hydros. He makes a distinction between the chelydros and the chersydros, but subsequent authorities confound them together. (See below.) He says it inhabits lakes and marshy grounds, feeding upon locusts and frogs. Its back is black, and its smell fetid. The symptoms occasioned by its sting are livid swelling, delirium, cutaneous pustules, dimness of vision, suppression of urine, coma, singultus, and vomiting of blood or bile.

Haly Abbas calls it adresa, and says that it emits a fetid smell, and brings on inflammatory redness with an aqueous discharge from the wound. (Theor. viii, 21.) Avicenna calls it *kedusu duras*. (iv, 6, 3.) Isidorus says, "Chelydros serpens qui et chersydros dicitur quia et in terris et in aquis moratur." (Origines.)

Virgil translates Nicander's account of this serpent into verses of inimitable spirit and elegance. It will be remarked by the curious reader that he mixes up together circumstances collected from Nicander's separate descriptions of the chelydros and dryinus. (Georg, iii, 425.) Though critical emendation of the text of ancient authors be foreign to the design of this work, we cannot omit the present opportunity of stating that, from a comparison of the descriptions given by the Greek and Latin poets, we are inclined to think that the 434th line of Virgil should run thus:

Sævit agris asperque siti atque exterritus œstro.

This is founded upon the 417th line of Nicander's Theriacs.

It seems to be the chersydros which Dante alludes to in the following verses:

"Come le rane innanzi alla nemica

Biscia per l'acqua si dileguan tutte,

Finch' alla terra ciascuna s' abbica."

Inferno, canto ix.

For an account of the hydrus, see the sixteenth section.

According to Sprengel, the dryinus is the *coluber lebetinus*. (Notæ in Dios.)

Agricola finds fault with Lucan for distinguishing the chersydros from the hydrus or natrix. He remarks that the boa is a species of hydrus. (De Anim. sub.) They are now generally held to be different. See, however, our commentary on the sixteenth section.

XV—ON THE HÆMORRHUS, PRESTER, OR DIPSAS

Those bitten by the hæmorrhus experience violent pains, and both longitudinal and lateral contractions of the porous parts of the body, occasioned by the persistence of the pains. From the bite there is a copious discharge of blood, and if there happen to be a sore on any part of the body it bursts out and discharges blood. The alvine evacuations likewise are bloody, and the blood which is evacuated is thrombous. When they cough they bring up blood from the lungs, and they die at last vomiting blood irremediably. Those bitten by the dipsas experience intolerable heat and intense thirst which is insatiable and unceasing, so that they swallow copious draughts, and yet they feel as if they had never drunk; and the whole system is affected, as in dropsy, owing to constant ingestion of drink. Hence the animal has been called prester, causon, and dipsas. By most of the ancients those bitten by the hæmorrhus and dipsas were given over as incurable. But if we have no particular remedies for this reptile we ought to make trial of the general applications, and immediately have recourse to scarifications and burning, and, if the part permit, to amputation of the extremities. Then acrid cataplasms may be applied. All kinds of acrid food are also useful, especially that from pickles, drinking undiluted wine, and using baths. These things are to be applied perseveringly, and repeated at short intervals, before the complaints make their attacks; for after they make their appearance no advantage can be derived from medical aid. We find these topical remedies described for their bites, namely, for those of the dipsas, the powdered leaves of purslain with vinegar, polenta, and bramble leaves powdered with honey, plantain, hyssop, white garlic, leeks, rue, and nettle; and for those of the hæmorrhus the same things, and, in addition, boiled vine leaves triturated with honey. By the mouth the burnt head of the animal itself may be taken in a draught, or garlic with oil of iris. They may likewise eat dried grapes.

Commentary. According to Nicander, the hæmorrhus is about a foot in length, of a black or fiery colour, with two horns on its head, and eyes like those of locusts. The symptoms brought on by its bite, as described by Nicander, appear to have been very similar to those of the disease called purpura hæmorrhagica, namely, a discharge of blood from the gums, nose, ears, bladder, bowels, or any open sore. Ælian gives exactly the same account of it. (H. A. xv, 13.)

It appears from Dioscorides that the dipsas was also sometimes called prester and causon. (vi.) See also Ælian (H. A. vi, 51.) Lucian and Isidorus, however, make a distinction between the dipsas and prester. Lucian says that it resembles the viper *de dipsadibus*. In fact the dipsas seems to have belonged to the viper kind. (See Bochart, Hieroz. ii, 367.) Galen states that he was informed by the Marsi, who made a living in Rome by dealing in serpents, that the dipsades were not a peculiar species of serpents, but a variety of the viper found on the sea-shores of Africa. (De Simpl. x.) Isidorus thus defines them: "*Hæmorrhois* aspis nuncupatur, eo quod sanguinem sudet qui ab eo morsus fuerit: ita ut dissolutis venis, quicquid vitæ est per sanguinem evocat." "*Dipsas* genus est aspidis quæ Latine *situla* quia quem memorderit siti perit." (Orig. xii, 4.) The effects produced upon the system by the sting of the dipsas seem to have been of a highly inflammatory nature. According to Nicander, it kindles a flame in the heart, the lips become parched, and the person is seized with an unquenchable thirst. These symptoms are strongly portrayed by Lucan:

"Ecce subit virus tacitum, carpitque medullas

Ignis edax, calidâque accendit viscera tabe.

Ebibit humorem circum vitalia fusum

Pestis, et in sicco linguam torrere palato

Cæpit....

Ille vel in Tanaim missus, Rhodanumque, Padumque,

Arderet, Nilumque bibens per rura vagantem.

Accessit morti Libye, *factique*[1] minorem

Famam Dipsas habet terris adjuta perastis."

Pharsal. ix, 754.

[1] Sic lege non *factiq*.

The Arabians give a similar description of its effects. Haly Abbas says, that it occasions great heat and burning. Dioscorides treats the wounds of the dipsas and hæmorrhus upon general principles, namely, by the external application of cauteries and cataplasms; and the internal administration of wine and acrid food. Actuarius, in like manner, recommends undiluted wine and acrid food, and also directs us to amputate the part, or apply acrid cataplasms according to the degree of danger. Most of the ancient authorities concur in recommending the theriac; for an account of the modus operandi of which in this case, see Alexander Aphrodisiensis (Prob. i, 152.)

We may mention that, after considering the descriptions given by Nicander, his commentator Eutecnius, Galen, Actuarius, and Avicenna, we are disposed to think that the text of our author at the beginning of this section must be corrupt; but we have not ventured to deviate from it, as we could not hit upon a conjectural emendation to satisfy us. None of the others mention contractions of the interstices or porous parts of the body, and all state that there is a discharge of blood from the pores of the skin. Now it is not probable that our author should have omitted a symptom so striking as this cutaneous hemorrhage, and substituted one which the others take no notice of.

Sprengel makes the dipsas to be the *coluber prester*, and the hæmorrhus the *C. cerastes*. That they were both vipers is quite obvious from the ancient descriptions of them, and more especially from the account of them given by Galen. (l. c.)

XVI—ON THE HYDRUS, OR WATER SERPENT

When a person has been bitten by a water serpent, the wound becomes broad, large, and pale, and a black, copious, and fetid discharge, as from a spreading ulcer, takes place, and the cure of the mischief is accomplished only after a length of time, and with difficulty. Wherefore powdered marjoram mixed with water is to be applied to their bites, or oak ashes mixed with oil, or barley-flour with melted honey is given to drink, and birthwort to the amount of two drachms in diluted wine, or two cyathi of oxycrate; and afterwards the juice of horehound, or its decoction with wine, or wild cresses, or the fruit of asphodel, or the flour or the seed of hog's fennel, with wine. A fresh honeycomb may also be eaten with vinegar.

Commentary. This section is taken almost word for word from Dioscorides. The chersydros, says Nicander, is like the asp, and its bite is followed by malignant symptoms. The skin about the wound becomes parched and putrid, along with heat and pains all over the body. Isidorus says of it: "Hydros aquatilis serpens a quo icti obturgescunt." (Orig. xii, 4.) See also Pliny. (H. N. xxix, 22.) Haly Abbas says, it occasions lividity of the part, from which a black fetid discharge takes place. (Theor. viii, 21.)

Bochart makes this to have been the serpent which so annoyed the children of Israel in the wilderness. (Hier. ii, 421.)

According to Sprengel, it is the *coluber natrix*. (Notæ in Dioscor.) Gesner and Dr. Milligan make it to have been the *coluber lutrix vel chersea*, L. It is now generally held not to be venomous. We have alluded in our commentary on the fourteenth section to the confusion of the hydrus with the dryinus. Schneider has a learned annotation on this subject in his 'Curæ posteriores' to Nicander's Theriacs, (l. 432.)

XVII—ON THE CENCHRINUS

When a person is bitten by the cenchrinus, the bite is like that of the echidna, mortification supervenes, and the flesh melts away, having been previously swelled as in dropsy, and he becomes lethargic and comatose. Erasistratus says that the liver, bladder, and colon are affected; for upon dissection these parts were found corrupted. Wherefore they are remedied by a cataplasm composed of the fruit of lettuce with linseed, and by pounded savory, and by wild rue, and by wild thyme triturated with asphodel; and two drachms of the root of centaury should be immediately given in a draught with three cyathi of nine, or the root of birthwort in like manner, and so also cresses and gentian.

Commentary. According to Nicander, the cenchrinus, called also the lion, has a body of varied size, and marked with punctated squamæ.

Dioscorides and Actuarius give exactly the same account of this serpent as our author. Haly Abbas in like manner describes it as occasioning mortification and putridity of the part. (Theor. viii, 21.) Isidorus says of it, "Cenchris serpens in flexuosis qui semper iter rectum efficit. De quo Lucanus: Et semper recto lapsurus limite cenchris."

Sprengel conjectures that it is a variety of the coluber berus, or viper, which is highly probable. According to Belon, it is three palms long, of the thickness of the little finger; of a cinereous colour, with black spots. Aëtius makes it to be the same as the acontias, which there can be no doubt was the same as the jaculus of Lucan. Yet Lucan treats of the jaculus and cenchris separately. (Phars. ix.)

XVIII—ON THE CERASTES AND ASP

According to Galen, there are three kinds of asps: that called the land asp, the chelidonian, and the third the ptyas, which is the most pernicious of all; for, stretching its neck, and measuring a convenient distance, with great sagacity, it disgorges the poison into the body. This is said to be the kind of asp which Queen Cleopatra, when Augustus, having vanquished Antony, wished to seize on her, took and applied to her left breast, and being bitten by it she died very quickly. When a person is bitten by the cerastes the part becomes tumefied, with hardness and blisters, and from the bite there flows an ichor which is sometimes black and sometimes pale, and like leeks; the whole system becomes of a dark pale colour, with erection of the privy member, and mental alienation; then dimness of sight comes on, and they die at last convulsed, as in tetanus. When a person is bitten by an asp, the bite resembles the prick of a needle, being very small in appearance, and without tumefaction, and it discharges blood not copiously but in small quantity, and of a black colour. Straightway dimness of the eyes seizes them, and various pains all over the body, which are altogether slight, and not without enjoyment, supervene; wherefore Nicander has properly said, "and without suffering dies the man." The colour is changed and becomes as green as grass, there is a gnawing pain at the orifice of the stomach, the forehead is constantly drawn upwards, the eyelids are moved insensibly as in sleep, and with these symptoms death cuts off the man before the third part of a day has passed over. In both these cases speedy amputation of the extremities averts the evil. Wherefore the bitten part is to be amputated without delay, if possible, or the flesh is to be cut off immediately down to the bone, in order that the poison may not pass through the parts which are bitten and the adjacent ones. Then what remains is to be seared by cauteries. For the poison of these, like that of the basilisk and bull's blood, quickly coagulates the blood and spirits in the arteries.

Commentary. According to Nicander, the most pestiferous asp is about an ell in length, its colour squalid, its eyes of a drowsy appearance, and when it bites a person it leaves a very small wound; neither swelling nor inflammation is perceived, "and the man without pain sinks into a profound sleep." This is the serpent which Cleopatra despatched herself with. See some curious remarks upon this event, and the nature of the serpent in Galen (Ther. ad Pison.), from which our author borrows his account of it.

Nicander says of the cerastes that it resembles the male viper, only that the latter has no horns, whereas the former has either two or four. Isidorus says of them, "*Aspis* vocata quod morsu venena immittat et aspergat: ἰὸς enim Græci venenum dicunt, et inde *aspis* quod morsu venenato interimat" (Orig. xii, iv); and of the cerastes, "*Cerastes* serpens dictus eo quod in capite cornua habeat similia arietum: sunt autem quadrigemina cornicula, quorum ostentatione, veluti escâ illiciens sollicitata animalia perimit." (Ibid.) Harris says, "The shephephon (Gen. xlix. 17) is probably the cerastes, a serpent of the viper kind." (Nat. Hist. of the Bible.) Bochart, however, has proved that the shephephon signifies both the cerastes and the hæmorrhus, which are very much alike, being both vipers. (Hier. ii, 416.) Sprengel, in fact, makes the hæmorrhus to be the same as the cerastes.

Our author's treatment is principally taken from Dioscorides. Aëtius, however, gives the fullest account of them. He says the sting of the most fatal species of asp proves fatal in three hours; and that those wounded by the cerastes generally live nine days. He represents the asp as occasioning great coldness, torpor, and at last convulsions. Besides the local remedies applicable in all such cases, he recommends in an especial manner vinegar, which is to be administered in great quantities. Celsus thus explains the way in which vinegar proves efficacious for counteracting the effect of a frigorific poison: "Credo quoniam id (acetum) quamvis refrigerandi vim habet, tamen habet etiam dissipandi. Quo fit ut terra respersa eo spumat. Eadem ergo vi verisimile est spissescentem quoque intus humorem hominis ab eo discuti, et sic dari sanitatem."

The author of the work 'Euporistôn,' usually published with those of Dioscorides, recommends, in the case of a person stung by the asp, constant shaking, beating, and movement of the whole body, with the affusion of hot salt water. (Euporist. ii, 120.)

Pliny says the poison of an asp proves immediately fatal when introduced into a fresh wound, more slowly when the sore is old, and that it is perfectly innoxious when swallowed by the mouth. (N. H. xxix, 18.)

The account which Avicenna gives of these serpents is mostly taken from Aëtius and our author.

Agricola describes the asp to be four feet long, and of the thickness of a spear. The cerastes, he says, in other respects resembles a viper, except that it has two or four substances on its head like horns.

Madden, a late traveller in the East, gives a different account of the horned serpent (coluber cerastes); he says that of two which he purchased from the Psylli one was a foot long, and the other a foot and a half. A lancet smeared with the venom of one of them killed a dog in three hours. The French naturalists who attended the expedition to Egypt found a viper, called *hage* by the inhabitants, which they held to be identical with the asp of the ancients. We need have no hesitation then in deciding that the coluber Ægyptiacus is the celebrated asp of antiquity. That the cerastes was a variety of the asp seems highly probable from the description which Nicander gives of both. (Theriac 177 and 259.) See also Wilkinson's 'Thebes,' p. 378. In fine, the asp and cerastes were merely varieties of the common viper of Egypt.

XIX—ON THE BASILISK

This reptile seldom comes under the sight of men; but Erasistratus says, when the basilisk bites one the wound becomes of a faint golden colour, and he also says that three drachms of castor taken in a draught proves a remedy in such cases, and in like manner the juice of poppy; but we have had no trial of these things.

Commentary. The basilisk, according to Nicander, has a sharp body about three palms in length, of a bright yellow colour, and is called the king of reptiles, because all the others flee from his hiss. Pliny, Solinus, and most of the ancient authorities seem to copy Nicander's description of the basilisk. The symptoms produced by his sting are said to be inflammation of the whole body, lividity and putrefaction of the flesh. (Theriac. l. c.) See also Galen (Ther. ad Pison.)

Avicenna states that the basilisk stupefies birds and other animals which approach him. He relates the case of a soldier who transfixed a basilisk with his spear, and the poison proved fatal both to him and his horse, whose lip was accidentally wounded with the spear. Lucan relates the case of a soldier in the army of Cato, who having wounded a basilisk with a spear, and having felt his hand affected with the poison, saved his life by immediately cutting it off with his sword. (Phars. ix, 830.) Similar histories are given by Pliny, Dioscorides, Actuarius, and Isidorus. Solinus affirms that it proves fatal to all beasts, birds, and vegetables.

For an explanation of the passages of scripture wherein mention is made of the basilisk, see Bochart (Hier. ii, 339.)

Sprengel says: "Linnæus omnem fabulam (de Basilisco) ad Lacertæ genus, capite cristato, *Iguanæ* proximum, reduxit." (Comment. in Dioscor.) M. l'Abbé Bonneterre also affirms that the basilisk is not poisonous. (Encyc. Méthod.) It may be doubted, however, if we be now acquainted with the basilisk of the ancients. It would appear to us almost certain that the ancient basilisk must have been either the *cobra di capello*, or one of the serpents described by an intelligent traveller under the names of *buskah* and *el effah* as being still found in Morocco. (Jackson's Account of Morocco, 109.) The former of these, indeed, judging of it from the drawing which he gives must be a variety of the *cobra* or *coluber naja*, L. We may add that a very intelligent modern authority on the toxicology of the ancients, Ardoyn, gives such a description of the basilisk as applies very well to the *cobra*. The crown (corona) on the head can refer to no other serpent than the hooded snake. (De venenis, vi.) It is now well ascertained that the *cobra* is indigenous in Africa.

XX—ON THE SEA PASTINACA AND MURÆNA

In the case of sea animals, such as the fire-flaire and murene, the diagnosis is obvious, for these fishes are well known. Those who are bitten by them are remedied by four drops of the juice of figs, or a little more, with three or four small branches of wild thyme in a draught, and those things used for echidna.

Commentary. Nicander says that the sting of the pastinaca occasions putridity in the flesh of a man who is wounded by it, and that it proves fatal to a tree in like manner. The same thing is asserted by Aëtius, Oppian, Phile, and Ælian. Our author and Actuarius copy from Dioscorides.

Avicenna recommends an embrocation of hot vinegar, and ointments composed of bay-leaves, oil of pellitory, and so forth; and in like manner recommends various calefacient medicines internally.

The murene of the ancients was that elegant species of eel to which the scientific name of *muræna helena* is now applied. It is rarely found on the British coasts but is common in the Mediterranean. The pastinaca marina of the ancients, was the *raia pastinaca*, L., i. q., *trygon pastinaca*, Cuvier, namely, the sting-ray or fire-flaire. Sprengel affirms that its sting is not venomous, as the ancients represent; but there can be no doubt that it is capable of producing inflammation. See Yarrel (British Fishes, ii, 588.) We may mention in this place that the account of the copulation between the viper and the murene which is given by Nicander, Oppian and other ancient authors, is held to be fabulous by Andreas, the physician, as quoted by the scholiast on Nicander. (Ad Theriac, 822.)

XXI—ON THE SEA-DRAGON

Rub the wound inflicted by the sea-dragon with lead, or apply a cataplasm of pounded wild thyme, or of boiled lentil, or of sulphur with vinegar, or the dragon itself may be torn in pieces and applied. Wash the part with human urine, and give potions of wormwood with diluted wine, or of sage, or of fig branches steeped in sweet wine, or of the brains of the fish itself. Commentary. A great variety of remedies for the wound of the sea-dragon are described by Nicander. For an account of the draco, see Dioscorides (vi, 45); Aristotle (H. A. viii, 13); Ælian (H. A. xiv, 12); Nonnus (276); Pliny (H. N. xxix, 20); Aëtius (xiii, 39); Phile (80); Avicenna (iv, 6, 3.)

We need have no hesitation in referring the sea-dragon of the ancients to the *trachinus draco*, L., Angl., the great weever or sting-ball. This is agreed upon by all the best commentators, as Rondelet, Artedi, Coray, and Sprengel. Fishermen are still very apprehensive of its sting. See Yarrel (Brit. Fishes, i, 25.)

XXII—ON THE SEA-SCORPION

The wound of the sea-scorpion is cured by a surmullet torn in pieces and applied, by sulphur vivum rubbed with vinegar, or by three bay-berries pounded and drunk.

Commentary. See Dioscor. (vi, 45); Nonnus (277); Aëtius (xiii, 40); Athenæus (353, ed. Casaubon.); Avicenna (iv, 6, 3, 23.)

Bochart says of the sea scorpion: "Is cum terrestri nihil habet commune præter venenatos aculeos, non in caudâ sed in capite et toto corpore sparsos." (Hierob. ii, 635.)

According to Sprengel, it is either the *scorpæna scrofa* or the *cottus scorpius* Bloch. (Comment. in Dios.) It is a fish still very much dreaded on account of its sharp spines. See Yarrel (Br. Fishes, i, 76.)

XXIII—THE PREPARATION OF THE BLOOD OF THE SEA-TORTOISE

The blood of the sea-tortoise is to be prepared for keeping in this way. Having stretched the tortoise with its belly upwards on a wooden or earthen vessel, cut off its head quickly, and when its blood is coagulated, divide it into many parts with a reed, put a sieve upon the vessel in place of a lid and lay it up in the sun. When dried take it and use for bites of vipers, as aforesaid; two drachms with one cyathus of vinegar, on the second day four drachms with two cyathi of vinegar, and on the third eight drachms with three cyathi of vinegar.

Commentary. This section is copied from Aëtius (xiii, 24.) In our translation we have followed the text of Aëtius, that of our author being manifestly corrupt.

XXIV—ON PERSONS BITTEN BY CROCODILES

For the bites of the crocodile apply levigated natron until the ulcer be cleansed, then fill it with honey, butter, stag's marrow, or the fat of geese. But Galen says, that he has known persons bitten by crocodiles manifestly relieved by the application of the fat of the crocodiles themselves to the wounds.

Commentary. This case is more fully treated of by Aëtius (xiii, 6.) His remedies are mostly of an acrid stimulant nature such as misy, pickle, salts, myrrh, verdigris, &c. The application recommended by our author upon the authority of Galen is ascribed by Aëtius to Apollonius.

XXV—ON PERSONS BITTEN BY A MAN

It will not be foreign to my subject along with venomous animals also to treat of persons bitten by men, since the bites inflicted by men are much more malignant than other ulcers, more especially if the person who bit happens to be fasting, or had previously eaten some pulse, particularly dried lentil. Wherefore, the general remedies for poisonous animals may be applied externally to the bite with advantage at the commencement, with the exception of such as are very acrid and caustic; in particular having first rubbed the bite with oil, apply a cataplasm of the roots of hog's fennel with honey, or apply the flour of beans with oxycrate, and vinegar and rose oil, sponging it frequently. And use the following plaster: Of squama æris, of galbanum, of verdigris, of each, oz. j; of wax, lb. j; of molybdæna, lb. ij; of oil, one sextarius. The molybdæna being first boiled in the oil receives the verdigris and squama æris, and when it thickens it receives the soluble substances. When the inflammation subsides treat it as a common ulcer.

Commentary. Similar treatment is recommended by Aëtius (xiii, 1); Apuleius (9, 2); Serenus (45); Pliny (H. N. xxviii, 4); Oribasius (de Morb. Curat. iii, 71); Avicenna (iv, 6, 4); and Haly Abbas (Pract. iv, 28.)

It may be proper to mention in this place that instances have not been wanting in modern times to confirm the accounts given by ancient authorities, of fatal effects being occasioned by the bite of a man. See Hildanus (Chirurg. i); Forestus (xxx, 12); Hoffman (Diss. de saliv. et op. morb. 5); Zacutus Lusitanus (Prax. adm. iii, 84, 89.)

XXVI—ON POISONS

Having given a compendious account of venomous animals, we shall next treat of deleterious substances, giving an exposition of the simple ones, and detailing the symptoms of them with their general and particular remedies. As to the compound ones we leave them to be treated of by any person who chooses; for some have described the compositions of certain deadly medicines which are more likely to prove injurious than beneficial to the reader. For neither are the exact symptoms which occurred in those who took them described, by which a suitable remedy might be found out; for the symptoms varying according to the nature of the prevailing ingredient, one might, from conjecture, vary the remedies accordingly. Wherefore here again we must begin with the prophylactics.

Commentary. We now enter upon the consideration of the second and most important division of toxicology; namely, alexipharmics, which treats of poisonous substances taken inwardly. All the writers on theriacs treat also of alexipharmics, and of these the most ancient, and one of the most interesting, is the Colophonian poet Nicander. Of the subsequent authors, Dioscorides and Aëtius among the Greeks, and Avicenna and Alsaharavius among the Arabians, are most particularly deserving of notice.

XXVII—ON THE PRESERVATIVES FROM POISONS

Of the doctrine of poisonous substances, the most difficult part is the prophylactic; because those who administer poisons in a concealed manner, prepare them so as to deceive the most skilful. Thus they take away the bitterness of deleterious substances by mixing them with sweet things, and the fetid smell by a mixture with aromatics. Sometimes in diseases, while appearing to administer such things as wormwood, southernwood, opoponax, and castor, for a beneficial purpose, they mix poisons with them; or they give them in the food, namely, in the harder and more complex articles, mixing the poisons with them. Wherefore a person who entertains suspicions, ought to avoid all prepared dishes and every intense quality, such as sweetness, saltness, and acidity; and in particular to take plenty of water, for when the appetite is satiated, the particular qualities are afterwards easily detected. There is likewise another efficacious mode of prophylaxis: for they who suspect anything of this kind should take such things as will blunt and take away the effect of the poisons, as dried grapes with walnuts, rue, a lump of salt, and citrons. Let them also take rape-seed to the amount of a drachm in wine, or the leaves of calamint, or Lemnian earth, and twenty leaves of rue, and they will not be hurt by any poison. And certain antidotes taken with wine every day to the amount of an Egyptian bean will protect completely, such as the one from skink, that from blood, and the Mithridate, which king Mithridates took every day as a preservative from deadly poison; and being captured by the Romans, he drank twice of a deadly poison, and not being able to despatch himself thereby, he killed himself with his sword. And since people are sometimes exposed to deleterious things accidentally in desert places without design, if they happen to take up their abode under certain trees, such as pines or firs, they ought to be on their guard against deadly animals, which fall from them and the roofs of houses, and keep the vessels in which their wine is contained, and in which they boil victuals, well covered up, as has been stated when treating of the preservatives from venomous animals.

Commentary. Nearly the whole contents of this section are taken from Dioscorides. (Præf.)

The account of the treatment given by Aëtius is somewhat fuller than our author's, but not materially different.

Avicenna makes mention of the same medicines as Dioscorides, and says nothing of any other remedies.

Of the substances mentioned by our author, and the others as preservatives from poisons, some are demulcents, and may be supposed to act by obtunding the acrimony of poisons, such as figs, walnuts, and rape-seed; some are simple absorbents, such as Lemnian earth, which probably resembled red ochre, and was also emetic: some are stimulants, such as rue, calamint, and wine; and some are refrigerant acids, such as citrons, which may be supposed to act as analeptics and restoratives. Virgil mentions this property of the citron:

> "Media fert tristes succos tardumque saporem
>
> Felicis mali: quo non præsentius ullum,
>
> Pocula si quando sævæ infecere novercæ
>
> Miscueruntque herbas, et non innoxia verba,
>
> Auxilium venit, ac membris agit atra venena."

Georg. ii.

See in particular Simeon Seth (in voce Κιτρὰ); and Athen. (Deip. ii.) Dr. Paris states that when a narcotic poison has been ejected from the stomach, citrons or any fruit containing a vegetable acid will produce the best effects. (See Pharmacologia i, 254.)

XXVIII—THE GENERAL TREATMENT OF THOSE WHO HAVE TAKEN ANY SORT OF DELETERIOUS SUBSTANCE

If any persons have already taken some deadly poison with the intention of despatching themselves, such as often happens in life, or from the wicked design of others, if it be obvious to us what substance has been taken, we can straightway apply the suitable remedy, as will be described in the account of them. But if the medicine is unknown to us, we must have recourse immediately to such things as are generally applicable to those who have taken any poison whatever; for to wait until the consequent symptoms have come on, is to render the case hopeless, since owing to the remedies being too long of being applied such symptoms can hardly be removed: wherefore, without delay, we must give warm oil by itself or with water, and force them to vomit, or if oil is not at hand, butter with hot water may be given, or a decoction of mallows, or of linseed, or of spelt, or of fenugreek, or of nettle seed. For these things will not only evacuate by vomiting, but will loosen the belly and counteract the bad effects of the poisons, by blunting their acrimony; and more especially oil will do this, as you may ascertain clearly from the following consideration. For if you wish to produce ulceration of the skin by means of cantharides, quicklime, or some such acrid substance, and the body has been previously rubbed with oil, no ulcers will take place, and neither also can you astringe the body if previously rubbed with oil. Besides, vomiting is not only useful by evacuating the offending matter, but by showing the poison which had been taken from its smell, particles, or colour. For by its smell and bitterness poppy-juice is known; by their colour, ceruse and gypsum; by their coagula, milk and fresh blood; by their heavy smell and quality, the sea-hare and toad: so that by these means we are enabled to have recourse to the remedies which are suitable to each. With the oil may be mixed the decoction of mallows, or the grease of geese, or broth prepared from fat flesh or fowls, or the cinders of wood. Natron also triturated with hydromel, much old wine, and those things which are prepared from fat or butter are efficacious. Having evacuated the contents of the stomach by emetics, we must bring away whatever had passed into the intestines by a stimulant clyster. After these things, we are to give milk to drink, for whatever is noxious and deleterious will be readily changed by it. We must also give those medicines which are generally applicable to all such cases, among which are the Lemnian vermilion, southernwood, agaric, hedge-mustard, the root of eryngo, the seed of parsnip or of calamint, the Celtic nard, castor, the inner part of green fennel-giant, the flowers of nerium (called also rhododendron and rhododaphon), the juice of leeks, laserwort or the juice thereof, sagapene, opoponax, the juice and root of hog's fennel, the long birthwort, the seed of wild rue, the leaves of that species of cestrum, called betony; of each of these a drachm may be taken in wine. The decoction of poley and liquid pitch in a linctus is also efficacious, and the aforesaid antidotes are excellent remedies, especially the theriac from vipers. But they have not the same power when taken after as before the poisonous substances, for a dose which would have been sufficient, if administered beforehand, to prevent any bad consequences, must be given in a fourfold or fivefold quantity, in order to prove effectual when administered afterwards, and that too not once, but twice a day. For such is the opinion of the celebrated Galen.

Commentary. Except the last two sentences the whole of this section is copied from Dioscorides. Celsus' directions, so far as they go, are excellent: "Commodissimum est tamen, ubi primum sensit aliquis, protinus oleo multo epoto vomere: deinde, ubi præcordia exhausit, bibere antidotum; si id non est, vel merum vinum." The directions given by Aëtius are to the same purpose as our author's, but somewhat fuller. He is particularly to be commended for the precision with which he lays down the rules of treatment, when any organ happens to be affected in an especial manner. Thus, if the poison attack the bladder, he directs us to put the patient into a hip-bath of oil or water, in which fenugreek, linseed, mallows, or some such emollient herbs have been, boiled and to give him to drink the decoction of some vegetable diuretic, such as parsley, fennel, or spikenard. If the bladder be corroded he directs us to give the seed of cucumber in diluted sweet wine. In the same manner when the intestines are corroded the same seed is to be given, and all heating articles are to be abstained from. When the poison is determined to the skin, he recommends the hip-bath of oil or water, friction with warm oil, and the like, evidently with the intention of evacuating it from the pores of the skin. Food of easy digestion, soups with honey, tender fishes, and the like are to be given. When the head is particularly affected he directs us to evacuate the bowels with a clyster of linseed, marshmallows, and a decoction of the root of the wild cucumber, after which sternutatories and odoriferous things are to be applied to the nose. Like our author, he strongly commends Lemnian earth with wine as an excellent and speedy emetic. This remedy is also mentioned by Avicenna. Galen assures us that he found it an excellent emetic in various cases of poisoning. (Simpl. ix.) It consists principally of silica, alumina, and oxyde of iron.

Avicenna directs us to give immediately as an emetic, oil of sesame or olive oil, impregnated if possible with the virtues of dill, and afterwards to use demulcents, such as the decoction of linseed, melted butter and milk. These emetics are to be followed by clysters, provided the mischief has spread downwards. If the disorder continue, another emetic is to be given, and draughts of milk repeated. When, after the emetic, inflammation supervenes, he directs us to give snow-water, or oil of roses, and to promote vomiting with them. When the poison is ascertained to be of an inflammatory nature the parts affected are to be cooled with camphor, rose-water, or that of coriander; or these things are to be congealed in snow and applied over the vital organs. If the poison is ascertained to be of a sharp penetrating nature, medicines are to be given to blunt its acrimony, such as milk, almond oil, melted butter, &c. Bloodletting, if indicated, is to be performed. When the poison is known to be of a stupefying nature, garlic is to be given, or the theriac and assafœtida in undiluted wine. When it is particularly deleterious, the cure is to be effected by means of the mithridate, theriac, musk, and other aromatics. He inculcates the necessity of preventing sleep and of rousing by every possible means. The patient is to be covered with aromatic cloths, the pit of his stomach is to be rubbed, his face is to be fanned, his hair pulled, and in short, everything is to be done to prevent him from sinking into a state of stupor.

Haly Abbas recommends the same plan of treatment. When the poison is discharged he recommends citrons, plums, and the like, as restoratives. Rhases gives the following directions: First, he says, produce vomiting with oil and water; then give food of a nauseating nature to continue this operation; if the bowels are inflamed give snow-water and rose-oil, and afterwards provoke vomiting once more: administer the theriac, rub the hands and feet, and when the poison appears to have descended to the intestines give clysters. (Contin. l. c.) Rhases and other of the Arabian authorities recommend the bezoar stone as an antidote for poisons.

XXIX—A CATALOGUE OF SIMPLE DELETERIOUS SUBSTANCES

Of deleterious substances, the following animals are destructive: cantharis, buprestis, salamander, pine-caterpillar, the sea-hare, the toad, the mute marsh frog, and leeches when swallowed; and, of seeds, the henbane, coriander, fleawort, hemlock, and gith; of juices, meconium, opocarpasum, thapsia, elaterium, and mandragora; of roots, chamæleon, wolfsbane, thapsia, ixia, hellebore, black agaric, ephemeron, which some call colchicum, because it grows in Colchis; of trees and potherbs, smilax, which some call thymium, but the Romans called taxus, the strychnus furiosa, which is called dorycnium, the Sardoan herb, which is a species of ranunculus, horned poppy, pharicum, toxicum, wild rue, and mushrooms; of animal productions, fresh bull's blood, coagulated milk, Heraclean honey; of metals, gypsum, ceruse, lime, arsenic, sandarach, litharge, adarce, lead, and that which is called mercury; and of domestic articles, much wine taken at a draught after the bath, or must, or cold water in like manner.

Commentary. Nicander, in his Alexipharmics, treats of the following deleterious substances:—1, Aconitum, or wolfsbane; 2, Argenti spuma, or litharge; 3, Buprestis; 4, Cantharides; 5, Ceruse, or whitelead; 6, Conium, or hemlock; 7, Coriander; 8, Dorycnium (see below); 9, Ephemeron, or meadow saffron; 10, Fungi, or poisonous mushrooms; 11, Hirudines, or leeches; 12, Hyoscyamus, or henbane; 13, Ixias, probably a species of chamæleon; 14, Coagulated milk; 15, The sea-hare; 16, Papaver, or poppy; 17, Pharicum, probably a composition from agaric (see Schneider's note); 18, the red toad and marsh frog; 19, the salamander; 20, Bulls' blood; 21, Taxus, or the yew-tree; 22, Toxicum, not ascertained. See Avicenna.

The lists of poisonous substances treated of by Dioscorides, Aëtius, and Actuarius are nearly the same as our author's. Those of Nonnus and Scribonius Largus are less numerous. The Arabians treat of several substances, the nature of which it is now difficult to determine. The catalogues of Avicenna and Rhases are the fullest; those of Haly Abbas and Alsaharavius scarcely contain so many articles; all of them, however, contain several substances which are not treated of by the Greek writers on toxicology. Among these we may just mention that they treat of the gall of the viper, of the leopard, of an animal called leunza (leæna?), of the shark, and also of the extremity of the stag's tail, and bad castor. The sweat of different animals is also included in their lists.

XXX—ON CANTHARIDES

The most grievous symptoms follow the administration of cantharides, for almost from the mouth to the bladder the parts are tormented with a gnawing pain. The taste resembles pitch or cedar rosin, and the patients have inflammation of the right hypochondrium, with dysuria, and frequently they pass blood by urine, and sometimes it is discharged by the intestines, as in dysentery: they fall into deliquium animi, nausea, and vertigo, and at last they become delirious. The proper remedies are vomiting with water and oil, drinking milk, taking four drachms of Cimolian earth with honied water, pine kernels, the seeds of cucumber, fat beef soup, or soup of geese or of mutton; the flesh of fowls, lambs, sheep, or pigs, being tender and fat, when boiled with linseed; much must; dr. iv of the bark of rosemary; and after the food inject by clyster the juice of rice, or of chondrus, or of spelt, or of ptisan, or of mallows, or of linseed, or of marshmallows, or of fenugreek. And sometimes having cleared out the intestine with honied water and nitre, we may then inject these things, and afterwards allay the inflammation with cataplasms of linseed and barley; for at first these things are pernicious. Then we may have recourse to baths of sweet water, and give the ointments of iris and of roses in a draught.

Commentary. The symptoms occasioned by taking cantharides, according to Nicander, are erosion of the whole intestinal canal, ulceration of the bladder, affection of the chest, and wild delirium. His remedies are emetics, such as fat, the oil of iris with rue, or Samian aster, laxatives, milk in clysters or taken by the mouth, and the decoction of vine-shoots with honey. Dioscorides describes the symptoms in the same terms as our author, and like him recommends emetics of oil and emollient clysters, such as the decoction of linseed or of mallows. Like our author, he disapproves of warm applications, such as cataplasms and the hot bath at the commencement, because by their heat they promote the distribution of the poison over the system; but after a time they are useful, he says, by allaying the pains and promoting the discharge of the poison by the cutaneous perspiration. His other remedies being the same as our author's, we need not enumerate them. Galen states that the wings and feet of cantharides prove useful for removing the deleterious effects occasioned by taking their bodies. His treatment otherwise, which is borrowed from Asclepiades, is very similar to that of Dioscorides. He in particular recommends the Lemnian earth, or terra sigillata, as an emetic in this case. (De simpl. ix.) He also speaks favorably of milk. (Ib. and de antidot. ii.) He approves very much of animal and vegetable oils given in sweet wine or tepid water to produce vomiting. Galen states decidedly that the viscus upon which the action of cantharides is exerted is the bladder. (Ad Pison.) The treatment recommended by

Scribonius Largus is little different. Aëtius, Oribasius, and Actuarius only copy from Dioscorides, without suggesting any improvement. Avicenna and Rhases mention that cantharides occasion inflammation of the penis and erections. They agree with the Greeks in recommending oily emetics, clysters of the same, and, what we believe is an improvement which we owe to the Arabians, injections of rose-oil into the bladder by means of a waxen tube (flexible catheter). Rhases approves of bleeding, provided it be long since the patient was bled, and violent pain be felt in the region of the thighs, that is to say, if the urinary organs are much affected. Haly Abbas mentions ardor urinæ, strangury, and bloody urine among the symptoms, and recommends oil by the mouth as an emetic and purgative, and by injection. Alsaharavius mentions swelling of the penis, bloody urine, and suppression thereof, and remarks that the same effects have been sometimes brought on by the external application of cantharides, in which case he recommends the tepid bath and emollient fomentations. His treatment is like that of his other countrymen; for example, he joins them in approving of injecting rose-oil into the bladder.

It would appear that cantharides were sometimes used by the ancients for the purpose of committing suicide. According to Cicero, it was by this means that C. Carbo destroyed himself. (Ad Familiar, ix, 21.)

Ambrose Paré, Matthiolus, and all the earlier modern writers on toxicology, follow the treatment laid down by the ancients. Notwithstanding the concurrent testimonies of all these authorities, Professor Orfila, in the last edition of his 'Toxicologie,' and Dr. Christison, in his late work on 'Poisons,' affirm "that oil is the reverse of an antidote." Yet, in a case lately published, the free administration of olive-oil was followed by copious discharges, both upwards and downwards, of cantharides mixed with the oil. (Edinb. Med. and Surg. Journ. No. 104, p. 214.) And surely, if laxatives are to be administered at all, oily ones are to be preferred, as producing least irritation, and not being likely to be absorbed.

It can scarcely admit of dispute, that the *mylabris cichorei* is the same as the ancient cantharis. It is still used in Turkey and India for the composition of blistering plasters, being possessed of much the same properties as the Spanish fly.

XXXI—ON THE BUPRESTIS

Those who have drunk of the buprestis experience a taste resembling fetid natron, which is followed by violent pain of the stomach and bowels; there is swelling of the abdomen, resembling dropsy, and the skin of the whole body is distended, the urine also being suppressed. They are relieved by the same remedies as are given to those who have taken cantharides; but they derive benefit in particular after evacuations by vomiting and by the bowels, from taking dried figs, and drinking the decoction of them with wine or milk, or a mixture of wine and honey, and they may eat all kinds of pears, and take a woman's milk. When the violence of the disease has subsided they may eat with advantage Theban palm-nuts boiled in wine.

Commentary. Isidorus says of the buprestis, "animal est in Italiâ parvum, simillimum scarabæo longipedi." (Orig. xii, 8.) See also Ælian (H. A. vi, 35); Pliny (H. N. xxx. 10.) The symptoms and treatment, as described by the other authorities, are nearly the same as in our author's description.

Among the remedies recommended by Nicander, the most efficacious are milk and emetics of tepid oil. (Alex. 360.) The Arabians do not treat of this article separately from cantharides, unless it be the stuphe of Alsaharavius. (Pract. xxx, 2, 8.)

We can have no hesitation in holding that the buprestis of the ancients was the *lytta vesicatoria*, or Spanish fly. See Sprengel (Comment. in Dioscor.) and Schneider (ad Nicand.)

XXXII—ON THE SALAMANDER

When a person has taken of salamander, inflammation of the tongue supervenes, with difficulty of speech, trembling, torpor, and ulceration. Certain parts of the body all around become livid, so that often, if the medicine remain, they mortify and drop off. In this case we should do the same things as for cantharides; but more particularly we must administer to them pine-rosin, or that of the pitch tree, or galbanum with honey, or pine-kernels with a decoction of ground-pine, or nettle-leaves boiled along with lilies in oil, the boiled eggs of land or sea tortoise, soup of frogs, having the root of eryngo boiled with them.

Commentary. The principal symptoms, as detailed by Nicander, are inflammation of the tongue, torpor, tremblings, aberration of mind, vibices, &c. He treats it like narcotic poisons, with stimulants and attenuants, such as pine-rosin, the leaves of ground-pine, nettle-seed mixed with the flour of tares, &c. Dioscorides, Avicenna, and most of the authorities direct us to treat this case of poisoning like that of cantharides; Alsaharavius recommends emetics, draughts containing pine-seed, honey, vinegar, wine, &c., with fat flesh. Oil and milk are recommended by most of the authorities.

Avicenna says the salamander is a species of lizard. Aristotle mentions the fabulous story of its being proof against fire as a circumstance which was related. Pliny (H. N. x, 67), Ælian (H. A. ii, 31), and Phile (c. 17) repeat it confidently. On the other hand, Dioscorides affirms that the story is entirely without foundation (ii, 56.)

It is the *salamandra terrestris*. Sprengel says it emits a cold mucus, which may extinguish a small lire. (Notæ in Dios. l. c.)

XXXIII—ON THE PITYOCAMPA, OR PINE-CATERPILLAR

When pine-caterpillar is drunk, there is straightway pain of the mouth and palate, strong inflammation of the tongue, pain of the stomach and intestines, with a prurient sensation of tension; and there is a fiery heat of the whole body, and anxiety. Such cases are to be relieved in like manner as those who have drunk cantharides; but in their case, instead of plain oil we may substitute the ointment of apples.

Commentary. Our author, and indeed all the others, only copy from Dioscorides.

Sprengel mentions several species of erucæ which infest pine-trees, such as the leparis monacha, lasiocampa pini, &c. (Notæ in Dioscor.) Virey remarks, that among the Romans there was an express law forbidding the administration of the hairy caterpillar of the pine, as it produces the most serious symptoms, and even loss of life, by its hairs. (Hist. des Mœurs des Anim.)

XXXIV—ON THE SEA-HARE

When the sea-hare has been drunk an ill-savoured taste, like that of a fetid fish, supervenes, and after a time the bowels are pained and the urine becomes obstructed, or if any is discharged it is of a purple colour. They loathe and detest all kinds of fishes, and have fetid perspirations mixed with blood. We must give them therefore asses' milk or must frequently, or a decoction of the root and leaves of mallows, or the root of hogs-fennel triturated with wine, or dr. j. of black hellebore, or of the juice of scammony in honied water, and the warm blood of a newly-killed goose, and river-crabs alone, if they can be borne, may be given. It is a symptom of recovery when they can eat fish.

Commentary. Nicander's description of the symptoms is like our author's, and his remedies are hellebore, and scammony, asses' milk, &c. Haly Abbas recommends only emetics at first, and afterwards milk. When there is continued oppression of breathing he directs us to bleed and give the syrup of poppies. (Pract. iv. 49.) Alsaharavius, like Nicander, depends principally upon drastic purgatives, such as scammony and hellebore. (See also Nonnus, 279.) Galen says it produces ulceration of the lungs. (See Ther. ad Pison. and de Med. sec. gen. i.) For an account of the lepus marinus, see

Ælian (H. A. ii, 45; ix, 51; xvi, 19); Pliny (H. N. ix, 48; xxxii, 1); Dioscorides (ii, 20; vi, 34,); Philostratus (vi, 32); Phile (93). According to Schneider, it is called *chat marin* in France. Gorræus says it is a species of lizard, and resembles the land hare only in colour. Sprengel inclines to think that it is the *aplysia depilans*. See also Paris and Fonblanque (Méd. Jurisprud. ii, 141.) Rondelet refers it to the class *mollusca*, and gives a drawing of it. (De Piscibus, xvii.) Bellonius and Gesner give the same account of it, and all agree respecting its poisonous qualities. They describe it as being a mass of nearly unorganized flesh. Virey says it has long appendages like the ears of the hare, but which are its eyes.

XXXV—ON THE RED TOAD OR MARSH FROG

When the red toad or marsh frog is taken, it brings on swelling of the body, with intense paleness resembling the colour of the box-tree; and dyspnœa supervenes with fœtor of the mouth, hiccough, and sometimes an involuntary emission of semen. They are easily remedied, however, after vomiting, by taking a large draught of undiluted wine, and two drachms of the root of sweet cane, or the same dose of cyperus. We must also compel them to exercise themselves strenuously in walking and running, on account of the torpor which is upon them; and they ought to take the bath every day.

Commentary. Nicander says the bufo apricans superinduces upon the body difficulty of breathing, fetid breath, and colour like that of the thapsus; he means probably jaundice. His remedies are, the flesh of frogs boiled or roasted, pitch mixed with sweet wine and the spleen of a marsh frog. Pliny says a decoction of marsh frogs in vinegar is an effectual remedy in this case and against salamanders. (H.N. xxxii, 5.) Dioscorides recommends emetics, wine, and active exercise. Avicenna, Rhases, and Haly Abbas recommend nearly the same treatment. Haly approves of friction, especially over the stomach. (Pract. iv. 49.) See a learned dissertation on the Poisonous Ranæ in Schneider's Notes on Nicander (Alexipharm.); see also Gorræus' Commentary on the same. Schneider inclines to think that it must have been the *bufo cornutus.*

Ælian states that when the blood of the phrynus is given with wine, it proves a very fatal poison. (H. A. xvii, 12.) It would appear from two passages in the Satires of Juvenal that in his time criminal acts of poisoning were generally performed by means of this substance. (See Sat. i, 510, and vi, 659.) Paris and Fonblanque, however, deny that any species of toad is poisonous. See also Pennant, (B. Z. iii, 17.) He calls the Rana rubeta the natter-jack.

XXXVI—ON LEECHES

If leeches have been swallowed with water, and have stuck to a part in deglutition, you may ascertain that this has happened from the mouth of the stomach being, as it were, sucked and bitten, which is a symptom of the leeches having been swallowed. Sometimes florid blood is spit up by hawking when the leeches have fixed to the windpipe. They may be rejected by swallowing brine, or the leaves of beet with vinegar, or by drinking snow with oxycrate. Let gargles of nitre (*soda*) with water be used, and of copperas with vinegar. When they have stuck to the throat, put the patient into a warm hip-bath and give him cold water to hold in his mouth, and they will readily come to the cold. Some give bugs to those who have swallowed leeches. I, says Galen, by using garlic in such cases, have not stood in need of bugs.

Commentary. Nicander judiciously recommends when leeches have been swallowed to drink vinegar, to take ice or snow, sea-water, fossil salt (sal gemmæ?), or salt prepared from sea-water. Dioscorides treats the case like our author. Celsus merely says, "acetum cum sale bibendum est." Bugs are recommended by Anatolius. (Geopon. xiii 17.)

Aaron, one of the authorities quoted by Rhases, directs us to lay the patient in the sunshine and examine his throat carefully; and if the leech can be detected to extract it with a forceps. If this cannot be effected he recommends him to gargle the throat with some bitter decoction or to swallow the same, if the leech has descended to the stomach. He also directs him to hold snow in the mouth. (Contin. vii.)

Avicenna recommends nearly the same plan of treatment, and, like our author, mentions the following device in order to get a leech extracted that is fixed in the gullet. The patient is to go into a hot bath and hold cold water in his mouth, which will have the effect of attracting the leech towards it. (iii, 9, 5.)

When a leech has fastened in the throat of a beast of burden and cannot be got at by the hand, Columella directs hot oil to be poured in by means of a pipe, or if it has passed into the stomach, it is to be killed with hot vinegar. (vi, 18.) The vapour from pounded bugs was also a popular remedy in such cases. (Ibid. and Geopon. xiii, 17.)

XXXVII—ON THE CHAMÆLEON

When one has taken the black chamæleon intense gnawing and pain supervene, and tremors with disturbance of the whole body; then convulsions attack, with pituitous and frothy vomiting, and in some cases hiccough with loss of speech, and distortion of the countenance. A fatty decoction of wheat taken hot will be applicable in such cases, and a sweet watery wine also hot, vomits, drinking of milk, emollient clysters, and fomentations by cataplasms. To that kind which occasions suffocation and lividity, a draught of wormwood or of natron with oxymel or of radishes will be proper, and also fomentations to the hypochondrium.

Commentary. Dioscorides and Aëtius give a similar account of the treatment and symptoms. On the chamæleon, see Apuleius (de Herb. 109.) The black chamæleon treated of in this section is the *carthamus corymbosus*. It is quite a different plant from the white chamæleon which is treated of in the 46th section.

XXXVIII—ON HENBANE

Hyoscyamos when drunk or eaten brings on disorder of mind like that of persons in intoxication; but is easily cured, being remedied by copious draughts of honied water and milk, especially that of asses or, if not, of that of goats or cows, and of the decoction of dried figs. Pine kernels are also serviceable in such cases, and the seed of cucumber taken with must, and salt wine with fresh axunge and must, and nettle-seed in like manner, or natron with water will be proper, also succory, mustard, cresses, radishes, onions, and garlic, each of these being taken with wine. They must then be made to remain in a state of rest in order that, like those who have drunk wine, they may digest what they have taken.

Commentary. The description of the symptoms in Nicander's Alexipharmics is imperfect owing to an hiatus in the text. His remedies are milk, fenugreek, nettle-seed, succory, cresses, mustard, the heads of garlic, &c.

This section is taken from Dioscorides. Celsus recommends hot water and milk, especially that of asses.

The description of the symptoms, as given by Aëtius, is somewhat fuller than our author's, but not otherwise different. He and Scribonius Largus mention lividity of the members. Alsaharavius says, it induces sleep, stupor, and coldness of the extremities. Avicenna and Haly Abbas recommend the theriac and antidote of Mithridates. Rhases speaks highly of milk. (Contin. ult.)

The general remedies which they all recommend are emetics, vinegar, milk, sweet wine, and at last, vegetable stimulants, such as mustard and onions, and the theriac.

See an account of the different varieties of henbane known to the ancients in Dioscor. (iv, 64.); Galen (Med. Simpl. viii); Pliny (H. N. xxv, 4); and in Schulze (Toxicol. vet. 20.) See also the Seventh Book of this work.

The Arabians, in this place, treat of another narcotic to which they give the name of *Derufitum* or *Darfion.* See Avicenna (iv, 6, 1, 4); Rhases (xxxix.)

XXXIX—ON CORIANDER

Coriander from its smell cannot be mistaken. When drunk it renders the voice thick, and brings on madness like that from intoxication. Wherefore those who have taken it talk obscenely, and the smell of the coriander is perceptible from the whole body. They are relieved after the removal of the poison by common oil or that of iris (as mentioned above), by undiluted wine with wormwood and drank by itself; by eggs emptied into one vessel and triturated with brine and swallowed; and brine also may be drunk, and salt broth from a hen or a goose, and sweet wine taken with lye.

Commentary. According to Nicander, the symptoms are violent delirium, and great derangement of the mind, as in intoxication. His remedies are principally emetics and wine, the intention of giving which is quite obvious. Dioscorides gives nearly the same account of the symptoms and treatment. Galen (de Simp. Med. viii) attacks Dioscorides in the most unmeasured terms for saying that the action of coriander is frigorific, while, on the contrary, he maintains that it is calefacient. Avicenna combats the reasoning of Galen and agrees with Dioscorides; as do Apuleius among the Latins, and Alsaharavius and Rhases among the Arabians. Pseudo-Macer calls it a cold austere medicine.

With regard to the treatment, the Arabians recommend oily emetics, with soda, pepper, salt, strong wine, &c. Avicenna (iii, 6, 2, 8); Rhases (Cont. xxi); Alsaharavius (Pract. xxx. 2.)

Schulze is satisfied that the corion or coriandrum of the ancients was the same as our coriander. He appears, however, to have rather overrated its deleterious properties. It is only in particular states of the body that it proves at all injurious. (Toxicol. vet. vii.) Sprengel also is satisfied as to the identity of the ancient and modern coriander. (Comment. in Dios.)

XL—ON PSYLLIUM OR FLEAWORT

Fleawort when drunk occasions coldness of the whole body and torpor, with relaxation and lowness of spirits, which are relieved by the same remedies as those given to persons who have drunk coriander.

Commentary. All the authorities agree in representing its effects as being similar to those produced by coriander. They treat the case then upon general principles with wine, pepper, and other such stimulants.

Schulze finds some difficulty in acknowledging that the *plantago psyllium*, L. is the true psyllium of the ancients, and yet he admits that no other plant has so good a claim to be identified with it. We see no grounds for scepticism on this point.

XLI—ON CONIUM OR HEMLOCK

Hemlock, when drunk, brings on vertigo and dimness of vision, so that the person can no longer see even to a small distance; there is hiccough, disorder of the mind, and coldness of the extremities, and at last he is suffocated in convulsions, the breath in the arteria aspera being stopped. At first, therefore, as in other cases of poisoning, we must bring it up by vomiting, and afterwards, by means of an injection, evacuate whatever part had passed into the intestines; and then, as our great remedy, we have recourse to undiluted wine, giving it at intervals, during which we must administer the milk of cows or of asses, or wormwood with pepper, wine, and castor; and rue and mint, with wine, and a dram of cardamom or of storax; or of pepper, with nettle-seeds in wine; or the tender leaves of bay tree; and in like manner laserwort, or the juice thereof, with common wine or must; and sweet wine drunk alone answers well.

Commentary. Theophrastus seems to have been acquainted with the sedative properties of hemlock, for he recommends pepper and rosemary as antidotes to it. (H. P. ix, 24); and Athen. (Deip. ii, 73.) The operation of this poison in the case of Socrates is well described by Plato in his 'Phædo.' Socrates, after swallowing the poisoned cup, walked about for a short time as he was directed by the executioner: when he felt a sense of heaviness in his limbs he lay down on his back; his feet and legs first lost their sensibility, and became stiff and cold; and this state gradually extended upwards to the heart, when he died convulsed.

The symptoms, according to Nicander, are dimness of sight, vertigo, a sense of suffocation, coldness of the extremities, impeded respiration, and death. His remedies are emetics of oil, or undiluted wine, clysters of the same, and undiluted wine taken by the mouth, with pepper, nettle, assafœtida, and the like. Dioscorides, and all the other authorities, recommend much the same treatment. Pliny and Aëtius mention lividity, after death, as a symptom of poisoning by cicuta.

Theophrastus (H. P. vi, 2) and Pliny (H. N. xxv, 95) have described the conium. Schulze is satisfied that it is the *conium maculatum*, L., and in this opinion we fully agree with him. He adds, that the ancients have made no mention of the cicuta virosa.

Dioscorides and most of the others enumerate convulsions among the symptoms. It will be remarked, that in the abstract given above of the symptoms of poisoning by hemlock in the case of Socrates, we have stated that the great philosopher died convulsed. This we think the true interpretation of the term used by Plato (ἐκινήθη), although it has not been so understood by most of his interpreters. Dioscorides, in another place, states somnolency, coma, stertor, lividity, torpor, coldness, stupor, insensibility, and pruritus of the whole body, as the common symptoms of poisoning by opium, mandragora, or conium.

Schulze ranks, among ancient mistakes, the assertion of Galen, that narcotic substances may, in some instances, become digested and prove nutritive. But Dr. Christison says, that both vegetable and animal poisons may become digested, of which he gives an interesting example with regard to opium (On Poisons, p. 52.)

XLII—ON THE JUICE OF THE POPPY

When one has drunk of the juice of the poppy drowsiness comes on, with coldness and intense itching, so that often when the medicine takes effect such an itching comes on that the person is roused from sleep thereby. The smell of the medicine too is emitted from the whole body. The remedies in such cases, after rejecting the substance taken by vomiting with oil, and evacuating downwards by a stimulant clyster, are oxymel drank with salts, or honey with warm rose-oil, and much undiluted wine with wormwood and cinnamon, and warm vinegar by itself, and natron with water, and marjoram with lye, the seed of rue and pepper given with castor, and oxymel, savory, or the decoction of marjoram with wine. We must also rouse by aromatics, put the person into a hot bath, and foment on account of the pruritus which supervenes; and after the bath we may use fat broths, with wine or must. Marrow also drunk with oil is useful.

Commentary. According to Nicander, the symptoms of poisoning by poppy-juice are coldness of the extremities, eyes fixed, heaviness of the eyelids, profuse and fetid perspiration, paleness, swelling of the lip, relaxation of the under jaw, slow respiration, cold breath, and the usual precursors of dissolution, namely, distortion of the nostrils, lividity of the nails, and hollow eyes. His remedies are emetics, such as the oil of iris or of roses, wine and honey; hot drink and rousing the patient by cries, striking his body in different places, and wrapping it in cloths smeared with oil and hot wine, and the hot bath as a restorative.

The symptoms mentioned by Dioscorides are lethargy, violent pruritus, and the perspiration smelling of opium. His remedies are the same as those of our author, namely, emetics at first, then clysters, and afterwards wine and vinegar, with various stimulant and strong-scented things; such as pepper, cinnamon, castor, marjoram, &c. The patient is to be roused as directed by Nicander; and baths and fomentations are to be used to relieve the pruritus.

Galen relates the case of a person reduced to the last stage of coldness, whom he saved by administering freely a strong, light-coloured, and fragrant wine. Yet, he remarks correctly, a small quantity of weak wine operates unfavorably by promoting the distribution of the poison over the system. He, in particular, recommends vomiting at first with wine and oil, and afterwards strong clysters.

Aëtius mentions, among the symptoms, violent pruritus and convulsions. None of the other Greek writers mention convulsions, but, among the Arabians, Avicenna, Rhases, and Alsaharavius, have mentioned them. Modern experience has determined that they are an occasional, but not a frequent symptom produced by the immoderate administration of opium.

Scribonius Largus directs us, after repeated vomiting, to apply embrocations of vinegar and roses to the head, to rub the feet, and to put sinapisms to them and the thighs. Simeon Seth strongly recommends vinegar.

Haly Abbas and Alsaharavius, and, in short, all the Arabians recommend nearly the same treatment; namely, emetics of oil and water, or oil and wine, hot clysters, acrid and strong-scented things, such as castor, assafœtida, savin, &c., and the warm bath, friction, sternutatories, and every means calculated to arouse, and to prevent sleep.

Serapion, Rhases, Avicenna, Haly Abbas, and Alsaharavius, agree in stating that the smallest dose of opium which will prove destructive to human life is two drachms. Modern authors are not agreed as to the smallest quantity which may prove fatal, but surely, as Dr. Christison remarks, Dr. Paris has fixed the minimum dose too low, when he affirms that four grains may be sufficient to produce this effect. On the other hand, we should think that a smaller dose than that mentioned by the Arabians might be sufficient to destroy life. Perhaps the ancient opium may have been weaker than that now in use.

It is worthy of remark, that most of the ancient authorities recommend vinegar in cases of poisoning by opium, but we are inclined to think that none of them administered it at the commencement, nor until the poison had been removed from the bowels. This practice agrees very well with the rule of treatment laid down by Orfila, Paris, and Christison, who state that vinegar is prejudicial, if given at first, by favouring the solution of the poison, but proves useful afterwards by acting as a restorative to the system.

None of the ancient authorities recommend venesection.

In another work we have thus explained the ancient theory of the action of opium upon the human frame. "In order to understand properly the ideas entertained by the ancients respecting the *modus operandi* of opium, it will be necessary to say a few words in explanation of their opinions upon certain points of physiology. Aristotle taught that the prime cause of all the operations of life is mind, and that the prime instrument by which it performs them is heat, which, therefore, he denominates the *co-cause* (συνάιτιον). He illustrates his meaning by comparing the mind to the artificer, and heat to the wimble or saw by which he performs his work. Having remarked, no doubt, that the heart is the warmest part of the body, he appears to have considered it as the spring which turns the whole machinery of the animal frame, the brain and nerves deriving their origin and influence from it. (I need scarcely mention how well these ideas accord with the ingenious hypothesis lately advanced by M. Serres.) Many facts, indeed, seem to point out the supreme importance of the heart. It is, as the ancients remarked, the *primum movens et ultimum moriens*; and, along with its accessory organ, the lungs, it is evidently the part which, in the higher classes of animals, renders them independent of the many variations of heat and cold to which they are subjected. It is this wonderful organ which, under the guidance of the principle of life, preserves the heat of the body unaltered in all the different gradations of temperature, from more than 100 degrees above the boiling, to as many below the freezing point of the thermometer. It seems, in fact, a real Prometheus that steals the fire from heaven. The connexion between heat and the vital actions is very apparent also in the inferior animals, who are not provided with such an apparatus for preserving an equability of temperature. Thus the zoophyta, insecta, et vermes, with the loss of heat, lose also sensibility and muscular energy, which they recover again when their heat is restored. In this case it is evident that heat is the cause (or at least the *co-cause*) of the vital actions, and not the vital actions of heat. It has always appeared to me a striking fact, illustrative of the great influence of heat over the vital actions, that the strength of all animals is, bulk to bulk, proportionate to the degree of their animal heat.

"This doctrine of the supreme authority of the heart, as being the focus of heat, thus maintained by Aristotle, was eagerly defended by the great Arabian commentator, Averrhoes, and by his countryman, Avenzoar, who keenly attacked Galen for having questioned its truth, and taught, as they represent, that the brain is the leading organ in the animal frame. After having, however, carefully ransacked every part of Galen's works, in which I could suppose it likely to meet with any allusion to this doctrine, I am led to believe that these Arabians, in the heat of controversy, have misrepresented the real opinion of their master's rival. Galen appears decidedly to have maintained with Hippocrates—'that there is in the body no one beginning, but that all parts are alike, beginning and end: for a circle has no beginning.' Agreeably to this idea, Galen remarks, that the brain cannot properly be said to derive its powers from the heart, since an animal will run, breathe, and cry after its heart has been taken out; nor can the heart be said properly to derive its powers from the brain, since it will palpitate and contract, after all communication with the brain is cut off, nay, after it has been removed from the body. In so far, then, the functions of the brain and the heart are independent of one another. But the brain is dependent upon the heart and its appendages for vital heat, without which it would be unable to continue its functions; and the heart, on the other hand, is dependent upon the brain for imparting nervous influence to the respiratory organs, without which it could not preserve its vital heat unaltered. Hence the mutual connexion and sympathy of important organs—a doctrine much insisted upon by ancient authors, and which bears some resemblance to the theory lately advanced by Mr. Morgan and Dr. Addison.

"We shall now have no difficulty in understanding the ideas of the ancients regarding the operation of opium. Galen and Avicenna believed that the poison exerts its primary influence upon the heart, and impairs its vital heat. Of course they considered its operation on the brain as secondary. They called the action of narcotics frigorific or congealing, no doubt because they remarked that it was attended with a diminution of vital heat, and to this they attributed the loss of sensibility and muscular energy. I leave it to the reader to judge whether this theory or the modification of it lately proposed by Messrs. Morgan and Addison be the more plausible." (Edinburgh Medical and Surgical Journal, No. 103.)

But although the ancient physiologists maintained that the prime organs of the animal frame suffer sympathetically in cases of poisoning, they did not hold, it will be remarked, that all poisons exert their primary action on the nervous system. This is the hypothesis lately advocated by Messrs. Morgan and Addison, but which is, in fact, only a revival of that maintained by Schulze in his 'Toxicologia Veterum.' He thus states his theory of the action of poisons,—"Omnia symptomata et lethales venenorum effectus hoc unum quam luculentissimè demonstrant, *ab omnibus venenis nervos ipsos graviter affligi.* Nervea igitur vis seu vitalis, a veneni stimulis commota, aut majori impetu agit, aut prævalente veneni vehementia prorsus silet, nexusque omnes sensorii communis cum reliquis nervis turbantur, vitâ animali aut graviter periclitante, aut prorsus interiturâ." (Toxic. Vet. vii.) Dr. Mead also, in his last edition of his work on Poisons, advocates this hypothesis.

It appears to us, however, that this theory, although very simple and plausible, is somewhat too exclusive. And that there are other modes by which poisons operate than through the brain and nerves appears to be demonstrated by the fact now clearly established, that poisons act upon vegetables as well as upon animals. (V. Annales de Chimie, t. xxix.) Now as vegetables are possessed of neither sensibility nor motion, it seems preposterous to suppose that they have any nervous system.

Perhaps, then, we cannot do better than revert to the old doctrine delivered by Alsaharavius. Sometimes, he says, poisons act upon the heart, and thereby prove instantly fatal; sometimes upon the liver, producing jaundice and phthisis; sometimes upon the brain, when they occasion delirium; and sometimes their action is local, giving rise to corruption and lividity of the part. (Pract. xxx. 2, 18.)

That the primary action of narcotics is upon the heart appears to us, upon the whole, the most probable theory hitherto advanced upon the subject.

XLIII—ON THE JUICE OF THE CARPESIA

When the juice of carpesia is drunk it brings on heavy sleep and acute suffocation. These are relieved by the same remedies as those given to persons who have drunk hemlock.

Commentary. This section is taken, almost word for word, from Dioscorides. Matthiolus confesses that he was quite unable to determine what substance it was. (Comment. in Dioscor. vi, 13.) It is doubtful whether the καρπήσιον of Galen and the κάρπασον of Dioscorides be the same substance, and whether either be the same as the ὀποκάρπασον. Sprengel can arrive at no certain conclusion respecting it. Valerius Cordus supposed it to be the *piper longum.*

XLIV—ON MANDRAGORA OR MANDRAKE

When mandragora has been drunk, stupor immediately comes on, with loss of strength, and a strong inclination to sleep, so that the affection differs in nothing from that which is called lethargy. Before any of these symptoms come on, vomiting will be proper in this case; and afterwards honied water, or natron and wormwood with must, or taken in a dulcified wine, embrocations to the head with rose-oil and vinegar, rousing by shaking the body, and by strong-smelling things, pepper, mustard, castor, and rue pounded with vinegar, liquid pitch, and the wicks of lamps lighted and extinguished, will be proper. When they are difficult to rouse we may also apply sternutatories, and have recourse to the general remedies in such cases.

Commentary. Our author, as usual, follows Dioscorides. Matthiolus, by the way, in his commentary, questions the propriety of applying rose-oil and vinegar to the head, as these things are of a cold nature, whereas stimulants and calefacients are indicated. Perhaps these things, when poured from a height upon the head, might prove restorative and stimulant. The other Greek authorities however, as, for example, Aëtius and Actuarius, approve of the practice. Alsaharavius recommends emetics, and also directs us to pour vinegar and rose-oil on the head, and to take vinegar in which hyssop and the like have been boiled.

Rhases recommends vomiting by means of water, honey, and fossil salt; after which sweet wine is to be given, and vinegar and rose-oil poured upon the head; castor, pepper, and rue are to be administered, along with sternutatories. He mentions, however, that he knew an old medical man who cured a young woman, who had fallen into a state of syncope, with flushing of the face, after swallowing the apples of mandragora, by the affusion of snow-water on her head. Avicenna properly directs everything to be done to prevent sleep.

Schulze is satisfied that it is the *atropa mandragora* of Linnæus. There seems no doubt, however, that the mandragora of Theophrastus is the *atropa belladonna*; while the mandragora mas of Dioscorides is the *mandragora vernalis*, Bertol.; and the M. femina of the same, the *mandragora autumnalis.*

Theophrastus, Dioscorides, Galen, Athenæus, Aëtius, Suidas, Hesychius, Apuleius, Pollux, and Frontinus, have made mention of the hypnotic property of mandragora. It is singular that it should now have fallen into neglect. It appears to have been used as a medicine in the days of Shakespeare. Iago says:

"Not poppy nor mandragora

Nor all the drowsy syrups of the world,

Shall ever medicine thee to that sweet sleep

Which thou owed'st yesterday."

Othello.

We will have occasion to treat of it in the Seventh Book.

XLV—ON ACONITUM OR WOLFSBANE

Wolfsbane immediately after being drunk occasions a sensation of sweetness on the tongue, with a little astringency; vertigo supervenes, more especially when the person attempts to rise up, and it brings on a watering of the eyes; there is heaviness of the chest and abdomen, with eructation of much flatus. In these cases the medicine must be brought up by vomits, and the contents of the bowels evacuated by a clyster. We must also give draughts from marjoram and rue, or from horehound with wine, or from wormwood, or from rocket, or from southernwood, or mezereon, or ground-pine. Opobalsam, too, taken to the amount of one drachm, with wine, will likewise answer with them; also the rennet of a kid, or of a hare, or of a fawn, with vinegar, and the dross of iron, or iron itself, or gold, or silver, may be dissolved in wine, and the liquid taken, and lye with wine, and the broth of a boiled cock, or the broth of fat flesh taken with wine. The ground-pine, which is said to be a specific in Heraclea of Pontus, where wolfsbane grows, is called holocleron, but ionia in Athens, and sideritis in Eubœa.

Commentary. The symptoms, as described by Nicander, are astringency of the lips, palate, and gums, gnawing pains at the stomach, singultus, flatulence, running from the eyes, double vision, as from intoxication. His remedies seem to have been principally emetics and calefacients. Thus he recommends a handful of quicklime to be drunk with a hemina of wine, also southernwood, spurge, ground-pine, marjoram, opobalsam, the metallic preparations mentioned by our author, and the like. The accounts of the treatment given by Dioscorides, Aëtius, and Actuarius agree exactly with our author's. Avicenna, Rhases, and Haly Abbas, in like manner, recommend emetics, clysters, and calefacient medicines internally.

Diogenes Laertius states, upon the authority of Eumelus the historian, that Aristotle the philosopher despatched himself with a draught of aconite. (Vita Aristot.) Pliny relates that this poison proves fatal when applied to the genital organs of women. (H. N. xxvii, 2.)

The ancients have described several varieties of aconite. See Theophrastus (H. P. ix, 19); Pliny (H. N. xxv, 75); Schulze (Toxicol, vet.); Schneider (in Nicand. Alexiphar.); and Sprengel (Rei. Herb. Hist.) These modern authors in general are disposed to think that it was the *iris tuberosa*. Sprengel, however, in the notes to his edition of Dioscorides, is decided that the second species of Dioscorides (Mat. Med. iv, 78) is the *aconitum napellus*; but respecting the first species, he is in great doubts. All agree that the aconitum of Theophrastus is different from the A. of Dioscorides and the other toxicologists. We may be permitted to add, that the symptoms of poisoning by aconitum, as given by Nicander, agree so well with those reported lately of cases of poisoning by the *aconitum napellus*, that we cannot doubt their identity.

XLVI—ON IXIA

Ixia, which is also called ulophonon, when drunk has some resemblance both in taste and smell to basil-royal. It brings on strong inflammation of the tongue, and disorder of the mind; it suppresses all the secretions, occasioning borborygmi and rumbling, with deliquium animi; but there are no alvine evacuations. After the greater part of the poison has been brought up by vomiting, or evacuated by the bowels, they will experience relief from drinking the decoction of wormwood, with much wine, vinegar, or oxymel, or the seed of wild rue, or the root of laserwort, and in the like manner the decoction of tragoriganum with some of the aforementioned, or with milk; or of turpentine, of nard, of castor, of laserwort, of each an obolus in wine. The fruit also of the walnut triturated with wine will be proper; or of rosin, of castor, and of rue, of each dr. j; and in like manner of mezereon, dr. ij; of the juice of thapsia, dr. ij, with honied water; and hot vinegar may be drunk by itself.

Commentary. Nicander's description of the symptoms is very similar to that given by our author, and his treatment seems to have been conducted upon the same principles; namely, by administering emetics and purgatives at first, and, afterwards, discutient and detergent medicines, to overcome the viscid nature of the poison. Our author's plan of treatment differs in no material respect from that recommended by Dioscorides, Aëtius, Actuarius, Avicenna, and Alsaharavius. Avicenna described it by the name of *aldabach*; Alsaharavius, by those of *alfos, aldolia,* i. e. arbor risi.

Apuleius make ixias, ulophonon, chamæleon, ocymoides, and various cardui synonymes (109.) The ixias, according to Gorræus, is a species of chamæleon, but what species cannot be determined. (See, also, Schneider's note on Nicander.) Matthiolus calls it a glutinous substance, found in the root of the chamæleon, or carline thistle. Schulze is decided that it was a species of carlina (Toxicol. vet., 22.) See Harduin's note on Pliny (H. N. xxii, 21.) After mature consideration, we have no difficulty in referring it to the *carlina acaulis*, or carline thistle.

XLVII—ON EPHEMERON, OR MEADOW SAFFRON

When one swallows ephemeron (which some call colchicum, because it grows in Colchis, or bulbus silvestris), pruritus takes place over the whole body, as if stung by nettle or squill; there is a gnawing pain within, and great heat of the stomach, with considerable heaviness; but when the affection gains strength, blood is discharged from the bowels, mixed with the scrapings thereof. The same remedies are to be applied as to those who have drunk salamander, in vomits and clysters. But before the medicine gain ground we must give a decoction of oak-leaves, or of acorns, or of the rind of pomegranate, or of wild thyme with milk, or the juice of bloodwort, or of vine-tops, or of brambles, or of the medulla of fennel-giant, or of myrtle berries, with wine; and when levigated myrtles themselves are pounded and macerated in water, the liquor thereof may be taken with advantage. And, in like manner, the middle pellicle of the chesnuts, called Sardian, may be taken with the aforesaid juices, and marjoram may be drunk with lye. Those affected are manifestly relieved by drinking hot cow's milk, and retaining it in the mouth, so that they who have plenty of it do not stand in need of any other remedy.

Commentary. Our author's detail of the symptoms is taken entirely from Nicander, and his treatment also is mostly derived from the same source. They seem to have depended principally upon vegetable astringents, such as oak-bark, pomegranate-rind, and chesnuts, for checking the hypercatharsis. Pliny, like our author, strongly commends milk (H. N. xxvii, 33.) Dioscorides recommends emetics, clysters, vegetable astringents, and demulcents. Alsaharavius says, that hermodactylus occasions pruritus of the whole body, swelling of the palate, pains of the stomach, and the like. He recommends emetics, clysters, cows' milk, and vegetable astringents, such as acorns with wine. This, it will be remarked, is similar to the account which the Greeks give of the symptoms and treatment of ephemeron, which is undoubtedly the *colchicum autumnale*; and this circumstance tends strongly to prove the identity of the ephemeron and the hermodactylus. We agree with Schulze, Prosper Alpinus, and Humelbergius, that they were unquestionably the same plant, notwithstanding that Sprengel, Matthiolus, and Dr. Murray are of a different opinion. Dr. Paris considers that there is no doubt of their identity. (See a learned dissertation on the Ephemeron in a note by Schneider, on Nicander's Alexipharmics.) We shall only further add, in this place, that the learned Ardoyn, in his elaborate work on Poisons, contends, that there is no doubt of the identity of the colchicum and the hermodactylus. We, in fact, are surprised that this should have been ever questioned.

XLVIII—ON THE SMILAX OR YEW

The tree called smilax is named thymium by some, and taxus by the Romans. When drunk it brings on coldness of the whole body, suffocation, and speedy death; the remedies for which are all those things which are given to those who have drunk of hemlock.

Commentary. The description of the symptoms and the plan of treatment are borrowed from Nicander, or, rather, copied direct from Dioscorides.

Different opinions have been entertained respecting the poisonous nature of the yew. Haller, Bulliard, and others, deny that it is poisonous; while Berkley, Ray, Matthiolus, and others, affirm that it is. Orfila holds it to be a narcotic poison (chap. iv, cl. 4.) We have known instances of its proving fatal to cattle. The newspapers lately contained a melancholy case of a boy poisoned by yew-berries at Winchester. Matthiolus is not pleased with Dioscorides for making it to be a frigorific medicine; but Orfila, it appears, gives it the same character; that is to say, he holds it to be narcotic. Virgil alludes to its poisonous qualities:

Sic tua Cyrnæas fugiant examina taxos.

See, also, Theophrastus (H. P. i, 5, and iii, 9); and Schulze (Tox. vet. 17).

XLIX—ON THE STRYCHNOS FURIOSA, CALLED DORYCNIUM, BY SOME

When one drinks of dorycnium, which some call strychnos furiosa, there follows a sensation, as it were, of milk to the taste; constant hiccough, watering of the tongue, and frequent ejection of blood; and there are mucous discharges by the bowels, as in dysenterical cases. They are to be remedied before any of these symptoms supervene, by those things which are taken for ephemeron, I mean emetics and clysters, and whatever else can evacuate the substance which had been taken. Honied water is a particularly good remedy; or the milk of asses or of goats and sweet wine, in a tepid state, may be drunk with a small quantity of anise. Bitter almonds also are proper, the boiled breasts of fowls, all the shell-fish eaten raw and boiled, crabs and crawfish, and the broth of them when drunk.

Commentary. Our author's detail of symptoms is taken mostly from Nicander, or, perhaps, direct from Dioscorides. The poet's plan of treatment seems to have been much the same as that of Paulus. He omits, indeed, to make mention of emetics and purgatives as being general remedies in all cases of poisoning; but he recommends milk, must, and the crustacea, such as the pinna, echinus, &c. The other authorities supply nothing additional. Avicenna treats of it under the name of uva vulpis stupefactiva mala; he copies from Dioscorides (iv, 6; i, 7.)

There is considerable difficulty about the nature of the dorycnium. Our author, Aëtius and Apuleius, make it to be the same as the strychnos furiosa, which is generally held to be either the solanum sodomeum, or the atropa belladonna. On this subject, see Galen (de Med. sec. loc. x, 3); Pliny (H. N. xxi, 105); Apuleius (de Herb., 22). Schulze affirms, that none of the ancient poisons is so little known as the dorycnium. He is undecided as to its nature, except that it belonged to the diadelphous or leguminous plants, and he is inclined to think that it was an astragalus. (Toxicol. Veterum, 2.) Sprengel inclines either to the convolvulus cneorus, L., or the con. dorycnium, L. But as far as we can see, the most probable conjecture that can be made regarding it is, that it was either the *solanum sodomeum*, or *atropa belladonna*.

L—ON THE SARDONIAN HERB

The herb called the Sardonian is a species of ranunculus, when drunk, or eaten, it brings on disorder of the intellect, and convulsions with contraction of the lips, so as to exhibit the appearance of laughter. From this affection that ill-omened expression, the Sardonian laugh, took its rise. In these cases, therefore, after vomiting, it will be proper to give honied water and milk, with embrocations and lubrications of the whole body, by calefacient remedies; and to have recourse to hot-baths of hot oil and water, and to anoint properly and rub them after the baths; and, upon the whole, to conduct the treatment as for convulsions.

Commentary. Dioscorides and our author are perfectly agreed as to the symptoms and treatment. Aëtius recommends, likewise, castor with sweet wine. Solinus, like our author, says that it brings on contractions of the muscles, and the risus Sardonicus. Avicenna acknowledges his ignorance of the nature and proper treatment of this herb, but supposes that it belongs to the class of acute poisons. There seems, however, no reason to doubt that it was a species of ranunculus. Schulze makes it the *ranunculus sceleratus*, L., which bears the English name of celery-leaved crowfoot; and we are clearly of the same opinion, although Avicenna seems to make a distinction between the Sardonian herb and the *kebekengi*, or apium risus, which is the βατράχιον of Dioscorides. See Alsaharavius (Pract. xxx, i, 39.)

LI—ON THE HORNED POPPY

Seeing that the species of poppy called the horned, when eaten or drunk, brings on the same symptoms as the juice of poppy, it is to be treated by the same remedies.

Commentary. Miller says that the glaucium is called horned poppy because it is a species of poppy having husks resembling horns. See some account of it in Apuleius (53.) Schulze remarks that Dioscorides has described several varieties of the poppy. 1, Papaver hortense; 2, P. opiiferum; 3, P.

agreste; 4, P. rhæas; 5, P. ceratites sive corniculatum; 6, Hypecoum. The fifth of these, or horned poppy, is the glaucium luteum, Scop. Dioscorides gives a distinct description, but treats of it as a medicine rather than as a poison. (M. M. iv, 66.) None of the Arabians treat of it separate from opium.

LII—ON PHARICUM

The substance called pharicum in taste completely resembles nard, and when drunk it brings on paralysis, with disorder of the mind and convulsion. After evacuation by vomiting, we must give the patient to drink, along with wine, some wormwood, cinnamon, myrrh, or Celtic nard (which some call saliunca), or of spikenard, dr. ij, or two oboli of myrrh mixed with must or iris, and the flower of saffron with wine. The head is to be shaven, and a cataplasm consisting of barley-flour, with levigated rue and vinegar, is to be applied.

Commentary. Nicander, like our author, compares its taste to that of spikenard, and says that it proves fatal in one day, inducing delirium. He recommends the same internal medicines, and also makes mention of applying a stimulant cataplasm to the head, evidently with a view of relieving the phrenitis. The other authorities recommend similar treatment.

There is great disagreement among the ancient writers on toxicology respecting the nature of the pharicum. (See the notes of Gorræus and Schneider on Nicander.) The former remarks that many suppose it a species of nard. Dioscorides (Præf. vi) and Galen (Antidot. ii) make it to be a herb. Scribonius Largus, and Hesychius consider it to have been a compound medicine. After balancing all the statements Schneider comes to the conclusion, that most probably it was a composition from agaric. Schulze is wholly undecided as to its nature. (Toxic. Vet. 21.) Sprengel, in like manner, can come to no certain conclusion respecting it. (Notæ in Dioscor. l. c.)

LIII—ON TOXICUM

The toxicum seems to be so called because the barbarians anointed their darts (τοξεύματα) with it. When a person has drunk of it, inflammation of the lips and tongue comes on, also irrestrainable madness leading to various fantasies, so that in the treatment of them they are difficult to cure, and it is rare that any of those who have drunk of it can be saved. However, they are to be forcibly bound with ligatures, and compelled to drink sweet wine with rose-oil, and to vomit. Turnip seed, also, drunk with wine will be proper for them, and the root of cinquefoil, the blood of a he or she-goat when taken, oak bark, that of the beech or ilex triturated with milk; also quinces when eaten, or triturated with pennyroyal and drunk in water; and ammomum, and the fruit of balsam with wine. But if any escape the danger they remain for a long time confined to bed, and when they get out of it they spend the rest of their lives in a state of timidity.

Commentary. The symptoms detailed by Nicander are much the same as those enumerated by our author, namely, swelling of the mouth and throat, with violent internal pains. His remedies likewise are much the same, namely, forcing the patient, after he is well secured, to drink wine until he vomit, and making him take bruised apples, rose-oil, oil of iris, &c. He says, that certain savage nations upon the Euphrates poisoned their arrows with it, which rendered their wounds immedicable, occasioning lividity and putrefaction. Dioscorides, Aëtius, Actuarius, and, in short, all the ancient authorities, copy his account.

It is very difficult to determine the nature of the toxicum. Theophrastus describes a species of calamus by the name of toxicus. (H. P. iii, 12.) Avicenna, however, admits that he was wholly unacquainted with its nature. (iv, 6; i, 29.) Some have supposed, with considerable probability, that it was a preparation from the rhus toxicodendron. Schulze is only decided that it was a vegetable poison. (Tox. Vet. 19.) But it even seems doubtful whether it was a simple or compound medicine, and whether of an animal or vegetable nature. (See Schneider's note on Nicander's Alexiph. 248.) Sprengel inclines to the opinion that it was collected from the venom of serpents. (Notæ in Dioscor.) All, however, is mere conjecture on this subject.

LIV—ON MUSHROOMS

Of mushrooms, some prove deleterious from their general nature, and some by the quantity taken. They all bring on suffocation resembling choking. The general remedy which is to be instantly applied is to compel the persons affected to vomit by means of oil. They are also wonderfully relieved by drinking of the lye from vine-shoots, or from the wood of the wild pear with oxycrate, salts, or natron. And wild pears or their leaves, if boiled with mushrooms, take away their suffocative quality, and if eaten they prove beneficial. Hen's dung, drunk in oxycrate, proves beneficial to them; likewise a drachm of birthwort, or of wormwood with wine, and honey when licked or drunk with water; and baum with natron, or the root and fruit of all-heal with wine, the burnt lees of wine with water, and copperas with vinegar, radish, mustard, or cresses when eaten. And since certain mushrooms having been tasted of by venomous animals occasion not only suffocation but also ulceration of the intestines, we must give in such cases plenty of wormwood, and the decoction of figs, and of marjoram, and honied water. Emetics, the hot hip-bath, and raw barley-flour when applied to the hypochondria, will also be proper.

Commentary. Nicander mentions suffocation as the common effect of taking mushrooms. His remedies are radishes, rue, the flowers of copper, natron, mustard, lixivial ashes, &c. Our author copies from Aëtius. Simeon Seth recommends honey with tepid water, and a moderate quantity of natron. Ruffus (ap. Oribas. Med. Collect, viii, 24) recommends clysters of natron, wormwood, the juice of radish, and the decoction of rue. Dioscorides recommends emetics of oil, natron, &c., and afterwards vinegar and stimulant decoctions. Avicenna's remedies are nearly the same as those of our author. Alsaharavius directs us to give at first emetics, and then calefacients, such as pepper, cumin, wine, and, if necessary, the theriac. Haly Abbas, in like manner, recommends emetics, and then wine with honey, the theriac, &c. The symptoms, he says, are cold sweats, faintings, and embarrassment of breathing. All the ancient authors affirm that mushrooms act upon the organs of respiration, and we remark that a sense of suffocation is generally mentioned in the cases reported by modern writers.

For a full report of fungi, or mushrooms, see Dioscor. (iv, 53); Pliny (H. N. xxii, 46); Schulze (Tox. Vet. 14); Sprengel (Comment. in Dioscor.); Schweighaeuser (in Athen. Deipnos. ii, 59); Schneider (ad Nicand. Alex. 521). Diphilus, as quoted by Athenæus, states that all mushrooms which are black, livid, and hard, or which grow hard after being boiled, are of a deleterious nature. He recommends us to give mulse, oxymel, natron, and vinegar, so as to produce vomiting.

Dioscorides gives the following characters of poisonous fungi: Such as grow near rusty nails, or putrid rags of cloth, or near the lodging-place of reptiles, or by trees which have bad fruits, are deleterious; such have a glutinous coagulum (membrane adhering to the cap?) and when gathered soon become putrid and melt away. (M. M. iv, 83). According to Sprengel, these characters are not universally applicable (l. c.); but considering the experience which the ancients had in the use of these articles, they are no doubt generally so. The *amanita muscaria*, the *agaricus necator*, and many other species, may be set down as belonging to the ancient list of poisonous mushrooms.—Schulze, who appears to have paid great attention to the subject, enumerates the poisonous mushrooms of the ancients as follows:—1, Agaricus muscarius; 2, Agaricus piperatus; 3, Agaricus emeticus; 4, Boletus versicolor; 5, Boletus laricis. (Toxic. Vet. xiii, 5.)

LV—ON BULLS' BLOOD

The blood of a newly-killed bull brings on dyspnœa and suffocation, obstructing the passages about the tonsils and the parts concerned in deglutition with violent spasms; the tongue, in such cases, is also found red; the teeth are stained, and there are clots between them. In this case we must avoid giving a vomit, because the grumous blood will be more firmly fastened in the stomach by being raised upwards with the contractions. We must give those things which are calculated to dissolve the coagulated blood and loosen the belly; green figs, therefore, are to be administered when filled with juice, along with oxycrate and natron. All kinds of rennet are also proper with vinegar, and the root of laserwort, with its juice in like manner; also cabbage seed, the lye of figs, and the leaves of fleabane with pepper, and the juice of bramble with vinegar. The bowels are also to be evacuated. Those who are going to recover have fetid and bloody discharges by the anus. Cataplasms, made of barley-flour with honey, are also to be applied to the regions of the stomach and bowels.

Commentary. Bulls' blood being exceedingly viscid and indigestible might prove deleterious by becoming quickly coagulated in the stomach: we do not find any mention of it, however, in modern works on toxicology. Themistocles is said to have despatched himself with it. Nicander makes no mention of emetics, and Dioscorides, like our author, condemns the use of them. Nicander recommends almost the same identical remedies as our author. It will be remarked that they are all of a penetrating, attenuant, and solvent nature, such as wild figs, natron, laserwort, the rennets of certain animals, &c. Galen mentions the pernicious effects of coagulated blood in the stomach, and recommends hot vinegar for it. (De Al. boni et mali succi.) Ruffus (ap. Oribas. Med. Collect. viii, 24) recommends clysters composed of natron, vinegar, the decoction of cabbage, and of its seed, with vinegar.

The Arabians treat the case in a similar manner. Alsaharavius directs us to give vinegar, natron, wine, and the like, also diuretics, but he forbids the use of emetics.

Sprengel inclines to believe that bulls' blood may prove deleterious, if allowed to remain long in the stomach, by evolving azotic gas. He therefore approves of the hot vinegar recommended by Galen. (Comment. in Dios. 25.) Ardoyn states that a large quantity of bulls' blood taken into the stomach may produce suffocation by stopping the action of the diaphragm. (De Venen. iv, 23.)

LVI—ON COAGULATED MILK

Those who take a large draught of milk containing rennet, experience a great feeling of suffocation from its becoming coagulated. In treating them, we may give as an antidote rennet with vinegar, compelling them often to drink of it; also the dried leaves of calamint, and its juice in like manner, or the roots of laserwort, or its juice with oxycrate, thyme with wine, and the lye used by bonnet-makers; but nothing saltish must be given, for thereby the milk becomes more firmly coagulated and is converted into cheese. Neither must we make them vomit, for thereby the coagula being lodged in the stomach will produce suffocation.

Commentary. Gorræus, in his notes on Nicander, remarks that milk only proves prejudicial when taken in great quantity, immediately after the rennet has been added to it, and before it has curdled. See also Matthiolus and Ardoyn (de Venenis). Nicander recommends the same remedies as our author, namely, such as are of a cutting and attenuant nature, as rennet, vinegar, wine, lasewort, &c. Dioscorides forbids all saltish things. Ruffus (ap. Oribas. Med. Col. viii, 24) recommends a clyster of vinegar and natron, or asses' milk with much salt. Celsus says, with his accustomed brevity, "Si lac intus coit, aut passum, aut coagulum, aut cum aceto laser." See also Galen (l. c.) Haly Abbas, Rhases, Avicenna and Alsaharavius also recommend rennet with pepper, assafœtida, vinegar, &c. For bad milk which has spoiled on the stomach, all the Arabian authorities concur in recommending first an emetic of hydromel, and afterwards wine with pepper.

Sprengel accounts for the deleterious effects of curdled milk in the same manner as he does for those of bulls' blood, and remarks, that the acid contained in the rennet of certain animals especially of hares, is well calculated for dissolving and evacuating the coagulum (Comment. in Dioscor. l. c.)

The Arabian authorities treat, among the deleterious substances, of flesh and fish which have been cooked and hung up in a wet place until they have become unwholesome. When eaten in this state, Rhases says they bring on violent vomiting and purging, and may prove fatal unless the proper remedies are applied. For these symptoms he recommends repeated emetics and then purgatives; after which wine and pepper is to be given; and, in the end, the remedies for poisonous mushrooms. (Ad Mansor. viii, 27, 28.) See also Alsaharavius (Pract. xxx, 2, 15); Haly Abbas (Pract. iv.) Haly Abbas recommends vomiting by means of tepid water, oxymel, and salt.

They treat, in like manner, of rancid fruits; which they state act as poisons when eaten in large quantity. For the cure of these they recommend emetics, the rob of bitter grapes, and medicines to whet the appetite. Rhases (ad Mansor. viii, 30); Avicenna (iv. 6; i, 30.)

Avenzoar relates, at considerable length, the history of a case in which delirium and other bad symptoms had been brought on and kept up by drinking out of a cup which had been poisoned with some putrid meat. (i, 9, 9.)

LVII—ON HERACLEAN HONEY

Those who eat or drink the honey formed in Heraclea, of Pontus, experience the same symptoms as they who have drunk of wolfsbane, and the same remedies will be applicable. They are readily relieved by drinking frequently of mulse, having the leaves of rue mixed with it.

Commentary. This section is taken from Dioscorides.

Avicenna makes mention of a poisonous kind of honey produced in Arabia, for which he applies much the same remedies as those recommended by our author. (iv, 6; i, 32.)

The effects of Pontic honey in occasioning madness is mentioned in the 'Anabasis' of Xenophon (iv, 8.) The same character of it is given by Aristotle, Pliny, Diodorus Siculus, and Ælian. Tournefort confirms the ancient accounts of its inebriating effects. See Sprengel (ad Dioscor. ii, 103.)

LVIII—ON GYPSUM

Gypsum, when drunk, produces suffocation, by being converted into stone; hence we must transfer the remedies applicable to those who have taken mushrooms, giving them in this case, and substituting the decoction of mallows for oil; for being of a fatty nature it lubricates the parts, and prevents them from being injured by the stony hardness of the gypsum. Oil, also, in honied water is proper; and the decoction of figs, and the lye of figs, or of the ashes of vine-shoots with much wine, and marjoram, or thyme with lye or vinegar. Clysters are also to be administered, consisting of must and the decoction of mallows.

Commentary. Our author copies closely from Dioscorides.

Rhases and Avicenna treat this case upon much the same principles as the Greeks, only they give scammony freely at first, and if dysentery supervene they recommend the remedies suitable for it. Aëtius, Dioscorides, and the other Greek authors, although they approve of clysters, say nothing about drastic purgatives. Avicenna says, gypsum in its action resembles ceruse, but is even more powerful than it in inducing strangulation. Haly Abbas says, gypsum occasions colic and ileus with dryness of the mouth, suffocation, difficulty of making urine, and so forth. He directs clysters at first, and afterwards an electuary of pepper and mustard to be given. Alsaharavius forbids emetics, recommends water mixed with honey, and olive-oil for drink, also emollient clysters, and sweet wine.

For an account of gypsum, see Pliny (H. N. xxxvi, 59) and Theophrastus (de Lapidibus.) Isidorus gives the following description of it:—"Gypsi plura genera: omnium autem optimum, lapis specularis: est enim signis ædificiorum, et coronis gratissimus." (Orig. xvi, 3.) The gypsum speculare was evidently selenite, or crystallized sulphate of lime. See Matthiolus (Com. in Dioscor.)

Dr. Kidd gives the following account of the varieties of the ancient gypsum:—"It was, by the general description of it, an earthy compound of lime; but the ancient naturalists seem to apply it to sulphate of lime, the gypsum of the present day, and sometimes to a calcined carbonate of lime, or quicklime, which they called calx." (Mineral. b. i, p. 70).

Sir John Hill gives a full account of the ancient gypsums in his notes on Theophrastus (de Lapidibus.) "Gypsum," he says, "is nothing more than a selenite less elegant than the rhomboidal or plated kinds." There can be no doubt that the γυψος διαφάνης of Philoponus (Com. in Aristot. de Anima. ii) was pure selenite. It is singular that our recent authorities on toxicology have not included gypsum in the list of poisonous substances which they treat of, although there is good reason to believe that the powder, if given in any great quantity, is highly deleterious. We know for certain that gypsum, or stucco, is often used for poisoning rats and mice. It is further deserving of remark that all the earlier modern authorities on medicine, down at least to the middle of the 16th century, treat of gypsum as an active poison. All the ancient authorities, it will be seen, represent it in this light. Pliny makes mention of a case of suicide committed by means of gypsum (H. N. xxxvi, 24.)

LIX—ON CERUSE

Ceruse, owing to its colour, cannot be mistaken, and when taken voluntarily it whitens the palate, tongue, and the intervals between the teeth. It also brings on hiccup and cough, dryness of the tongue, and coldness of the extremities, with disorder of the intellect and difficulty of moving. In this case it will be proper to give honied water or the decoction of figs, or of mallows, or hot milk, or sesame triturated with wine, or the lye of vine-shoots, or the oil of marjoram, or of iris; also the bones of peaches, with a decoction of barley or frankincense, or the gum of prunes, or the juice of the elm which is contained in its follicles, along with tepid water; but let them immediately vomit. The juice of thapsia will also be proper for them, or three oboli of the juice of scammony, when drunk with honied water.

Commentary. Nicander compares the colour of ceruse to frothy milk. The symptoms of poisoning by it are constriction of the palate and gums, asperity of the tongue, singultus, a dry cough, nausea, heaviness of the head, unnatural vision, and torpor. His remedies are emetics of oil, thin milk, decoctions of mallows, sesame triturated with wine, prunes or elms, which are to be given partly as emetics, and partly with the intention of their being digested; for which purpose the patient is to be put into the warm bath. See the Paraphrase of Eutecnius; also Dioscorides, Aëtius, Avicenna, and Rhases, who recommend similar treatment. Aëtius, like our author, directs us to give scammony, evidently to counteract its astringency. Alsaharavius recommends emetics of the decoction of figs with mead or common oil, the infusion of wormwood as a diuretic, scammony with hydromel, and hot milk. Rhases recommends emetics of the decoctions of figs and oil, with drastic purgatives and diuretics. (Ad Mansor. viii, and Contin. xx, 2.) Avicenna's principles of treatment are quite similar, that is to say, he trusts to emetics, diuretics, and clysters, and prevents the patient from sleeping. (iv, 6, 1.) Haly Abbas recommends an emetic consisting of honey with hot water, vinegar and salt; he also gives diuretics, such as the infusion of parsley, fennel, anise, and southernwood. (Pract. iv.)

Dr. Alston says, "our white lead is certainly the ψιμύθιον of Dioscorides and the cerussa of Pliny." It was prepared by exposing the carbonate of lead to the vapours of vinegar. See Milligan (Ad Cels. p. 112.)

LX—ON LIME, SANDARACH, AND ARSENIC

Lime, sandarach, and arsenic, when taken in a draught, bring on pains of the stomach and bowels, with violent corrosion. Wherefore we must administer all things of a diluent and solvent nature, such things as will produce ready vomiting and lubricate the bowels, as the juice of the marsh or common mallows, and a decoction of linseed, or of spelt, or of rice, copious draughts of milk and honied water, broths which are fatty and contain wholesome juices.

Commentary. Nicander has not treated of poisoning by these substances. Dioscorides, Aëtius, and Actuarius give almost the same account of the symptoms and treatment as our author. Their remedies are emetics, lubricants, and laxatives. The Arabians copy their descriptions and follow their treatment. Thus Alsaharavius directs these cases to be treated by giving emetics of oily and fatty things, emollient clysters, and unctuous articles, to prevent ulceration of the intestines. Avicenna orders, in the first place, an emetic of warm water and oil, then emollient decoctions, such as those of linseed and mallows, and fat broths and milk. The cough is to be soothed by demulcents. (iv, 6, 1.) Rhases states that quicklime and arsenic occasion putrefaction of the intestines. (Cont. xxxvii. tr. 1.) Galen, however, has stated that arsenic is not, properly speaking, a septic, but a strong caustic. (De Simp. 1.)

However meagre this account of these important medicines may appear, it will be seen, upon reference to the standard works on toxicology, that the treatment at the present day scarcely differs, in any one point, from the ancient mode of practice. Emetics, demulcents, consisting of decoctions of emollient herbs, or copious draughts of milk, laxatives and clysters, form the present practice.

The ancient arsenicum, or auripigmentum, was orpiment; the sandarach was realgar, or the orange-red sulphuret. Our oxide of arsenic is a factitious substance, prepared by sublimation from cobalt: it is much more deleterious than auripigmentum or orpiment. Servitor and Avicenna have described the factitious arsenic, or oxide of arsenic of the moderns. The Arabian chemist Geber treats largely and ingeniously of orpiment, which he holds to be closely allied to sulphur. He also speaks of sublimed arsenic. (iii. 29.)

LXI—ON LITHARGE

Litharge, when drunk, brings on heaviness of the stomach and bowels, with intense tormina; sometimes by its weight it wounds the intestines, occasions retention of urine and swelling of the body, which becomes of a leaden hue, and assumes an unseemly appearance. In such cases it will be proper, after vomiting, to give the seed of the wild clary (horminum) to drink with wine, three oboli of myrrh, wormwood, parsley-seed, pepper, the flower of privet with wine, and the dried dung of wild pigeons, with nard and wine.

Commentary. The symptoms which Nicander mentions as being superinduced by litharge are borborygmi, pains resembling those of ileus, retention of urine, and discoloration of the skin. His remedies are carminatives, warm stimulants, and diuretics, such as myrrh, clary, St. John's-wort, hyssop, pepper, hedge mustard taken in wine, the green shoots of privet, and the fruit of pomegranate. Scribonius Largus recommends emetics and calefacient medicines, such as pepper, myrrh, parsley. The Arabians, namely, Rhases, Avicenna, and Alsaharavius, concur in recommending emetics, drastic purgatives, and calefacient medicines.

The ancient litharge was prepared like the modern. It is a semi-vitrified peroxide of lead.

LXII—ON LEAD

When a person has drunk the shavings of lead or its soil, he experiences the same symptoms as those from litharge, and is to be treated in the same manner.

Commentary. We need scarcely say that litharge is now ascertained to be a preparation of lead. (See the preceding section.) Most of the ancient authorities state, like our author, that the symptoms and treatment of poisoning by lead and litharge are exactly the same. It appears singular that it should be asserted in some modern works on the materia medica that the ancients were unacquainted with the deleterious properties of lead. Galen even mentions that water conveyed in leaden pipes sometimes proves deleterious by occasioning dysentery. (Med. sec. loc. vii.) Aëtius makes the same observation. (xi, 45.) Palladius, the writer on agriculture, speaks of it in the following terms: "Ultima ratio est, plumbeis fistulis ducere, quæ aquas noxias reddunt; nam cerusa plumbo creatur attrito, quæ corporibus nocet humanis." (ix, 11.) Vitruvius also mentions that water impregnated with lead is deleterious. (Arch. viii.) Pliny notices the deleterious effects of the exhalations from lead mines. (H. N. xxxiv, 50.)

The Greek writers on toxicology do not treat of copper as a poison; but the Arabians have done so in brief terms, all agreeing in recommending the same treatment as in cases of poisoning with arsenic. (See Avicenna, Rhases, Haly Abbas, and Alsaharavius.) These authorities, likewise, lay down in very succinct terms the treatment of poisoning by iron, which they direct to be conducted upon general principles. They in particular recommend laxative and demulcent medicines. (See Avicenna iv, 6, 18.) As a slight novelty in their practice we may mention that he recommends the affusion of vinegar with oil of roses, violets, &c., upon the head. Averrhoes recommends from ⅓ to 1 dr. of balsam. (Coll. v.)

LXIII—ON MERCURY

Mercury, when swallowed, brings on the same symptoms as litharge, and the same remedies are to be used in this case. A copious draught of milk seems to be beneficial, and vomiting ought to be produced.

Commentary. Dioscorides, Galen, and Aëtius give the same imperfect account of this important medicine and poison as our author gives, and supply no additional information of any importance. The Arabians were better acquainted with its properties, having ascertained that it might be taken in its metallic state with impunity. Rhases says, "I do not think that any great harm will result from drinking mercury when it is pure, unless it be pains in the stomach and intestines. It afterwards passes out in its natural state, especially if the person who swallowed it moves about. I gave a draught of it to an ape, nor did I perceive any inconvenience arise from it, except, as I have mentioned, that it appeared to be pained in its belly, for it often bit it with its mouth, and grasped it with its hands." (Ad Mansor. viii, 42.)

Haly Abbas gives a similar account. Mercury, he says, in its natural state, is not poisonous, and merely occasions some tormina in the belly; but when killed (oxydised?) it is deleterious, and is to be remedied by giving emetics of oil and dill, and afterwards oily clysters, &c. (Pract. iv, 53.) See a similar account in Avicenna (iv, 6, 1, 2.) Mercury that has been killed, or sublimed, that is to say attenuated, produces, he says, grave symptoms, such as pain of the bowels, a bloody flux, retention of urine, and so forth. He recommends, after vomiting, myrrh in wine, with honied water, &c.

Serapion mentions that fumigations with mercury are very prejudicial by superinducing nervous affections and paralysis. (De Simpl. 385.) Alsaharavius is, we believe, the only ancient author who has mentioned that rubbing the body with mercury occasions swelling of the mouth, tongue, and throat, with erosion of those parts. He directs us to wash or gargle with the decoction of dill, camomile, or mint. (Pract. xxx, 3.) Pliny mentions milk as a remedy against gypsum, ceruse, sulphur, and mercury. (H. N. xxviii.)

Not having access to the unpublished mss. of the ancient 'Scriptores Chemici,' we cannot pretend to determine whether or not they had acquired any considerable skill in analysing and detecting poisonous substances. See an interesting account of these mss. in Fabricii 'Bibliotheca Græca,' xiii, p. 747. Consult also Vossius 'De Naturâ Artium,' v. 9; Sir William Drummond's Papers in the 'Classical Journal' on the Literature of the Ancient Egyptians; and Doutens 'Dec. de Modern.' p. 176. The only original work on the chemistry of the ancients which we have read with any attention is the 'Chemia' of Geber, which contains much curious information regarding the metals, although nothing that suits our present purpose.

LXIV—ON WHITE HELLEBORE, THAPSIA, ELATERIUM, BLACK AGARIC, WILD RUE, GITH, AND THE DOWN OF THE CACTOS

We must be guarded in the administration of certain medicinal substances, which often occasion as great danger as poisons themselves. Such are the following, namely, white hellebore, thapsia, elaterium, and the black agaric, for these bring on either suffocation or hypercatharsis, in which cases we may cure the suffocation in the way described for mushrooms, and such like substances, and stop the hypercatharsis by such things are as calculated to suppress immoderate discharges. Likewise certain substances which might seem not injurious to any considerable degree, will sometimes occasion dangerous symptoms, and should not be neglected. Such are the wild rue, gith, and the fresh poppy, which are the flowers of the thorn called cactos. In such cases the administration of a vomit alone relieves those who have taken them.

Commentary. This section is taken from Dioscorides. Of the pappus Actuarius says, like our author, that it is the flower of the thorn called cactos, and that vomiting relieves those who have taken it. (Meth. Med. v, 12.) See Avicenna (iv, 6, 1); and Rhases (ad Mansor. viii, 49.) Alsaharavius directs us in the case of hellebore to clear the stomach by emetics, and to apply cooling plasters of citrons, apples, and roses. For the wild rue he recommends emetics of oil, emollient clysters, and the ashes of vine tops taken with water and vinegar.

In the Seventh Book we shall have occasion to state the opinions which have been entertained respecting the helleborus albus of the ancients. Schulze is very undecided. (Toxic. vet. iv.) The thapsia he makes to be the same as the T. fœtida of Linnæus. Theophrastus has described it (H. P. ix, 23). Pliny says it occasions swelling of the body, with erysipelas. (N. H. xiii, 43.)

We shall treat of the elaterium also in the Seventh Book. Hippocrates uses the word as a general term for all drastic purgatives, but by Dioscorides, and the subsequent writers on the materia medica, it is applied to the fæcula of the *momordica elaterium*.

The agaricus muscarius is a well-known poisonous mushroom. Schulze properly remarks that its effects are narcotic; and Dr. Christison places it in the class of narcotico-acrid poisons. See sec. liv.

Schulze is much inclined to believe that the πήγανον ἄγριον here treated of is the *peganum harmala* of Linnæus, a plant intermediate between the ruta and melanthium. He is also disposed to think that the melanthium of the ancients was the *nigella sativa*, L. We are inclined to adopt this opinion from the text of Avicenna. (iv, 6, 1, 16.) Sprengel agrees with Anguillara and Dalechampius in opinion that the cactos was the *cynara carduncculus*, L., or cardoon artichoke, a variety of the C. scolymus. (Comment. in Dioscor.) Schweighaeuser inclines to the opinion of Villebrun, the French translator of Athenæus, who makes it to be the C. sylvestris latifolia, which he says grows commonly in Sicily at the present day. (In Deipnos. ii, 83.)

Under this head we may notice the treatment of poisoning by gum euphorbium, and the spurges, of which no mention is made by the Greek authorities on toxicology. For the Arabians, see Avicenna (iv, 6, 1, 4, 5); Rhases (Contin. xx, 2; ad Mansor. viii, 48); Alsaharavius (Pract. xxx, 1, 19.) The symptoms as given by them all are, violent pain and heat in the primæ viæ, with bloody discharges, and death, unless timely relief be given. Their remedies are immediate vomiting with hot water and oil, then administering demulcents, barley-water, and in the end, the theriac. Galen and Haly Abbas, in their treatises on the Theriac, recommend it in this case of poisoning.

The mezereon is not noticed by the Greeks or Romans either as a poison nor as a medicinal substance. The Arabians treat of it under both these heads. See Avicenna (iv, 6, 1); Rhases (ad Mansor. viii, 53.) The symptoms as given by them are violent vomiting and purging, for which they recommend sweet milk, butter, juleps, in the first place, and in extreme cases the theriac and sealed earth. The Arabian authorities confound their mezereon with the chamæleon of the Greeks, treated of in the thirty-seventh section of this book. The *dende* of Avicenna and Serapion was the strychnos colubrinus, according to Sprengel. (R. H. H. i, 250.)

Rhases classes the nux vomica along with the articles treated of in this section. He recommends us in all these cases to give warm water to promote the vomiting, and render it easier, and if violent convulsions come on, he directs the patient to be put into a warm bath, and anointed with hot oils. (Ad Mansor. viii, 49.) Serapion treats of it in his Materia Medica (163.) The Arabians also treat of the methel-nut.

We are unable to determine satisfactorily the nature of the *condisi*, which is treated of by the Arabians, under the present head. See Rhases (ad Mansor. viii, 49); Avicenna (iv, 6, 1, 16.) Alsaharavius calls it *cundes*. The symptoms, he says, are dryness of the nose, throat, and palate, sneezing, muttering delirium, pain of the stomach, and, unless speedy relief be brought, death. (Pract. xxx, 1, 24.) Ardoyn mentions that some referred it to the struthium; but the above characters do not at all apply to the soapwort (*saponaria officinalis*, L.), which is the στϱόυθιον of Theophrastus and Dioscorides. See further Sprengel (Comment. in Dioscor. i, 192.)

The sow-bread (*cyclamen Europæum*) is also treated of by the Arabians under this head. See Avicenna (iv, 6, 1, 16); Rhases (ad Mansor. viii, 59); Alsaharavius (Pract. xxx, 1, 24.) The symptoms, according to Alsaharavius, are swelling of the throat, and strong pain of the bowels. The sow-bread is treated of as an article of the Materia Medica by Dioscorides (ii, 193.)

Dioscorides (M. M. iv, 82) does not reckon the oleander (*nerium oleander*, L.) destructive to man, but the Arabians rank it among the deleterious substances, of a heating and desiccant nature; and recommend for it emetics, with the decoction of fenugreek, figs with honey, and the like. See Avicenna (iv, 6, 18); Alsaharavius (Pract. xxx, 1, 27); Rhases (ad Mansor. viii, 36.)

The anacardium, or Malacca bean, is treated of as a poison by Rhases (Contin. xx, 2; ad Mansor. viii, 35); Avicenna (iv, 6, 1, 9); Alsaharavius (Pract. xxx, 1, 42); Haly Abbas (Pract. iv, 50.) They all describe it as an irritant poison, and recommend emetics of animal and vegetable oils, with demulcents, to obviate the bad effects of it.

The apocynum, although not treated of by the ancient authorities on toxicology, is described as a deleterious substance by Dioscorides (Mat. Med. iv, 81); by Galen (De Simpl.); and by Pliny (H. N. xxv, 83.) It appears to be the *periploca Græca*, L.

Dioscorides and Pliny likewise reckon saffron, or the *crocus sativus*, a deleterious plant. Its deleterious action is very weak.

The atramentum sutorium, which was a solution of vitriol, was used as a poison. See Cicero (ad Familiar. ix, 21.)

LXV—ON DOMESTIC ARTICLES, SUCH AS WINE AND COLD WATER

Cold water when drunk in a great quantity, and much undiluted sweet wine, more especially after the bath, running, or violent exercises, bring on suffocation and pains. In such cases, venesection quickly had recourse to, and evacuation by clysters, remove the impending danger.

Commentary. Galen says, "Some by taking an immoderate draught of cold water have been instantly seized with dyspnœa, convulsions, and tremors; in a word, their whole nervous system has become affected." (Meth. Med. ix, 5.)

Dioscorides, Aëtius, and Actuarius concur in recommending the same mode of treatment as our author. The Arabians, however, treat those who have taken a draught of cold water unseasonably in a very different manner from the Greeks. Thus Rhases and Avicenna recommend undiluted wine internally, and the application of a plaster over the liver. The difference between the practice of the Greeks and Arabians may be thus accounted for. A large draught of cold drink may either threaten to prove fatal at once by producing a violent impression upon the nerves of the stomach, or it may superinduce symptoms resembling those of gastritis. In the former case the practice of the Arabians may seem most proper in order to support the heat and powers of the system, whereas that of the Greeks will be indicated when inflammatory symptoms have come on; and, indeed, even the Arabians bled under these circumstances. (Avicenna, iv, 61, 31.) For an immoderate draught of pure wine which has been taken unseasonably, the Arabian authorities concur with the Greek in recommending immediate evacuation of the stomach and venesection, to which they add cold water or whey, with troches of camphor. See in particular Avicenna (iv, 6, 1, 31.)

APPENDIX TO BOOK V

As no better opportunity is likely to occur, we shall in this place give a short notice of two subjects connected with medical practice, which are entirely omitted by our author.

ON FEIGNED DISEASES, AND THE DETECTION OF THEM

Galen, we believe, is the only ancient author who has treated professedly of the detection of simulated diseases. He begins his short treatise on this head with remarking, that persons feign diseases from various motives, and that it is expected the physicians should detect such impostures. That, for example, inflammation, erysipelas, and œdema, when produced artificially, ought to be distinguished from the same diseases when they originate in constitutional causes. He adds, that hæmoptysis, hæmatemesis, and bloody discharges from the bowels, are often simulated. Hæmoptysis is simulated by opening a vein in the gums, and sucking blood from it while one affects to cough. Others, he says, affect dementia, fatuity, and insanity, all which cases the vulgar expect that the physician should detect. Inward pain, such as that of colic, he had often known to be simulated, and relates briefly an interesting case in point. He remarks, that experience and natural sagacity will enable a man to expose all impositions of this nature. He gives a very interesting account of the manner in which he detected the nature of a swelling at the knee, that had been produced intentionally by the juice of thapsia (*thapsia garganica*, deadly carrot?) Feigned inward pains, he remarks, may often be distinguished from the real by the aversion which the *malingerer* discovers to swallow medicines, which he would be anxious to have given him if he were actually in acute pain; and adds, that the state of the pulse, and the other symptoms of intestinal diseases, will assist in making the detection. (Quomodo coarg. sint qui fing. se Ægrot. t. iii, 388, ed. Basil.)

ON PROFESSIONAL IMPOSTORS

Rhases has an interesting chapter on this head. The frauds of impostors, he says, are more numerous than could be contained in his whole work. Some of them, he adds, pretend to be able to cure epilepsy, and having made a crucial incision in the back part of the head, they extract from the wound something which they hold in their hands, and thus impose upon people. Others, in like manner, cause it to be believed that they extract a small lizard by the nostrils. Some of these characters, he says, make it be believed that they remove films from the eye, by secretly introducing a small membrane into the eye, and taking it out again. Others manage to create a belief that they suck water from the ear with a reed. Others also make it be believed that they extract worms from the ears or teeth. Others practice a trick by which they obtain the credit of extracting the ranula below the tongue. Why should I mention those, he adds, who introduce pieces of bone into wounds and ulcers, and afterwards extract them? He says, it is not uncommon for these impostors to sound a man for the stone, pretend to find one, perform the operation, and exhibit a calculus which they themselves had introduced secretly into the incision. Others pretend to cure piles, make incisions about the anus, and form ulcers there which did not exist before. Certain of them affect by scarifications and other means to suck the vitreous humour from the hip-joint, while they exhibit something of the kind which they themselves have introduced. There are some who undertake to collect all the infirmities of the body into one spot, and then extract them; for this pretended object they raise an itching and violent heat in some place by means of *alkekengi* (winter cherry); and having accomplished this they exact a fee for removing the uneasiness from the spot, which they do by anointing it with oil. There are others who will make a man believe that he has swallowed hairs, glass, or the like; and then tickling his throat with a feather, and making him vomit, they exhibit the substance in question as if it had been brought up. Thus, he adds, they often do much mischief, and sometimes are guilty of culpable homicide. He concludes by warning sensible people to be upon their guard against such wretches. (Ad Mansor. vii. 27.)

BOOK VI

SECT

I—PREFACE TO THE SURGICAL PART

Having divided the treatise on the surgical matters into what relates to manual operations on the flesh, and the account of fractures and dislocations of bones, we shall begin with what relates to the flesh, observing there our accustomed brevity. Beginning therefore, again with the upper parts, we shall first give an account of the operations on the head, more particularly of the burning of the vertex.

Commentary. This book contains the most complete system of operative surgery which has come down to us from ancient times. We shall have occasion also to refer frequently to Celsus, who, in the last two books of his work, has treated of surgical operations with considerable accuracy. Our author appears to have been wholly unacquainted with him; but when did a Greek writer ever acknowledge himself under obligations to a Roman? Haly Abbas, in the 9th book of his 'Practica,' copies almost everything from Paulus. Albucasis gives more original matter on surgery than any other Arabian author, and yet, as will be seen from our commentary, he is indebted for whole chapters to Paulus. In the 'Continens' of Rhases, that precious repository of ancient opinions on medical subjects, if there be any surgical information not to be found in our author, it is mostly derived from Antyllus and Archigenes. As to the other authorities, although we will occasionally have to explain their opinions upon particular subjects, no one has treated of surgery in a systematical manner; for even Avicenna, who treats so fully of everything else connected with medicine, is defective in his account of surgical operations; and the descriptions which he does give of them are almost all borrowed from our author. The account of fractures and dislocations given by Hippocrates and his commentator Galen may be pronounced almost complete; but the information which they supply upon most other surgical subjects is scanty.

II—ON BURNING OF THE HEAD FOR OPHTHALMIA, DYSPNŒA, AND ELEPHANTIASIS

In ophthalmia, occasioned by a defluxion from above, and in dyspnœa, produced by a redundance of a recrementitious humour which is sent from the head down to the chest, and by lodging there proves injurious to the parts contained in it, they burn the middle of the head in this manner. Having first shaven the parts about the vertex, they apply cauteries shaped like olive-kernels and burn the skin down to the bone, scraping the bone after the falling off of the eschar. Some by burning even the bone itself make a small scale exfoliate from it, in order to allow the humours of the head to perspire and be evacuated the more readily; and for this purpose they keep the ulcer open for some time and then allow it to cicatrize. In treating elephantiasis some burn five eschars in the head, one anteriorly above the part called the bregma; another, below this, a little above the forehead, at the extremity of the hairs; another, at the part called the occiput; two others at the parts called the squamous plates, above the ears, one on the right side and another on the left; and thus, by the removal of several scales, they procure the evaporation and discharge of the collection of thick humours in the deep-seated parts of the head, and prevent the sight from being injured. They also apply another cautery on the spleen, in order to remedy the prime organ in the formation of the melancholic humour by the eschar formed in the skin.

Commentary. See Hippocrates (de Visu); Aretæus (de curat. Morb. Chron. i, 1); Celsus (iii, 23, and vi, 6); Cælius Aurelianus (Morb. Acut. i, i, and Morb. Chron. i, 4); Aëtius (vi, 50); Actuarius (Meth. Med. iii, 2); Rhases (Cont. xxvii, 1, 24); Albucasis (Chirurg. i); Mesue (de Ægr. Capitis); Avicenna (iii, 1); Haly Abbas (Pract. ix, 69); Avenzoar (I, 9, 17).

The use of the actual cautery in surgical practice is often alluded to by the classical authors. See a collection of these passages in Dr. Blomfield's edition of the 'Agamemnon' of Æschylus (822.) Consult also Gataker's 'Marcus Antoninus' (v. 193); and Boissonade's 'Anecdota Græca' (vol. ii, p. 311.) A very elaborate and sensible account of the use of the cautery in the practice of surgery is given by Vegetius. (Malomed. i, 28.)

Hippocrates, or whoever was the author of the work referred to above, applied the cautery to the head very freely in diseases of the eyes and other complaints.

Aretæus directs us, in cases of cephalæa and epilepsy, to perforate the bone as far as the diploe, and afterwards to burn it until the dura mater is separated from the bone. He admits, however, that it is a harsh remedy.

Celsus directs us, as an ultimum remedium in epileptic cases, to form issues with a burning iron upon the occiput and at the juncture of the first vertebra with the head.

Aëtius speaks of burning the head in nearly the same terms as our author. He directs us to avoid the muscular parts. Actuarius does the same.

Cælius Aurelianus, however, disapproves of this practice in cases of cephalæa and epilepsy.

The Arabians were even more partial than the Greeks to burning the head in these and other complaints. See in particular Albucasis, whose description is very minute. In cases of cephalæa he recommends the cautery to be applied to the occiput, but cautions against touching the bone lest it produce violent pain. He directs us to be careful to avoid muscles, nerves, and arteries. Avicenna, Rhases, Mesue, and Haly Abbas recommend the operation, in the most unqualified terms, as a powerful remedy in the cases mentioned by our author. Avenzoar, however, condemns the unguarded application of the burning iron to the head.

Guido de Cauliaco recommends the cautery in cases of hydrocephalus (ii, 2, 10). Brunus also applied it for hydrocephalus, (ii, 17.) But see in particular Lanfrancus (III, iii, 18.)

Fabricius ab Aquapendente states that from the most ample experience he had ascertained the good effects of applying the cautery over the sutures of the skull in various complaints, especially asthma, consumption, and all cold defluxions from the head to the chest. He gives a full account of the operation. (Œuvres Chirurg. ii, 1.) But see De Haën. (Rat. Méd. t. iii, p. vi, c. 6.)

III—ON HYDROCEPHALUS

The hydrocephalic affection is so named from the peculiarity of the fluid, it being of a watery consistence. It occurs in infants, owing to their heads being improperly squeezed by midwives during parturition, or from some other obscure cause; or from the rupture of a vessel or vessels, and the extravasated blood being converted into an inert fluid; or from rarefaction, the matter exuding and lodging between the skin and the pericranium. For the fluid is formed either between the pericranium and the skin, or between the pericranium and the bone, or between the bone and the meninx. In those cases, therefore, in which the fluid is formed between the skin and the pericranium, there is a soft tumour, all of one colour, and without pain, accompanied with an elevated swelling, having only a thin substance intervening between it and the fingers, readily yielding and again resuming its form. When it is seated between the pericranium and the bone, all the other appearances are the same, but the swelling is harder, yields more slowly, seems to be felt through thicker substances, and is more painful. When the fluid is seated between the meninx and the bone, there will still be a swelling, but not of so yielding a nature, nor so easily felt, only it yields to the application of strong pressure; for the bones of infants, being recently formed, are of a more yielding nature; and this is more especially the case when, owing to enlargement of the sutures, the fluid escapes outwards. This is readily ascertained from the circumstance, that by pressure of the fluid it retreats to the deep-seated parts. In such cases the pain is greater, the whole head is distended, the forehead projects outwards, the eyes are fixed and shed tears frequently. In these cases we reprobate any surgical interference, although some remove a piece of the bone by trepanning, as will be described in the section on fractures of the bones of the head. But if the fluid be formed between the skin and the pericranium, and the swelling be small, we may make one transverse incision through the middle. But if the fluid is seated between the pericranium and the bone, and the tumour is large, we make two incisions intersecting one another in the middle; or if it is still larger we may make three imitating the form of the Greek letter H. After the operation, having evacuated the fluid and applied suitable compresses, we bind it up, and soak it with wine and oil until the third day; after which, having loosed the bandages, we may cure it by the application of pledgets; or, if the bone is long of incarnating we may scrape it lightly.

Commentary. See Hippocrates (de Morbis, ii, 15); Celsus (iv, 2); Aëtius (vi, 1); Galeni (ut aiunt) Isagoge; Antyllus (apud Nicetam); Avicenna (iii, 1; iv, 2); Avenzoar (I, 9, 17); Albucasis (Chirurg. ii, 1); Haly Abbas (Pract. ix, 16); Rhases (Contin. xxvii; and ad Mansor. ii, 25.)

Hippocrates gives an interesting account of water in the brain, the symptoms of which, as described by him, are pain in the opening of the head and temples, rigor, fever, double vision, impatience of sounds, vomiting of phlegm, &c. He recommends emetics, caputpurgia, and afterwards purgatives. He also makes mention of hellebore and sternutatories, and even directs us to perforate the skull, or, in other words, to trephine it.

Celsus describes only the hydrocephalus externus. He recommends us to use stimulant applications to the head, such as sinapisms, and if this treatment does not succeed, he directs us to use the scalpel. The case, otherwise, is to be treated like dropsy, with sudorifics, exercise, friction, and diuretics.

Our author's description is mostly abridged from Aëtius, who gives an extract from Leonidas. Even when the fluid is collected within the skull he directs us to let it out, provided it is in such quantity as to occasion a separation of the suture.

The account of the disease, given by Antyllus, in the Collection of Nicetas is nearly the same as our author's. He speaks favorably of the operation only in cases in which the water is collected externally to the bone.

In the 'Isagoge,' generally ascribed to Galen, it is directed, when the water is collected below the skin on the pericranium, to evacuate it by making two or three straight incisions; and when immediately below the bone, to perforate it; but the case in which the fluid is seated between the membrane and the brain is pronounced to be utterly incurable.

Rhases borrows his account mostly from Antyllus and our author. Upon his own authority, however, he recommends bandages with compresses. He also approves of applying the actual cautery over the sutures. He further recommends friction and burning the temporal veins.

Avicenna borrows freely from Aëtius and our author, and supplies no new views of practice. When water is collected in the anterior ventricles of the brain, Avenzoar, although in general no advocate for the actual cautery, directs us to apply it over the sutures.

Albucasis says that he had only known hydrocephalus internus in infancy, and in every case it had proved fatal. However, he describes the operation of evacuating the collection in much the same terms as the Greeks. He warns the operator to avoid wounding an artery, lest the evacuation of blood should occasion immediate death. Alsaharavius mentions the frequent occurrence of the disease in sheep. Haly's treatment is the same as our author's.

The hydrocephalus externus is now scarcely mentioned, and the existence of such a case has been even questioned. Van Swieten allows the reality of it, but says that it is of rare occurrence. (Comment. 1217.) We are disposed to think that the cases described by our author must have been collections of lymph, or pus occasioned by external injuries forming between the integuments and the bone. Modern pathologists admit the reality of collections of serum and pus between the bone and the dura mater. We may further mention that the earlier modern authorities approve of the cautery in the present case. See Guido de Cauliaco (ii, 2, 10.)

The late Baron Larrey was a decided advocate for the application of moxa in this complaint. Henricus Regius directs us to evacuate the water slowly by making a small incision and introducing a silver canula. (Animad. Medic. 13.) Though recent experience does not give much encouragement to the operation, it sometimes happens that it is attended with success.

Fabricius gives the same account of these cases as the ancients. (Œuv. Chir. ii. 22.)

IV—ON ARTERIOTOMY

In chronic defluxions of the eyes, and in the affection of vertigo, we are in the practice of dividing the arteries behind the ears. Having, therefore, shaven the hind part of the head, and marked with the fingers the position of the artery, which is easily discovered by its pulsation, and then having marked out the line of an incision two fingers in length with black ink, we cut down to the bone. When this does not succeed we must measure a distance of three fingers' breadth from the ears, and then operate by making a transverse division of the artery until blood flow *per saltum*, and the instrument strike the bone. After a moderate evacuation of blood, the pericranium is to be divided, lest it become inflamed from the distension; and having scraped the bone we apply a wedge-like tent of linen to the wounds, and accomplish the cure by pledgets. But if, after all, the bone remain bare, we must have recourse to scraping it in like manner.

Commentary. Our author's description is mostly abridged from Aëtius (vi, 90), who copies from Severus.

This operation is minutely described by Albucasis. (Chirurg. ii, 2.) He directs us to shave the head, and rub the parts behind the ears with a rough cloth until the arteries become visible. The course of the vessels is to be marked with ink, and they are to be divided with a sharp scalpel, the incision penetrating down to the bone. He says, however, that if the surgeon choose, he may introduce the scalpel below the vessel, and cut upwards. The length of the incision is to be two fingers' breadth. Blood, he remarks, springs from an artery per saltum. About six ounces, more or less, may be taken.

The operation is likewise mentioned by Avicenna (Cantic. iv,) and Averrhoes (in Cantic.); by Rhases (ad Mansor. vii, 21); and is described in exactly the same terms as our author's by Haly Abbas. (Pract. ix, 4.)

V—ON ANGIOLOGY, OR SECTION OF THE TEMPORAL VESSELS, AND ON BURNING THE SAME

In hemicrania and in chronic or acute defluxions, when the eyes are affected with a hot and acrid defluxion, so as to occasion heat of the temporal muscles with swelling, every one approves of angiology for the cure of them. Having, therefore, first shaven the hairs of the temples, and noted the part with our fingers, we must use warm fomentations, and apply a bandage round the neck; and, when the vessels become visible, having marked their course with ink, we must draw the skin aside with our left hand or the fingers of an assistant, and make a superficial incision along the vessel; then cutting quite through, and stretching the parts with hooks, and exposing the vessel by means of the instruments used in operations on membranous parts, we must raise it up when it is separated all around. If it be small, having stretched and twisted it with a blind hook, we may divide it through, so as to be able to seize upon part of it. But if it be large, we must apply a double ligature under it with a needle, either a piece of raw flax, or some other strong thing; and, in the first place, making a straight opening into the vessel with a scalpel used in venesection, and taking away a moderate quantity of blood, we must tie the ligatures at both extremities of the exposed vessel, and cutting the intermediate part, we may remove it either immediately, or at the time of loosing the dressings. Some, without dividing the vessels at all, burn them to a sufficient depth with burning-irons shaped like olive-kernels. After the operation we must use pledgets of dry charpie, and put on an oblong compress (*splenium*) with a bandage. After the removal of these dressings, we must accomplish the cure by incarnating powders, applications on pledgets, and cicatrizing remedies; the threads and ligatures having previously dropped out from putrefaction.

Commentary. The author of the Hippocratic treatise (de Morbis in Homine, c. 49) recommends us to open the temporal veins for obstinate headaches; and, if this does not effect a cure, he directs us to burn them.

Celsus describes both operations very distinctly. He directs us to apply a ligature round the neck, so as to make the vessels swell, and then, having marked the course of the vessels with ink, to remove the ligature, and open the veins. When a sufficient quantity of blood is discharged, the part is to be burnt with slender irons cautiously about the temples, for fear of wounding the temporal muscles, but more boldly between the forehead and the vertex, so as to produce exfoliation of a scale of the bone. He also speaks favorably of cutting the vessels in the temples and upper part of the head. (vii, 7.)

Aëtius gives nearly the same description as our author. The part which relates to the burning is taken from Leonidas (vii, 93.)

Angiology is briefly described in the 'Isagoge' of Galen. A minute description is given by Albucasis. He recommends the operation as a remedy for inveterate cases of hemicrania, catarrh, and cephalæa. He directs us to shave the hairs about the temples, and to continue to do so until the artery appears. It is known, he remarks, by its pulsation. When it does not readily make its appearance, he recommends us to apply a cloth round the patient's head, and to rub the place with a rough towel. Then, he says, take a scalpel, and make an incision so as to lay bare the artery, which seize with a hook, and separate from the surrounding parts, and if the vessel is small, cut out a proper piece of it, and allow from three to six ounces of blood to flow. But if the vessel is large, bind it in two places with strong silk threads, or strips of raw cloth (*alhohod*), so that it may not drop out before the wound is consolidated. Then cut out the part between the two ligatures. He directs us to dress the wound as recommended by our author. He also mentions the operation of burning the temporal veins as being one that is less serious than angiology. (Chirurg. ii, 3.)

Jesu Haly's account of the operations of tying and burning the temporal arteries is very distinct. (iii, 25.)

Haly Abbas describes the operations of cutting out and burning the temporal vessels in nearly the same terms as our author. (Pract. ix, 70.)

Rhases mentions that the celebrated Archigenes recommended the temporal veins to be burnt for epilepsy. (Contin. i.)

The veterinary surgeons burnt the temporal veins in diseases of cattle. See Vegetius (Mulomed. ii, 16.)

We are inclined to think that it was the temporal veins and not the arteries which were cut out and burnt by the Greek surgeons in this operation. It will be seen, however, that the Arabians direct us to cut out a portion of the artery; at least this is sufficiently clear in the description of Albucasis, for he states decidedly that the vessel to be secured will be recognized by its pulsation, and he further recommends us to apply beforehand a ligature about the head, and not about the neck as directed by our author, whereby it is obvious that the arteries and not the veins would become distended; these observations apply also to Jesu Haly's description. As Celsus, like our author, directs the ligature to be applied round the neck (cervix ante modice deliganda est), we may suppose that his operation related to the veins. From his using the word venæ indeed no inference can be drawn, as he applies it indiscriminately to arteries and veins. We are at a loss what to determine respecting the description given by Haly Abbas, for although the vessel that is secured be called arteria, the ligature or strip of cloth is directed to be applied round the collum. Where the mistake lies in this case we cannot venture to conjecture, and leave it to be found out by some person who has access to the MS. of the original. For our part we may exclaim with a celebrated German scholar,—"Felices sæpe prædicavimus Bochartum, Plempium, Celsium, Hydium, Casirium, quibus usus codicum Arabicorum concessus erat." (Sprengel, Rei Herbariæ Historia, i, 239.)

Fabricius ab Aquapendente describes the operation as relating to the veins (Œuv. Chir. ii, 3.) Tagliacozzi, however, seems to refer it to the arteries. It thus appears that there is a good deal of uncertainty regarding this ancient operation.

VI—ON HYPOSPATHISMUS

This surgical operation derived its name from the kind of instrument used in it. We have recourse to it when a copious and hot defluxion is determined to the eyes. The face is ruddy, and about the forehead there is a sensation as of worms or ants passing along it. Having therefore first shaven the hairs about the forehead, we must permit the lower jaw to move, and avoiding the place where the temporal muscles are seen to act, we are to make three straight and parallel incisions on the forehead, each having the length of two fingers, and descending to the bone, and being at the distance of about three fingers' breadth from one another. After the incision we apply the instrument called hypospathister, and extend the division from the left temple to the middle incision, dividing all the intermediate substance along with the pericranium; then we push a spatula from the middle one to the rest, and applying the point of a sharp-pointed knife to the first division, so that its sharp side may be turned to the flesh within the skin, and the blunt one to the bone, we push it as far as the middle division, cutting through all the vessels which descend from the head to the eyes, but not comprehending the external skin. And again we push it from the middle to the last incision, cutting through the vessels in like manner. After a moderate evacuation of blood, having squeezed out the coagula, and made three twisted tents, we are to put one into each division, and applying a compress soaked in water, we must secure it with a bandage. Next day we bathe not only the ulcers, but likewise the temporal muscles, and the ears with wine and oil, on account of the inflammation; and on the third day having removed the dressings, we must have recourse to copious affusion, and afterwards complete the cure suitably with tents out of basilicon dissolved in rose-oil.

Commentary. See Aëtius (vii, 92); Albucasis (Chirurg. ii, 4); Haly Abbas (Pract. ix, 7.) This operation is better described by our author than by any of the others. Celsus, although he describes several grave operations for the relief of defluxions on the eyes, makes no mention of it. Aëtius barely alludes to it in general terms. It must have been a very formidable operation, and for that reason perhaps, has been entirely abandoned in moderate times. Even Albucasis speaks of it as being an operation which was performed by the ancients; from which language we may suppose that it had been given up in his time. His description of it is evidently taken from our author. Haly Abbas describes the operation very distinctly. Three longitudinal incisions at the distance of three fingers' breadth from one another are to be made in the forehead down to the bone, then a knife, or some such instrument, is to be introduced so as to divide the parts between the longitudinal incisions, sparing only the outer skin.

VII—ON PERISCYPHISMUS

When many deep-seated vessels send a copious defluxion to the eyes, we have recourse to the operation called periscyphismus. These cases are attended with such symptoms as these: in the first place you will find the patient's eyes atrophied and small, weak of sight, the canthi corroded, and the eyelids ulcerated, the hairs falling off, with a discharge of very thin, acrid, and hot tears; there is a deep-seated pain in the head of an acute and violent character, and there is frequent sneezing. Having first shaved the head as aforesaid, and avoiding the place where the temporal muscles play, we make a transverse incision, beginning at the left temple and ending at the other. The incision must have its terminations where there are no muscles, its direction being a little above the forehead, and we must avoid the coronal suture. Leonidas directs the incision to be made along the middle of the forehead. When the bone is laid bare we may keep the parts asunder with tents and plenty of pledgets, and bind the extremities of the division; and, as we formerly stated, bathe with wine and oil. After loosing them, if the inflammation is on the decline, we may scrape the bone until it begin to incarnate, and accomplish the cure by a mode of practice calculated to promote incarnation, using the incarnative powders; among which is that containing of wheaten flour, p. ij; of colophonian rosin, p. j; and that called the cephalic, and those incarnatives prepared from pumice-stone. For, when the skin is thickened by a dense cicatrix, and the mouths of the vessels constricted, the defluxion is prevented from being determined to the eyes as before.

Commentary. See Aëtius (vii, 93); Pseudo Galen (Isagoge); Albucasis (Chirurg. ii, 5); Haly Abbas (Pract. ix, 18.)

It is evident that this operation is neither more nor less than a complete division of the integuments of the head from temple to temple; of course it must even have been more dangerous than the operation treated of in the last section. Aëtius, Haly Abbas, and Albucasis describe it in the same terms as our author. The periscyphismus and hypospathismus are briefly noticed in the 'Isagoge.'

Fabricius ab Aquapendente treats of these operations among those of the ancients, *qui ne sont plus en usage* (Œ. C. ii, iv); even Tagliacozzi speaks of them as being cruel and dangerous. However, a surgical operation, similar in principle, called the "long issue of the scalp," is still practised in certain hospitals of Great Britain. See the 'Transactions of the Provincial Association,' (vol. xi.)

VIII—ON SUTURE OF THE UPPER EYELID, AND OTHER MODES OF OPERATING FOR TRICHIASIS

Distichiasis is a preternatural growth of hairs, superadded to the natural order of hairs of the eyelids; and derives its origin from a defluxion, when there happens to be a flow upon the part of a humour which is not pungent or acrid; for that which is more acrid, saltish, or otherwise pungent, when it lodges in these parts, consumes the natural series of hairs. For this state then we sometimes have recourse to the suture of the upper eyelid, and sometimes also for phalangosis when the eyelid inclines inward, the phalanx or row of the hairs being inverted; and sometimes for relaxation of the eyelid, when the natural row of hairs hurts the ball of the eye. Having placed the patient on a seat, either before us or on the left hand, we turn the upper eyelid outwards, and, if it has long hairs, we take hold of them between the index-finger and thumb of the left hand; but if they are very short we push a needle having a thread, through the middle of the tarsus from within outwards; then stretching the eyelid with the left hand by means of his thread, with the point of a scalpel held in the right hand, having folded out the eyelid and everted it, behind the thread we make the under-incision within the hairs which irritate the eye, extending from the larger canthus to the smaller, along the tarsus. After this subsection, having extracted the thread, and putting a small compress under the thumb of the left hand, we stretch the eyebrow upwards. Then arranging other small compresses on the canthi at the extremities, we direct the assistant who stands behind to stretch the eyelid by means of them. Then by means of the scalpel used for sutures we make the first incision, called the veruted (shaped like a verutum or short dart) a little above the hairs, which are in their natural state, extending from canthus to canthus, and penetrating only the depth of the skin; and afterwards we perform the incision called the lunated, beginning at the same place as the former, and carrying it upwards to such a height as to comprehend the whole redundant skin, and ending in like manner as it did. Thus the whole skin comprehended within the incisions will have the shape of a myrtle leaf, of which portion, having perforated the angle on the right hand with a hook (tenaculum), we dissect away the whole skin: then washing away the clots with a sponge, we unite the lips of the incision by three or four sutures, beginning at the middle, and passing the needle itself through the under-section. The thread should be made of wool; and having cut away the superfluity of the thread, not close to the sutures, but so as to leave a superfluity of three fingers' breadth, we stretch this remainder along the forehead and fasten it by means of any of the agglutinative plasters. But the hairs of the eyelid are to be freed from the sutures with the point of a needle. Such is the common and safe mode of performing this surgical operation. Some avoid the dissection of the skin, and therefore after the under-incision, having stretched the redundant skin by means of the forceps used in operations on the eyelids, they cut it off with a scalpel, and apply sutures as described above. But if the irritation from the hairs is produced only by a part of the eyelid, it will be proper to confine the operation to that part. Then soaking the compresses in oxycrate, and laying them on the part, we secure them with bandages, continuing to moisten the dressings with diluted oxycrate until the third day; after which we remove them, and cutting away the superfluous parts of the threads, we anoint the eyelids either with saffron, glaucium, or some of the anti-inflammatory collyria, such as that formed of saffron and roses. But if the sutures inflame, we apply some one of the softening plasters, and soothe the eye by an injection of eggs mixed with milk. When the ligatures slacken we cut and extract them. I know a certain person who having made the dissection of the skin of the eyelid, as mentioned above, did not have recourse to sutures, but effected the cure with a healing ointment. For when the wound cicatrised, the eyelid being somewhat contracted, forced the hairs to incline outwards. In like manner, another person not practising the dissection of the eyelid, nor the two external incisions, but only making the under-incision, stretched with his fingers or by a hook the fold of the eyelid, two reeds or plates of the same length as the eyelid, and as broad as for venesection, he twisted a ligature round it at both its extremities; and thus the whole skin behind not being nourished, and on that account being deprived of life, fell off within ten, or at most fifteen days along with the reeds or plates, so as to leave scarcely any scar.

Commentary. On suture of the upper eyelid, and other methods of operating for distichiasis, see Hippocrates (de Victu acut. 66); Aëtius (vii, 71, 72); Celsus (vii, 7); Albucasis (Chir. ii, 11); Rhases (Divis. i, 30; ad Mansor. ix, 26; Contin. ii, 3); Avicenna (iii, iii, 3, 32); Avenzoar (i, 8, 6); Serapion (ii, 7); Mesue (ii, 18); Jesu Hali (ii, 10); Canamusali (vi, 26); Haly Abbas (Pract. ix, 19); Vegetius (Mulom. ii, 15.)

The description of the operation given by Aëtius from Leonidas being nearly the same as that described by our author, we shall confine ourselves to an abridged account of it, and merely make a few remarks to illustrate the description of Paulus. In order to facilitate the operation, he recommends the operator to have two assistants instead of one, as directed by our author. He also recommends him, in the first place, to mark with ink the portion of skin which requires to be cut out. He then directs him to make the under-incision, by which he seems to have meant an incision within the ciliary hairs along the tarsus, and extending from canthus to canthus. He recommends it to be made pretty deep, and even in certain cases suggests the propriety of making two under-incisions, one as above described within the ciliary hairs, in order to relax the tarsus; and the other upon the preternatural hairs. He next directs first a transverse incision to be made along the eyelid above the ciliary hairs, and then a lunated one beginning and ending like the other, after which the skin, thus separated, is to be dissected out. He recommends the edges to be united by means of five sutures, one in the middle and two at each extremity of the incisions. The other steps of the operation are exactly the same as those described by our author, and cannot be misunderstood. Hippocrates describes an operation for trichiasis, which Heister thought the same as that recommended by Aëtius, but the description is so obscure that we must confess our inability to explain it.

Celsus describes three methods of cure for trichiasis. 1. By burning the roots of the hairs. 2. The anabrochismus, which will be explained in the 13th section. 3. The anarrhaphè or suture, as described by Aëtius and our author. As the steps of the operation described by him are almost exactly the same as those of Aëtius, we need not dwell upon the explanation of them. Lest, however, there should be any misapprehension about the under-incision, we shall give his directions about it in his own language: "præter hoc, in superiore palpebrâ sub pilis ipsis incidenda linea est ut ab inferiore parte diducti pili sursum spectant; idque si levis inclinatio est, solum satis est." Instead of five sutures, as directed by Aëtius, he recommends only three.

Albucasis states that there are four modes of curing trichiasis. 1. By the actual cautery. 2. By the potential cautery. 3. By incision and the suture, which operation he describes at great length. He directs us in the first place to evert the eyelid, either by taking hold of the ciliary hairs, or by passing a needle, armed with a hair, through the tarsus, and raising the eyelid with it. He then, like the others, directs us to make the under-incision within the ciliary hairs, from the greater canthus to the smaller, to cut out the redundant skin of the eyelid, and unite the surfaces with sutures. In short, his operation is exactly the same as our author's. He mentions, however, another method of making the incision by elevating the redundant fold of the skin with hooks or a trident, and cutting it off with a pair of scissors. 4. The fourth method consists of making the under-incision, as in the last operation, and then twisting the redundant skin firmly about reeds or small pieces of wood until it mortifies: after which the wound is to be cured upon general principles.

Serapion's account of the operation is defective, and need not be particularly noticed. Canamasuli directs us to cut out the hairs and burn the part with a cautery of gold.

Avicenna merely mentions, in very general terms, that the cure may be accomplished by agglutinative applications, by the cautery, or by excision.

Mesue briefly describes four modes of cure: 1. By means of agglutinants. 2. By passing a needle, armed with a hair, through the tarsus, as will be explained in the 13th section. 3. By plucking out the hairs and cauterising the part. 4. By applying medicines calculated to prevent the renewal of the hairs after they have been plucked out.

Jesu Hali's description of these operations is very circumstantial; he speaks of cutting out the piece of skin with a fine pair of scissors.

Rhases states that the cure of trichiasis may be effected by burning the roots of the hairs with a red-hot needle, or by making the excision of the superfluous skin of the eyelid. He also makes mention of the treatment by agglutinants. In his great work, the 'Continens,' he briefly notices the four operations described by Albucasis. He appears to have approved very much of the burning. He also describes the operation with the reeds or pieces of wood.

Avenzoar mentions four methods of curing inversion of the ciliary hairs. 1. By everting the upper eyelid and securing it with agglutinants until the roots of the hairs have been cauterised with a rod of gold. This method he does not approve of. 2. By extirpating the offending hairs and applying the blood of a bat to the places from which they were torn. 3. By making an excision of the superfluous skin of the eyelid, and afterwards applying sutures. He alludes, we suppose, to the operation of Aëtius. 4. By twisting the skin about small reeds or tubes, in the manner described by our author and Albucasis.

Haly Abbas accurately describes the four following operations: 1. By excision and the suture. He directs the under-incision not to be made deep. 2. By twisting the hairs into the fold of a silk thread and flattening it to the forehead. 3. By the actual cautery. 4. By the potential cautery.

We will give the description of the veterinary surgeon, Vegetius, in his own words: "Non longe a pilis ab interiori parte scalpello plagam dabis in cute palpebræ, post forficibus per longum ad mensuram oculi fasciolam præcides, et impositis fibulis consucs palpebram foris versus, ut oculus sine deformitate recipiat visum et gratiam naturalem."

It is to be remarked that Albucasis, Jesu Hali, and Vegetius speak of cutting out the superfluous skin of the eyelid with a pair of scissors, as was done by Scarpa.

All the ancient operations for trichiasis are described by Guido de Cauliaco (vi, 2.) The mode of cure by twisting the skin about small reeds until the parts slough is still generally practised in China. The Chinese surgeons grasp the fold between two slips of bamboo, which being tightly fastened at their ends perform the office of a ligature.

IX—ON BURNING OF THE EYELIDS BY MEDICINES

The burning of the eyelids with caustic medicines was reprobated, in a word, by all the ancients, lest the acrimony of the application should prove injurious to the eyes; and because when the burning was carried to too great an extent the affection called lagophthalmos was produced, in which case the eyelids cannot be shut, and the vision is apt to be injured by everything that comes in the way. But since many who suffer from the irritation of the ciliary hairs are not able to endure even the name of the operation by suture, we are compelled from necessity, against our will, to have recourse to burning by medicine. The following is a composition of that kind: of quicklime, p. ij; of Gallic or common soap, p. ij; and some add of aphronitrum, p. iv. These things being pounded with strained ley, or soap ley, or some other ley, as that of figs or of oaks, and being mixed with the urine of a young man not come to maturity, we apply to the eyelid, upon the knob of a specillum, the part touched having the shape of a myrtle leaf; and we burn to the extent comprehended in the operation by suture. The skin being burnt at the first application, we remove so much of it with a sponge, and apply the medicine a second time, allowing it to remain until the part blacken; and if it does not blacken we apply it a third time. When the skin is blackened and the eschar also formed, we must clean away the medicine and have recourse to bathing and washing until the eschar drop off; after which it will be proper to complete the cure by means of pledgets of charpie and emollient collyria.

Commentary. None of the other authorities describe this method of cure so minutely as our author, except Haly Abbas, who evidently copies from him. (Pract. ix, 71.) Rhases and Albucasis, however, also mention the operation. They direct us to burn the part with a preparation of quicklime and soap, with the addition of some caustic lixivia, *or* leys. These ancient leys, *or* lixivian ashes, appear to have been preparations of potass more or less pure. We need scarcely remark that these applications must have resembled the caustic paste, now used for forming issues. The method of treatment here described is, in principle, much the same as that performed by Quadri with sulphuric acid. A caustic paste very similar to that now used is described by Guy of Caulico. (vii, 1.)

The strained ley, of which mention is made by Paulus, was probably the same as the calx colata of Cælius Aurelianus. (Tard. Pass, v, 1.) It appears to have been an impure preparation of potass with the addition of some lime.

It is the same, we suppose, as the πρωτόστακτον mentioned in the Third Book of this work. The calx colata would seem to have been identical with the Vienna paste now used in the treatment of varix. A composition for burning the eyelids, mentioned by Jesu Hali, contains lime, prepared beans, nitre, and sal ammoniac, formed into a paste with the water of soap and pure myrrh. Jesu, however, does not much approve of this method of treatment.

X—ON LAGOPHTHALMOS OR HARE-EYE

Those persons are said to have hare-eyes who have the eyelids drawn upwards. This complaint arises either naturally or from the cicatrix of a wound, and this may have occurred spontaneously, or from the operations of the suture or burning (as just mentioned) having been improperly performed; in which case even a moderate relief can only be accomplished when the eyelid is sufficiently thick. For we must divide the cicatrix, and having separated the lips with a tent, use bandages until the cure is completed, avoiding such things as are very desiccative, and having recourse to those which are fatty and relaxing, such as the juice of fenugreek poured on the part, and the ointment prepared with four ingredients called basilicon, applied on a tent.

Commentary. See Celsus (vii, 7); Aëtius (vii, 71); Albucasis (Chirurg. ii, 13); Avicenna (iii, 3, 3, 12); Haly Abbas (Pract. ix, 20); Rhases (Cont. ii, 4.)

Celsus directs us to make a lunated incision below the eyebrows, the horns of the incision being turned downwards, and care being taken not to wound the muscles. A tent or pledget of lint is to be put into this incision to prevent the edges of it from uniting. This simple operation is described in nearly the same terms by Aëtius, Albucasis, Avicenna, Haly Abbas, and Rhases.

Fabricius ab Aquapendente informs us that the operation had fallen into disuse in his time. It is now sometimes practised. See Scultet, (Arsen. de Chirurg. Tab. xxxiv, 8.)

XI—ON THE SUTURE OF THE UNDER EYELID, AND THE BURNING OF IT BY MEDICINES

The under eyelid is subject to the same complaints from the ciliary hairs as the upper; for, when larger than natural, it is everted; and it is subject likewise to phalangosis and distichiasis. We must, therefore, perform the operation of the suture in the same manner as for the upper eyelid, but in an inverted order, beginning with the *lunated* incision on account of the obstruction occasioned by the blood, and then making the *veruted*. But the *under-incision* is to be omitted altogether, because the lower eyelid, by its natural weight, is readily everted. The rest of the treatment to be completed as in the suture of the upper eyelid, except that the extremities of the ligatures are not to be glued to the forehead. If in this case the patient is averse to an operation, and prefers burning by medicines, you have already got a description of this process.

Commentary. This section requires no commentary.

XII—ON ECTROPION, OR EVERSION OF THE LOWER EYELID

Ectropion of the under lid is occasioned by the same causes as lagophthalmos of the upper, only that it does not occur naturally, but arises sometimes from relaxation produced by medicines possessed of this property, which have been applied for inflammation; and sometimes the eversion is occasioned by the suture or burning having been improperly performed. Taking, therefore, a needle, armed with a double thread, we perforate the fleshy mass, pushing it through from the left canthus to the right, and then by means of the thread fastened to both of its extremities, we stretch the skin with the needle, and cut down upon it with a scalpel, removing the needle at the same time. Then, if the eyelid resume its proper shape and is turned inwards, this operation will be sufficient. But if the eversion continue after the removal of the flesh, we apply the back of the specillum to the divided eyelid; and on the inside of the eyelid, having made two incisions, beginning at the two angles of the incision formerly made, and terminating in an acute point, and meeting together like the Greek Λ, we remove this substance, so that its acute point may be below at the eye, and the broad above at what is called the tarsus. Afterwards we unite the separated parts with a needle containing a woollen thread, being satisfied with two sutures. But if the ectropion be occasioned by the operation of the suture or burning we make a simple incision along the first cicatrix below the hairs of the tarsi, and having separated its lips, we fill up the wound with pledgets, using the same methods as for lagophthalmos (except fomentations) until the parts which have been stitched unite.

Commentary. See Aëtius (vii, 74); Celsus (vii, 7); Albucasis (Chirurg. ii, 14); Haly Abbas (Pract. ix, 20.)

Aëtius gives a full account of the treatment of ectropion from Demosthenes and Antyllus. When the disease is occasioned by fungous flesh on the inner membrane of the eyelid, he recommends us to burn it down with escharotics, such as misy, chalcitis, &c. (See the Third Book.) He describes the surgical operation in the following terms:—when the fleshy excrescences are very large they are to be dissected out with a scalpel, and the part touched with burnt copper or the like. When the eversion is greater, he directs us to perform an operation upon the inner part of the eyelid, making two incisions, which unite below like the Greek letter Λ, and afterwards dissecting out this lambdoid or triangular piece, and along with it the flesh below, which, he remarks, is not cartilaginous like the upper eyelid, but taking care to preserve the skin untouched. The edges of the incisions are then to be united by one suture at the eyelids. When the ectropion is occasioned by an external cicatrix, we are to operate upon the inner surface of the eyelid in the manner just now described, only avoiding to make deep incisions, and uniting the edges of the incisions as before directed. Then stretching the cicatrix with a hook, and pushing a needle armed with a double thread, under the thickened flesh from the smaller canthus to the larger, we are to cut down upon the needle and divide the thickened flesh. A pledget of lint is then to be put into the external incision, and a compress, moistened with cold water, applied with a bandage. He directs us to avoid warm fomentations until the ligatures drop out. When ectropion arises from the excrescence called encanthis, he recommends us to dissect it out. When the disease is occasioned by paralysis, or arises from too large a portion of the eyelid having been cut out in the operation for entropion, he pronounces it to be incurable. It is also said to be incurable when occasioned by the sloughing of carbuncles.

Celsus says that ectropion arises either from an operation for inversion improperly performed or from old age. In the former case he directs us to make an incision like that for lagophthalmos, only with this difference, that the horns of it are to be turned to the jaws (maxillas) and not to the eye. When it arises from old age he recommends us to burn the excrescence with a slender piece of iron, and then to anoint it with honey.

Albucasis describes the operation in nearly the same terms as Aëtius. Thus, he directs us to pass a needle armed with a double thread, below the fleshy excrescence from the left canthus to the right, and stretching it by means of the threads to cut it out with a broad scalpel. If this incision does not relieve the eyelid, he directs us to take the specillum (radius) and applying it to the incision, to evert the eyelid with it, and then to make two incisions in the inner surface of the eyelid so that they may meet at an angle below, like the Greek letter Λ. Then this triangular portion is to be dissected out, and the edges united by a suture with a woollen thread. When the disease arises from a cicatrix he directs us to divide it, and then to keep the lips of the wound separate by the application of a pledget. He concludes with the remark that, as the disease puts on various forms, a prudent surgeon will show his skill by restoring the parts to their natural state.

Haly Abbas evidently borrows his description from Aëtius or our author.

The operation here described is very similar to the one practised by the late Sir William Adams. In the days of Fabricius this operation was condemned as cruel and troublesome. It will be remarked that the V operation of modern times is a modification of the operation now described.

XIII—ON ANABROCHISMUS AND BURNING WITH IRON

When the hairs which irritate the eye are not numerous, but only one, two, or at most, three, close to one another, we approve of the operation called anabrochismus. Taking, therefore, a very slender needle, we pass through its ear (eye?) a woman's hair or a fine flaxen thread, and unite the two extremities together in such a manner that the thread or hair which is passed through may have a double loop; and we pass another such thread or hair through the loop, and pushing the needle through the tarsus where the preternatural hairs appear, we introduce the hair or hairs into the loop by means of an ear-specillum, and draw it upwards. And if the hair of the eyelash be fixed in it, we draw up the loop; but if one or more, fall out, we again, by means of the one at first introduced, draw down the loop, and once more introducing a hair or hairs, draw them upwards. But if there is only one slender hair that irritates the eye we draw up another of the ciliary hairs along with it, anointing them with gum or some other glutinous substance, and bending them until they unite to the skin. Some preferring burning to the operation of anabrochismus, turn the eyelid outwards, and with a hair-forceps dragging out the offending hair, if there is but one, or two, or three; if there be as many, they apply a double-headed specillum, or an ear-specillum, or some such small instrument heated, to the place whence the hair or hairs were removed. For the skin being thus constricted, no other hair is produced.

Commentary. We will give Celsus's description of this operation in his own words: "Quidam aiunt, acu transui juxta pilos exteriorem partem palpebræ debere, eamque transmitti duplicem capillum muliebrem ducentem, atque ubi acus transiit, in ipsius capilli sinum, qua duplicatur, pilum esse conjiciendum, et per eum in superiorem palpebræ partem attrahendum, ibique corpori agglutinandum, et imponendum medicamentum quo foramen glutinetur; sic enim fore, ut is pilus in exteriorem partem postea spectet." However, he does not much approve of the operation. He also describes the operation of cauterising the roots of the hairs. (vii, 7.)

Albucasis, Haly Abbas, and Rhases describe the operation in much the same terms as Celsus and our author. Most of the Arabian authorities, likewise, describe the operation of burning the roots of the hairs by means of a specillum or any such instrument. Canamusali gives a short account of both operations, that is to say, the anabrochismus and burning the roots of the hairs.

This operation is described by the earlier of the modern writers on surgery. The agglutinative composition recommended for this purpose by Guido de Cauliaco consists of mastich, frankincense, aloes, sarcocol, and tragacanth, dissolved in the white of an egg. (vi, ii.)

XIV—ON HYDATIDS

The hydatid is a fatty substance, naturally lodged under the skin of the eyelid, which, in some persons, more especially in children of a more humid temperament, increases until it become the cause of disagreeable symptoms by encumbering the eye, and thereby occasioning defluxions. The eyelids, therefore, under the brows appear watery and cannot be raised in a becoming manner; and if, when we press upon them with our fingers, we separate the fingers, the intermediate space swells up. They are most troubled with defluxions about day-break, and cannot look direct against the rays of the sun, but shed tears and are subject to continued ophthalmies. Wherefore, having placed the patient in a proper position, we compress the eyelid with the index and middle fingers a little separated from one another, so as to form a collection of the watery contents between the fingers, and direct the assistant, who stands behind and holds the head, to stretch the eyelid moderately at the middle of the brow; then taking a lancet used for bleeding, we make a transverse incision through the middle, not longer than that made in venesection, and of such a depth as to divide the skin or even to touch the hydatid itself; but this is to be done with due circumspection. For many plunging the instrument too deep, have either divided the cornea or wounded some muscle of the eyelid. If the hydatid immediately appear, we draw it out, or if not, we again make a slight incision. When it comes in sight we seize on it by the fingers, with a soft cloth, and moving it hither and thither and round about, we draw it out. After the removal of it we soak a double compress in oxycrate, and bind it on the part. Some apply levigated salts, upon the knob of a specillum, to the incision, in order that if any part of the hydatid remain it may be dissolved. After the removal, should there be no inflammation, we accomplish the cure with collyria in the form of liniments, or with lycium, horned poppy, or saffron. But when there is inflammation we treat it with suitable cataplasms and the other remedies.

Commentary. Celsus describes them by the name of vesicæ pingues gravesque. It is clear that they are different from the tumours to which modern surgeons apply the name. They appear to have been encysted tumours, or perhaps enlargements of the sebaceous glands. Celsus directs us to apply pressure with two fingers, and the skin being stretched to make a transverse incision, taking care not to wound the bladder or cyst. The tumour is then to be seized with the fingers and pulled out. He remarks that when the cyst is opened, and its contents evacuated, it renders the operation more difficult. When such a thing happens he recommends us to encourage suppuration.

To this class of tumours we may perhaps refer the white rough bodies resembling chalk-stones, on the inner surface of the eyelid, which are described by Aëtius. He directs us to evert the eyelid, and, making an incision along the vertex of the tumour, to scoop it out with an earpick, and apply burnt copper, finely triturated, to the part. When extracted outwardly he recommends a dressing with tetrapharmacum. (vii, 82.)

See Albucasis (Chirurg. ii, 10); Avicenna (iii, 3, 3, 18); and Haly Abbas (Pract. ix, 21.) They evidently copy from our author. Rhases professes to borrow his description of the operation from Antyllus and Paulus. (Cont. ii, 3, 2.)

Fabricius ab Aquapendente, describes under the name of hydatid, two kinds of encysted tumours, the contents of the one being of a thick and heavy nature, and the other, an atheroma. He approves of the ancient modes of operating. (O. L. ii, 9.) Heister incorrectly calls them vesiculæ aquâ plenæ. (Ch. ii, 2, 9.) Tumours similar to those which we have here treated of are described by Scarpa, in the third chapter of his work on the Eye, and every practical surgeon must be familiar with them.

XV—ON ADHESION OF THE EYELIDS

The upper eyelid undergoes adhesion sometimes to the lower tarsus, sometimes to the tunica adnata, and sometimes to the cornea itself. This disease obstructs the motions of the eye. Wherefore, applying an ear-specillum to the broad margin of the eyelid, or stretching it with a hook-like instrument, we free the adhesion with the scalpel used in the operation for pterygia, taking care that the cornea be not wounded, lest we give rise to procidentia. After the incision, having bathed the eye, we separate the eyelids with tents, lest adhesion again take place, and applying wool, soaked in an egg, after the third day we have recourse to attenuant and healing collyria.

Commentary. See Aëtius (vii, 66); Celsus (vii, 7); Albucasis (Chirurg. ii, 15); Avenzoar (i, 8, 5); Avicenna (iii, 3, 8, 10); Haly Abbas (Pract. ix, 22); Alsaharavius (Pract. iv, 5); Rhases (Cont. ii); Jesu Hali (ii, 7.)

The description given by Aëtius is exactly the same as our author's.

Celsus correctly remarks that the disease is the consequence of neglected ulcers. He describes the operation in the following terms:—"Igitur aversum specillum inserendum deducendæque eo palpebræ sunt: deinde exigua penicilla interponenda, donec exulceratio ejus loci finiatur." He mentions that Heraclides of Tarentum directed the eyelid to be dissected from the white of the eye when there is adhesion between them; but recommends us to do it cautiously with an averted specillum (dos de la spathule, Fabr. d'Aquapen.), taking care to wound the eyelid rather than the ball of the eye. Suitable ointments are afterwards to be applied. Yet he says that he never saw a case thus cured; and states, that Meges likewise thought the disease incurable.

In order to understand the above description of Celsus it may be useful to give from Fabricius some account of the ancient specillum. "Il nous suffit scauvoir que *specillum* (qui est le mot Latin de Celse) est un instrument long et rond, de cuivre, d'argent, ou de plomb, duquel on sonde les fistules, ayant un de ses bouts plus large, et l'autre plus étroit, en vulgaire Italien *stilo*." (Œuv. Chir. ii.) It was, therefore, a sort of sound.

Avenzoar directs us to make the separation by means of a golden rod or probe, and then to apply the white of an egg broken with oil of roses and oil of almonds. When the eyelid adheres to the white of the eye he advises us in like manner to make the separation gently with a golden spatula, and then to apply the oil of roses and of almonds. But the latter case, he says, is difficult to cure.

Of the other Arabians, Albucasis and Haly Abbas evidently copy the description of the operation given by Paulus; and Rhases and Avicenna supply no additional information. Jesu Hali's description is accurate, but similar to that of Celsus.

XVI—CHALAZIA OR TUMOURS RESEMBLING HAIL-STONES

The chalazion is a concretion of inert fluid in the eyelid. If it occur on the external side of the eyelid, having divided the outer part of the eyelid transversely with a scalpel, we extract the chalazion with an ear-pick, or some such instrument, and when the incision is large and the lips thereof separated, we unite them with a suture, and have recourse to some plaster. But if it be small we omit the suture and effect the cure in the same manner otherwise. But if the chalazion be internal, so as to appear through the cartilage, having turned the eyelid outwards, and divided it transversely within, we extract it and use an injection of salt water.

Commentary. Aëtius says that the contents of the chalazia, in some cases, resemble the white of an egg. These he directs us to open, and, having evacuated their fluid contents, to touch the part with a powder consisting of verdigris, burnt copper, and other such escharotics. When the contents are harder he recommends complete excision, like our author. (vii, 83.)

Celsus describes the mode of operating with his usual terseness:—"Hæc incidi debent, si sub cute sunt, ab exteriore parte, si sub cartilagine, ab interiore, dein scalpelli manubrio deducenda ab integris partibus sunt." (vii, 7.)

The descriptions of the operation given by Albucasis and Haly Abbas, if not literally copied from our author, are altogether to the same effect.

Rhases and Avicenna approve most of the treatment by medicines. See Book Third. Jesu Hali directs us to avert the eyelid and extract the tumour. Fabricius ab Aquapendente says that the fluid contained in the chalazion (gresle) is "blanche et transparente, en quelque façon comme de la gresle." He repeats the directions given by Celsus. (Œuv. Chir. ii, 11.)

The chalazion is evidently an encysted tumour of a soft nature, and is not identical with the hordeolum, as Scarpa makes it to be. The treatment here recommended is such as admits of no improvement.

XVII—ON ACROCHORDON AND ENCANTHIS

Acrochordon of the eyelid and that tumour at the greater canthus called encanthis we seize with a flesh forceps, and cutting them out with a scalpel, apply levigated chalcitis.

Commentary. The nature of the acrochordon is explained in the Fourth Book.

Celsus, like our author, directs us to seize the encanthis with a hook, and cut it out, taking care not to interfere with the angle of the eyelid. He then recommends us to apply a pledget sprinkled with calamine or atramentum sutorium (sulphate of copper?) between the eyelids. (vii, 7.)

Aëtius recommends us either to use a forceps, or if the tumour is large, to transfix it with a needle armed with a thread, and to tie it at its base, and to twist the thread round it.

Albucasis and Haly Abbas evidently copy from our author. Avenzoar prefers reducing the fleshy tumour with septics. Rhases mentions that some recommend septics in cases of encanthis, but he prefers excision. After the operation he recommends squama æris to the part. (Cont. ii.) Jesu Hali directs us to remove it with septics. (ii, 33.) It will be remarked that our author's operation is the same as that recommended by modern authorities.

XVIII—ON PTERYGIA

This disease is occasioned by a nervous (tendinous) membrane beginning for the most part at the great canthus, and gradually spreading inwards. It proves injurious to the eye both by obstructing the motion of the ball, owing to the contractions it produces, and because when it advances forwards it covers the pupil. Those therefore which are thin and of a white colour being easiest to cure, we operate upon in this manner: having separated the eyelids, and seized upon the pterygia with a hook-like instrument, having a small curvature, we stretch it, and taking a needle having a horse-hair and a strong flaxen thread in its ear (eye?), and a little bent at the extremity, we transfix it through the middle of the pterygium, and with the thread we bind the pterygium and raise it upwards, while with the hair we separate and saw as it were the part at the pupil away unto its extremity; but the remainder of it at the great canthus we cut off from the base with the scalpel used for the operation by suture, but leaving the natural flesh of the canthus, lest there be a running of the eye when it is taken away. Some stretching as aforesaid with a thread, dissect away the whole pterygium with the instrument called pterygotomos, taking care not to touch the cornea. After the operation, having applied some levigated salts to the part, we bind on it some wool dipped in an egg. After the removal of this we inject into the eye salt water for a long time. But if inflammation supervene we have recourse to the remedies described for it.

Commentary. Celsus gives an excellent account of the pterygium. He correctly states that the membrane generally begins at the inner angle of the eye. His description of the operation is very precise. The patient being properly seated, the surgeon is to raise the membrane with a sharp hook somewhat bent at the extremity, and is then to pass below it a needle armed with a thread, the two ends of which he is to lay hold of and separate the membranes everywhere from the ball of the eye. The membrane is then to be cut out with a scalpel, care being taken not to hurt the angle of the eyelid. He directs us to apply to the part a piece of sponge, or some wool, or a pledget spread with honey. (vii, 7.)

Aëtius also describes the operation very correctly, but in the same terms as our author; that is to say, he directs us to use the needle armed with a flaxen thread and a horse-hair, and afterwards to cut out the membrane, using the precautions here mentioned. (vii, 60.)

Albucasis recommends the same mode of procedure as Aëtius (Chirurg. ii, 16.) Haly gives similar directions. (Pract. ix, 25.) Both caution us not to carry the incision too near the inner canthus. Haly Abbas recommends the use of the scissors, and not of the scalpel (in the translation read *forficibus* and not *forcipibus*.)

Avicenna likewise recommends the scissors. (iii, 3, 2, 23.) Rhases gives directions for passing a needle below the membrane, and for cutting it off. He speaks of using a pair of scissors. He mentions that he had seen a surgeon perform it with a pen. (Divis. 25, and Cont. ii, 3.)

Jesu Hali directs us to operate either with a scalpel or pair of scissors. (De Oculis ii, 38.)

The modern methods of treatment do not appear to differ in principle from the ancient. Scarpa operates with a pair of scissors; but Beer prefers the scalpel. Scarpa seems to approve of the direction given by the ancient authors, not to carry the incision too far towards the inner angle of the eye. See also Fabricius ab Aquapendente (Œuv. Chir. ii, 18), and Brunus (Chir. Mag. ii, 4.)

XIX—ON STAPHYLOMA

Staphyloma is an incurvation of the cornea, and of the tunica choroides, arising from debility, and being produced sometimes by a defluxion, and sometimes by ulceration. We operate upon it not in order to restore the eyesight, for that is impossible, but to moderate the patient's deformity. Wherefore having passed a needle from below upwards through the base of the staphyloma, we are to push another needle, having a double thread, from the canthus next the hand to the other, through the base of the staphyloma; and the first needle remaining, we cut the double of the thread, and tie part of the staphyloma upwards and part downwards with the threads, and then removing the needle we apply wool dipped in eggs. After the removal of the dressings we soothe the eyes with emollient injections until the ligatures fall off along with the staphyloma.

Commentary. Celsus thus describes the disease: "In ipso autem oculo nonnunquam summa attolitur tunica, sive ruptis intus membranis aliquibus, sive laxatis: et similes figura acino fit: unde id σταφύλωμα Græci vocant." He describes two methods of cure: the first of which is by ligatures, as recommended by our author; and the other consists in cutting from the apex a circular portion equal in size to a lentil.

Scarpa and Guthrie concur in recommending the latter operations, the merits of which, as they state, have not been generally appreciated properly.

Aëtius directs us to introduce the cross threads, as recommended by our author, and then to cut out the apex of the tumour. He is at great pains in directing us to introduce the threads obliquely, and not at right angles to one another. He also recommends general bleeding and emollient fomentations, (vii, 37.)

The operation with the ligatures is briefly described in the 'Isagoge,' generally ascribed to Galen.

Haly Abbas and Albucasis describe the operation with the cross threads in nearly the same terms as our author. The latter, however, makes mention of puncturing the apex of the tumour after the application of the ligatures. Jesu Hali gives nearly the same account of the operation.

Although Scarpa condemns in strong terms the use of the needle and ligatures, this method of treatment is sanctioned by the authority of Mr. Travers. This operation was approved of by William of Saliceto.

Scultet explains the descriptions given by Celsus and Paulus, but they are sufficiently plain of themselves. (Arsen. de Chirurg. tab. 32.)

It will be perceived that the ancients applied the name staphyloma to two distinct, or at least considerably different diseases, namely, to enlargement with protrusion of the cornea, and to prolapsus of the iris connected with ulceration of the cornea. Heister, Wenzel, and other continental writers, use it in the same sense as the ancients. Scarpa and our English oculists apply it only to protrusion of the cornea, without ulceration.

XX—ON HYPOPYON OF THE EYE

Regarding hypopyon of the eyes it will be sufficient to deliver Galen's account, which is to this effect:—"A certain oculist of our time, named Justus, cured many cases of hypopyon by shaking the head. Placing them, therefore, erect upon a chair, and grasping their head on both sides obliquely, he shook them so that we could see clearly the pus descending downwards; and, owing to the weight of the substance, it remained below, although cataracts will not remain unless fixed carefully." And again, he says below, "oftentimes we evacuate the pus freely by dividing the cornea a little above the place where all the coats of the eye unite. This place is called by some the iris, and by others the corona." These are the words of Galen in his work, 'On the Method of Cure.' After the discharge of the pus, we clean the ulcer with injections of honied water, or of the juice of fenugreek with the addition of some honey, and then apply the other treatment conformably.

Commentary. Galen recommends three methods of treatment for the cure of hypopyon; namely, by discutients, shaking, and incision. (Meth. Méd. xiv.)

Aëtius, Albucasis, and Haly Abbas, like our author, are advocates for shaking and incision. Neither of these methods is now much in use, but both have had their advocates in modern times.

XXI—ON CATARACTS

The cataract is a collection of inert fluids upon the cornea at the pupil, obstructing vision, or preventing distinct vision. It arises most commonly from a congelation and weakness of the visual spirit, and on that account the disease rather attacks old persons, and those who are debilitated by protracted illness. It is occasioned also by violent vomiting, a blow, and many other causes. Those kinds of cataract which are but commencing, as not being proper objects of surgery, have been treated of in the Third Book. We shall now give the characters of those which are fairly formed and have acquired consistence. All those, therefore, who have cataract see the light more or less, and by this we distinguish cataract from amaurosis and glaucoma; for persons affected with these complaints do not perceive the light at all. Wherefore, again, Galen well instructs us as to the consistence and difference of cataracts and which kinds ought to be operated upon. Having shut the eye affected with the cataract, and with the large finger pressing the eyelid to the eye, and moving it with pressure to this side and that, then opening the eyelids and observing the cataract in the eye; if it has not yet acquired consistence, a certain flow takes place from the pressure of the finger, and at first it appears broader, but straightway resumes its former figure and magnitude. But in those which have acquired consistence no change takes place as to breadth or figure from the pressure. But since this appearance is common to those which are of moderate consistence, and those which are over-compacted, we distinguish these cases from one another by their colour. For those which are of an iron, cœrulean, or leaden colour, are of moderate consistence, and fit for couching; but those which resemble gypsum and hailstones are over-compacted. After ascertaining these circumstances, as directed by Galen, having placed the patient opposite the light, but not in the sun, we bind up carefully the sound eye, and having separated the lids of the other, at the distance from the part called the iris towards the small canthus, of about the size of the knob of the specillum, we then with the point of the perforator mark the place about to be perforated; and if it is the left eye we operate with the right hand, or if the right eye with the left; and turning round the point of the perforator, which is bent at its extremity, we push it strongly through the part which was marked out, until we come to an empty place. The depth of the perforation should be as great as the distance of the pupil from the iris. Wherefore, raising the perforator to the apex of the cataract, (for the copper of it is seen through the transparency of the cornea,) we push down the cataract to the parts below, and if it is immediately carried downwards, we rest for a little, but if it reascends we press it back again. After the depression of the cataract we turn round the perforator and extract it gently. After this, bathing with water and injecting into the eye a little Cappadocian salts, we apply externally some wool soaked in the white of an egg with rose-oil, and bind it up, and at the same time bind up the sound eye, that it may not move. Then lodging the patient in an apartment below ground, we order him to remain in a state of perfect rest, and upon a spare diet; and the bandages are to be kept on, if nothing prevent, until the seventh day, after which we loose them, and make trial of the sight by presenting him with some object: but this we disapprove of during the operation and immediately after it, lest by the intense exertion the cataract reascend. If the inflammation become urgent we loose the dressing before the seventh day, and must direct our attention to it.

Commentary. See Celsus (vii, 7); Galen (Ars Medica, 35; Isagoge); Aëtius (vii, 53); Albucasis (Chirurg. ii, 23), Canamusali (vi); Avenzoar (i, 8, 19); Mesue (de Ægr. Oculi; 15); Haly Abbas (Pract. ix, 28); Jesu Hali (Tract. de Oculis, 68); Avicenna (iii, 3, 4, 20); Rhases (ad Mansor. ix, 27, and Cont. ii); Vegetius (Mulom. ii, 17.)

This disease is called *suffusio* by the Latins, and *aqua* by the Arabians.

We have stated in our commentary on affections of the eye, in the Third Book, that the ancients were aware that the crystalline lens is the seat of one of the species of cataract. This opinion is clearly delivered by Galen, Aëtius, Oribasius, Haly Abbas, and some of the others. As a proof that this notion prevailed generally, we will give the words of Psellus literally translated: "Glaucoma is a grievous and incurable affection, being a certain change of the crystalline humour, and transmutation of its colour to a sea-green. The suffusion is a concretion of the fluid between the cornea and crystalline humour." (Opus Medicum.) The other species then, as Psellus states, was held to be a concretion between the crystalline lens and the cornea. That such a disease, although of comparatively rare occurrence, is sometimes met with seems undeniable.

Celsus lays it down as a rule, that when the suffusion is small, immovable, and of the colour of sea-water, or of shining iron, and if a small degree of light can be perceived at the side, there is reason to hope well of the case. He forbids us to operate until the disease has attained a proper consistence. He directs us to place the patient opposite the operator, who is to sit on a higher seat, while the patient's head is firmly held by an assistant. The sound eye is to be previously covered up with wool. If the left eye is affected the operator must use his right hand, and vice versa. A needle which is sharp and not too slender is to be passed direct through the two coats at a place intermediate between the temporal angle and the black of the eye, and towards the middle of the cataract. When the needle has perforated far enough, which is readily known by the absence of resistance, it is to be gently turned so as gradually to remove the cataract below the region of the pupil, and this object being attained it is to be strongly pressed to the lower part. If it remain there the operation is completed; but if it return it is to be cut and torn by the needle into many pieces, in which state they are easier depressed, and prove less troublesome. The needle is then to be drawn out direct, and soft wool smeared with the white of an egg, and other anti-inflammatory applications are to be used. Quiet, restricted diet, and soothing treatment will be proper.

Galen, in his 'Ars Medica' alludes to the operation, but does not describe it.

Paulus is the only Greek author who describes the operation. Sextus Platonicus, however, just mentions that the diseased part is sometimes to be depressed with a specillum. (De Medic. ex Animalibus.)

Mesue describes the operation of couching briefly, but nearly in the same terms as our author. He directs us to put the patient upon a spare diet, and to bleed him before the operation. He recommends us to be careful to depress the cataract (aqua) properly.

Albucasis describes the operation of Paulus very minutely, and gives drawings of the couching-needles, called by him almagda. The instrument is to be passed down into the eye to as great a space as the pupil of the eye is distant from the end of the black part called the corona. He says nothing of tearing the cataract into pieces when it proves difficult to depress. He mentions that he had heard of a certain oculist who, it was said, sucked out the cataract through a small tube. He adds, however, that he had never seen any person who performed this operation, nor had read anything about it in the works of the ancients.

Avenzoar briefly mentions that when a cataract cannot be got discussed it must be depressed. He gives directions to press it well down, but says nothing about tearing it into pieces. He recommends retirement, abstinence, and rest afterwards.

Avicenna's description is evidently copied from our author. He also mentions that some surgeons open the lower part of the cornea, and extract by it. However, he does not approve much of this procedure.

Canamusali briefly mentions that cataract must sometimes be removed by a surgical operation. When convulsions come on after the operation he directs us to apply castor to the nose.

Rhases describes accurately the operations of couching, extracting, and sucking out the cataract. He is the only ancient author, except Celsus, who recommends the cataract to be torn in pieces when it cannot be got properly depressed. He mentions that the famous surgeon Antyllus practised extraction by opening the lower part of the cornea. He also speaks of a certain surgeon who sucked it out through a glass tube.

Haly Abbas describes distinctly the operation of couching, but evidently copies from Paulus. He makes no mention, however, of extraction, as far as we can discover, in any part of his works. The operation of couching the cataract is minutely described by Jesu Haly, but he makes no mention of extraction. He was the son of Haly Abbas.

Sprengel, in his 'History of Medicine,' refers to Haly Abbas as one of the ancient authorities who make mention of the operation of extracting the cataract; but if this be the case the edition from which they quote (Venetiis, 1492) must be considerably different from the one with which we are acquainted. (Lyon, 1523.) Haly forbids examinations of the eye after the operation, to ascertain whether or not the patient has recovered his sight.

We will give the description of Vegetius in his own language: "Jumentum igitur pridie temperabis a cibo vel potu maximè prohibebis, in loco molli elides caputque ejus et cervicem aptè collocabis: ita patentem oculum facies ut claudere non possit: deinde ab ipsâ fronte paracenterium inter tunicas oculares subjicito, ne pupillam tangas, aut aliquid lædas interius. sed ipsum album de superiori parte ubi hypochysis posita est, capitello paracenterii deorsum deprimis ad palpebram inferiorem subtiliter. Quod si depositum fuerit, non prius paracenterium eximas, nisi clausum oculum penicello calido diutissime vaporaveris. solet enim resilire. Quod si evenerit, reprimito, donec ita componatur ut resilire non possit. Cum itaque intellexeris claritatem pupillæ sine illo obstaculo hypochysis, tunc eximes ferrum, et invenies animal videre."

Sprengel affirms, but not quite correctly, as will be perceived from the account of the ancient opinions given above, that it was towards the beginning of the 18th century that it was first discovered that the crystalline lens is the seat of the cataract. Otherwise he gives an admirable history of the operation, in which he does ample justice to the ingenuity and inventive genius of the ancients. (Hist. de la Méd. xviii. 2.)

Fabricius's description is altogether borrowed from the ancient authors. (Œ. C. ii, 16.) Guy of Cauliac, and the other surgical writers of that age, describe the operation in the same terms as the ancients. Guy mentions the operation of sucking out the cataract through a cannula, but does not approve of it. (vi, 2.)

XXII—ON ÆGILOPS, OR FISTULA LACHRYMALIS

The ægilops is an apostematous swelling between the great canthus and the nose; and it is an affection difficult to cure, owing to the thinness of the bodies, and the fear of injuring the eye by sympathy. If, therefore, the abscess burst at the surface, we remove the whole protruberance as far as the bone; and if the fistulous sore incline towards the cheek, we must lay it all open, and if the bone be sound, we must scrape it; but if diseased, we must burn it with cauteries, applying to the eye a sponge soaked in cold water. Some, after the excision of the flesh, use a perforator, and make a passage for the fluid or matter to the nose; but we are contented with burning alone, using the cauteries for ægilops, and burning down until a lamina of bone drop off; and after the burning we have recourse to lentils and honey, or to the application consisting of pomegranate-rind with honey, and other such desiccative remedies. If the ægilops incline to the canthus, and do not tend at all towards the surface, then, with a lancet for the operation on ptrygium, or one for bleeding, we may dissect out the body between the canthus as far as the abscess, and remove the deep-seated flesh, and have recourse to moderately desiccative applications. Glass reduced to a fine powder is wonderfully desiccative, and aloes with manna, in like manner. The rest of the treatment of fistula lachrymalis we have delivered in the Third Book.

Commentary. Celsus remarks that the ægilops is sometimes of a carcinomatous nature, in which case he recommends us not to interfere with it. He refers here, no doubt, to lupus, which is of not uncommon occurrence near the inner angle of the eye. In recent cases which are not of this kind, he directs us to proceed in the following manner: the whole cavity of the abscess, as in fistulæ, is to be laid open down to the bone, which is to be burned with a red-hot iron, more especially if the bone be carious. Others, he says, instead of the cautery, use caustics, such as atramentum sutorium, chalcitis, or verdigris; but these things, he adds, are more slow in their operation, and less effectual. (vii, 7.)

When the bone is diseased the celebrated Archigenes recommends it to be pierced with a slender perforator, or a hole is to be burnt in it with a red-hot iron. He mentions that others burned it by means of a funnel and melted lead. (Apud Galen. sec. loc. v; and Rhases Contin. ii, 4.)

Aëtius gives a full and lengthy account of ægilops. He recommends us to attempt the cure first with medicines (see Book Third); and if these do not succeed, he directs us to open the abscess freely, and apply to the fungous flesh medicines possessed of strong stypticity, such as powdered glass, stone alum, and the like. A pledget of lint is to be placed over the medicines. When this method of practice does not succeed, he recommends burning, and for this purpose directs us to make a triangular incision in the flesh, and then to touch the bone with a heated iron, so as to produce exfoliation. Alum with turpentine is then to be applied to the bottom of the sore. (vii, 77.)

When the disease does not yield to medicines, Albucasis directs us to open the abscess freely, so as to make an outlet for the matter, and expose the bone. If it is found to be diseased, he recommends us to scrape it with an iron instrument, and then to apply styptic and desiccative medicines to it. When this treatment does not succeed, he directs us to perforate the bone with a triangular instrument of iron. When air issues from the nose by the opening we know, he says, that the operation is completed.

For the cure of ægilops, Mesue recommends the removal of all the diseased flesh by means of strong caustics, such as arsenic, sal ammoniac, chalcitis, alum, &c. When the bone is carious, he directs us to scrape off the carious part. Some, he adds, perforate the bone; but the operation had not succeeded well in his hands. He makes mention of the cautery in the same terms as the others. (De Ægr. Oculi, 12.)

Jesu Hali approves decidedly of perforating the bone with a specillum, or any suitable instrument. He also speaks favorably of the actual cautery. (De Oculis, ii, 32.)

Haly Abbas directs us to lay open the swelling, and apply the cautery. We have mentioned in another place that he was acquainted with the lachrymal duct. (Pract. ix, 29, and ix, 72.)

It will be unnecessary to give a particular account of the treatment recommended by Avicenna, as it does not differ from that of Albucasis. According to circumstances he approves of perforating the bone, and of applying the actual cautery to it. He also speaks of introducing a thread into the lachrymal passages and of using injections. (iii, 3, 2, 14.)

Avenzoar recommends compression and injections, but does not describe the operation. He speaks of the matter passing into the nose, from which it may be inferred that he also was acquainted with the lachrymal duct. (i, 8, 10.)

Rhases likewise makes mention of the lachrymal duct. He recommends us very particularly to make incisions down to the bone, to perforate it, or to apply the actual cautery to it. He makes mention also of escharotic applications containing arsenic, quicklime, and vitriol. He relates a case of apostema lachrymale in which he effected a cure by the ligature and friction. (Contin. ii, 2.)

The practice of perforating the bone as recommended by Albucasis, was approved of by Pott, and the use of the cautery for this purpose is also supported by the high authority of Scarpa. M. A. Severinus, Hildanus, and Garengoit, were likewise advocates for the actual cautery. Fabricius seems to have understood the disease very well, and treated it in the way recommended by the ancients. (Œuv. Chirurg. ii, 21.)

Guy of Cauliac, Theodoricus, and Lanfrancus describe and appear to have performed the ancient operations for the cure of fistula lachrymalis.

XXIII—ON IMPERFORATE MEATUS AUDITORIUS

This affection is sometimes congenital, being occasioned by a membrane which blocks up the entrance into the ear; and it is sometimes superficial and sometimes deep-seated. And it is formed in after life by a preceding ulceration in the meatus; for a growth of fungous flesh taking place blocks up the passage. If, therefore, the membrane which obstructs the opening be deep-seated, the attempt at cure is hazardous; and yet we may try with some slender instrument to divide it, but if it is superficial we divide it with a sharp knife, and if necessary cut it out. If there be a fleshy excrescence it may be dissected out with the scalpel used for the operation in pterygium, or that used for polypus; then making a twisted tent of the size of the meatus from a linen rag, we soak it in water, and sprinkling it with levigated chalcitis, or some such powder, we introduce it into the meatus to prevent the flesh from growing again. Should inflammation come on we must soon take it out. If there be a discharge of blood from the meatus we may soak a sponge in cold water, and apply it along with other appropriate remedies.

Commentary. Celsus describes this case with his usual terseness: "Solet tamen evenire vel a primo natali die protinus, vel postea factâ exulceratione, deinde per cicatricem aure repletâ ut foramen in eo nullum sit, ideoque audiendi sensu careat." He directs us to make an examination with a sound (specillum) in order to ascertain whether the membrane be superficial or deep-seated, and in the latter case recommends us not to interfere with it, but in the former, directs us to make an opening by means of caustics, burning iron, or scalpel. (vii, 8.)

Albucasis describes the nature of the case and the operation in nearly the same terms as Celsus and our author. If the obstruction is occasioned by a superficial membrane he directs us to perforate it with a slender instrument. If a fleshy excrescence obstruct the passage he approves of seizing it with a hook, and dissecting it out. If the obstruction be more deeply seated he directs the membrane to be opened by means of a heated iron, taking care not to hurt the nerves. It is to be kept open with a tent. (Chirurg. ii, 7.)

Avicenna mostly borrows his account of the case from Paulus. When the obstruction is occasioned by a fleshy excrescence he directs it to be burnt down with arsenic or some other escharotic. He also approves of perforating the membrane. (iii, 4, 1, 17.)

The account given by Haly Abbas accords very well with our author's. (Pract. ix, 30.)

Fabricius ab Aquapendente describes correctly the treatment recommended by the ancients. He admits that he had never attempted to perforate the membrane when deep-seated. (Œuv. Chirurg. ii, 41.)

XXIV—ON SUBSTANCES THAT HAVE FALLEN INTO THE MEATUS AUDITORIUS

Not only do stones fall into the meatus, but also glass, beans, and the stones of carob nuts. Of these the stones and glass retain their original magnitude, but the beans and stones of carobs being swelled with the natural moisture of the body, occasion very severe pains. They must therefore be extracted by an earpick, a hook, or tweezers, or by using powerful shaking of the head, while the ear is placed upon some circular board. In like manner we extract bodies frequently by sucking them through a reed; and do the like with water when it falls into the ear, covering up the outside of the reed with wax when it is applied to the ear in order that there may be no outlet to the breath. Stones and such like bodies we extract by wrapping wool around an earpick, and smearing it with turpentine-rosin, or some glutinous substance and introducing it gently into the meatus auditorius. If it does not yield we introduce a sternutatory into the nose and close the mouth and nostrils. If it yield to none of these, before inflammation, convulsions, and dangerous symptoms supervene, we must bring it away by a surgical operation. Wherefore, having placed the patient in a proper position with his ear turned upwards, at the base of the ear, behind what is called the lobe, we make a small lunated incision, and with the circular part of an earpick we extract the body which is lodged there. After the extraction the wound is to be sewed up, and the cure completed by the treatment applicable in cases of recent wounds.

Commentary. See Celsus (vi, 7); Aëtius (vi, 87); Alexander Trallianus (iii, 6); Oribasius (Loc. Affect. iv, 36, 39); Galen (de Med. sec. loc. iii); Avicenna (iii, 5, 1, 23); Mesue (ii, 7, 8); Serapion (ii, 12); Rhases (ad Mansor. ix, 36; Contin. iii); Haly Abbas (Pract. ix, 31.)

Celsus gives nearly the same directions as our author, recommending us to use wool wrapped round a specillum, and smeared with turpentine-rosin, or a hook slightly bent, or an ear-syringe, or sternutatories, or shaking the patient's head. The last-mentioned operation he directs us to execute in the following manner: "Tabula quoque collocatur, media adhærens, capitibus utrinque pendentibus, superque eam homo deligatur in id latus versus, cujus auris eo modo laborat, sic, ut extra tabulam non emineat: tum malleo caput tabulæ, quod a pedibus est, feritur: atque ita concussa aure, id quod inest excidet."

The treatment recommended by Aëtius is exactly the same as our author's. Alexander and Oribasius also deliver similar directions. However, Aëtius, Oribasius, Alexander, and our author, copy from Galen, who in his turn acknowledges his obligations to Archigenes and Appollonius. (De Comp. Med. sec. loc. iii.)

Albucasis's directions are so judicious that we regret our limits do not allow of our giving them fully. For the extraction of a piece of stone he recommends us among other means to use a slender forceps, of which he gives a drawing. It resembles the modern dissecting forceps. He also gives a drawing of a hook slightly bent, which he commends; and also of a brazen tube to be used for sucking out bodies. When other means do not succeed, he directs us to make an incision at the under part of the ear, having previously let blood in order to avert inflammation and convulsions. Animals are to be sucked out with a tube narrow below and wider externally, or they are to be extracted with a forceps or hook. When these means do not succeed, an oil, to which some substance destructive of these animals has been added, is to be injected with an instrument, of which he gives a drawing.

The reader may likewise consult Mesue with advantage. Serapion also recommends the same remedies as the Greeks. Avicenna supplies no new views. Haly recommends incision when other means have failed.

Rhases directs us to pour tepid oil into the ear, and to put the patient into a warm bath in order to lubricate and produce relaxation. His translator, however, remarks that if the substance lodged in the ear be a bean or a pea there may be danger of the water occasioning a swelling of it.

XXV—ON POLYPUS

The polypus is a preternatural tumour forming in the nose; so called from its resemblance to a sea polypus, because it resembles its flesh, and because, as the animal with its fibrils resists those who would seize on it by catching at their hands, so does this affection, in like manner, block up the nostrils, occasioning inconvenience both in breathing and speaking. Wherefore those kinds of polypi which are hard, unyielding, somewhat livid and malignant, inasmuch as they partake of a carcinomatous nature, are not to be meddled with; but such as are more friable, spongy, insensible, and not malignant, are to be subjected to a surgical operation. Having placed the person on a seat exposed to the rays of the sun, and opened the nostrils with the left hand, and holding in the right hand a polypus scalpel, having its extremity shaped like a myrtle-leaf, we cut around the polypus or sarcomatous tumour, applying the extremity of the instrument to the parts where it adheres to the nose. Afterwards, turning round the instrument, we bring out the separated fleshy body with its concave part. And if we see that the nasal passage is perfectly cleared, we proceed to the cure; but if any part of the polypus be left behind, we take another instrument for eradicating polypi, and, with the extremity thereof, we bring away what remains by stretching, twisting, and scraping it strongly. Malignant polypi we burn with cauteries, knob-shaped; and, after the burning, we have recourse to the treatment for burnt parts. After the operation, having sponged the parts carefully, we inject oxycrate or wine into the nose, and, if the fluid descend by the roof of the mouth to the pharynx, the operation will have been rightly done; but if it does not descend, it is clear that about the ethmoid bones, or the upper parts of the nose, there are fleshy bodies which have not been reached with the polypus instruments. Taking, then, a thread moderately thick, like a cord, and having tied knots upon it at the distance of two or three fingers' breadths, we introduce it into the opening of a double-headed specillum, and we push the other extremity of the specillum upwards to the ethmoid openings, passing it by the palate and mouth, and then drawing it with both hands, we saw away, as it were, with the knots the fleshy bodies. After the operation, we keep the opening separate by means of a tent resembling the wick of a lamp; and after the third day we consume whatever is left behind by the trochisk of Musa or the like, and at the same time use desiccative applications to the part. Afterwards, we have recourse to epulotic trochisks, and, if necessary, during the whole treatment we keep leaden tubes in the nose.

Commentary. For an account of the treatment by medicines we refer to section xxiv of the Third Book.

The author of one of the Hippocratic treatises, according to circumstances, recommends sawing it out, consuming it with septics, tying it with a ligature, and burning it with a red-hot iron. (De Morbis, ii.)

In the 'Isagoge' of Galen, it is merely recommended to cut out the tumour, and to scrape its roots.

Celsus, like our author, recommends excision with a sharp instrument of iron, and directs us to apply afterwards to the part a tent smeared with some styptic. A proper dressing is then to be applied for cleansing the sore. (vii, 10.)

Oribasius briefly mentions excision as a proper remedy when medicines fail.

Albucasis describes minutely the operations of excision and sawing out the tumour. Like our author, he directs us to seize the tumour with a hook, to pull it down, and cut it out. If any part remain, he recommends us to scrape it out with a slender instrument, and then to apply styptics, such as vinegar, water, or snow. The operation of sawing it out with a thick knotted thread is minutely described by him. He also speaks of cauterizing the part from which the tumour has been removed.

Mesue describes the process of sawing out the tumour, with some slight differences. He recommends us to use three horse-hairs, which, being tied together with knots, are to be introduced into the nose with a leaden needle, and one end conveyed out by the openings of the palate; and then, by pulling at both ends, the tumour is to be sawed out.

Avicenna, Haly Abbas, and Rhases make mention of excision and the process of sawing out the tumour. Rhases relates the history of a case of polypus, unusually large, which he had seen extracted in an hospital. He and Albucasis recommend the part to be dressed with green ointment.

The veterinary surgeons appear to have depended principally upon the actual cautery. See Vegetius (Mulom. ii, 38.)

The method of curing polypi of the nose, by sawing them out, seems to have now fallen completely into disuse, whether deservedly or not we cannot, from our own experience, venture to decide. Fabricius ab Aquapendente disapproved of it; but he was evidently much prejudiced in favour of the operation with a new forceps of his own invention. (Œuv. Chir. ii, 24.) Sprengel informs us that this method was practised by the surgeons of the middle ages. It is described by Brunus (Chir. Mag. ii.)

Sprengel thus explains the other operation described by our author: "Il se servait d'un instrument particulier auquel il donnait le nom de σπάθιον πολυπικὸν et qui était garni à l'une de ses extrémités d'un ciseau, κυκλίσκος" (Hist. de la Méd. viii, 4.) Why does he substitute κυκλίσκος for κυαθίσκος? That the instrument had a chisel (ciseau) at its extremity is altogether improbable, and this supposition is unwarranted by the context. Κυαθίσκος means the cup-like or concave end of the instrument.

XXVI—ON MAIMED PARTS

When the ears or the lips have been mutilated, we restore them by first dissecting the skin below, and afterwards bringing together the lips of the wounds; then removing the callous parts, and afterwards sewing and glueing them together.

Commentary. This section is taken from Galen. (Meth. Med. xiv.) See, also, the 'Isagoge.'

Celsus's observations are too minute and lengthy for our limits. Suffice it to say, that he directs the edges to be pared, and then united with sutures. (vii, 9.)

Rhases' directions for the treatment of mutilated ears and noses are to the same effect as our author's. (Cont. xiv.) Similar ones are given by Albucasis. He directs us to make the suture either with needles, as in gastroraphe, or with a thread. (Chirurg. ii, 26.)

Celsus has been supposed, but, as we think, incorrectly, to touch on the operation for the hare-lip. (vii, 10, 6.) See Sprengel (Hist. de la Méd.)

XXVII—ON EPULIS AND PARULIS

Epulis is a fleshy excrescence which forms upon the gums beside one of the teeth; but parulis is an abscess which forms near the gums. The epulis, then, we raise with a flesh forceps or a hook, and cut out; but the parulis we divide circularly and fill the incision with tents. I am aware that often when opened only with the common lancet used for venesection and the matter evacuated, the disease has ceased. After the operation we give orders to gargle with wine, then with honied water, and afterwards apply to the wound the Flowery powder, until the cure is completed. But if mortification attack the gums, and do not yield to the suitable applications, we must burn the part with knob-shaped cauteries.

Commentary. Parulis is the gum-boil. Epulis is a soft fleshy tumour which forms on the gums. Aëtius treats fully of them. To the former he directs us to apply at first such things as promote suppuration, after which it may either be allowed to break of itself or may be opened with a lancet. Styptic applications will then be proper. For the epulis he recommends us at first to apply alum, verdigris, &c., and if these have not the desired effect he directs us to cut it off with a scalpel. (viii, 24, 25.)

Celsus treats of both at considerable length by the name of parulides. For that species which corresponds to the gum-boil, among other remedies, he recommends us to hold in the mouth a decoction of figs, and directs to open it before it is ripe, lest the matter should hurt the bone. Larger tumours are to be cut out entire. (vi, 13.)

Haly Abbas recommends excision for the epulis, and to open the parulis in due time with a lancet. (Pract. ix, 33.)

It appears to us that of all the ancient authorities Albucasis lays down the best rules for treating the epulis. He directs us to cut it out with a forceps and scalpel, and then to apply styptic powders to the part, or if the tumour grow again, the actual cautery. For our own part, we have generally found that no permanent cure could be effected without the cautery. See Chirurg. (ii, 28, and i, 22.)

It is unnecessary to detail the treatment recommended by the other authorities.

XXVIII—ON THE EXTRACTION OF TEETH

Having scarified around the tooth down to the socket, we must by degrees shake the teeth with a tooth-extractor, and draw it out. But if it is carious we must first plug up the hole with a small tent, that it may not break when compressed by the instrument. After the extraction we may consume the flesh that is left by sprinkling it with finely levigated salts, and afterwards gargles of wine or oxycrate may be used until the completion of the cure. And since sometimes supernumerary teeth are formed, those that are fixed in the socket we must scrape down with a graving-tool, but those that are not so fixed we must extract with a tooth-extractor. If any tooth grow to an unnatural size, or is broken, we may scrape away the projecting or redundant part of it with a file. The laminæ which unite to them we may remove as may appear proper, with the concave part of a specillum, a raspatory, or a file.

Commentary. Cælius Aurelianus disapproves of extracting teeth, except in cases of extreme necessity. Herophilus and Heraclides Ponticus, he says, have related cases in which the operation had proved fatal; and in modern times we hear sometimes of such occurrences. (Pass. Tard. ii, 4.)

Celsus directs us, when the pains of toothache cannot be got otherwise alleviated, to separate the gums from the tooth by free scarifications, and then to shake it until it is loosened, and forbids us to proceed rashly to perform extraction, for fear of occasioning dislocation of the jaw-bone, or, if the tooth belong to the upper jaw, of hurting the temples or eyes. If loose, it is to be taken out with the hand, but otherwise with a forceps, and, if eaten, the hole is to be filled with a tent, or with lead, to prevent it from breaking during extraction. The instrument is to be pulled direct, lest the spongy bone to which the tooth is fixed should be broken. Of this accident occurring there is, he adds, considerable danger; and not unfrequently when the tooth is short and its roots long, the instrument takes hold of a piece of bone and breaks it; in which case he directs us to extract the broken piece with a pincers. When the teeth are carious he directs us to scrape them, and apply to them a mixture of the flowers of roses, galls, and myrrh, and to hold undiluted wine in the mouth. When the teeth are slackened by any accident, he directs us to fasten them to the surrounding ones with a golden thread, and then to hold some stringent decoction in the mouth. When in young persons a second tooth appears before the first has fallen out, he recommends us to scarify around the latter and pull it out, and to endeavour to force the other gradually into its proper place. Stumps of teeth are to be taken out with a stump-extractor. (vii, 12.)

Scribonius Largus makes some ingenious observations on the extraction of teeth, but disapproves of the operation, except in extreme cases. (De Comp. Med. i, 10.)

Galen, and the medical authorities subsequent to him, direct us to file down teeth when they are diseased and project, but disapprove in general of extraction.

Albucasis is particularly full in treating of the operations on the teeth. Like our author, he recommends us to perform extraction by first making free scarifications, and then pulling the tooth direct with a forceps, the patient's head being held between the knees of the operator. When the tooth is hollow he directs us to stuff it beforehand with a tent of cloth. When a piece of the alveolar process has been broken, he properly recommends that it be taken out. He gives suitable directions for filing down the teeth, and for fastening them with gold threads. He gives drawings of instruments for extracting roots. (Chir. ii, 30.)

The other Arabians describe the operation, but less precisely than Albucasis. Haly's directions are judicious. He recommends the operator to use a forceps, and to stuff the tooth when it is hollow. (Pract. ix, 31.)

XXIX—ON CONSTRICTION OF THE TONGUE, OR TONGUE-TIED PERSONS

The affection called ancyloglossus is sometimes congenital, the membrane which fastens the tongue being originally harder and more constricted than ordinary; but sometimes is acquired from some hard cicatrix formed under it by ulceration. Those therefore who have this affection naturally are distinguished by being slow in beginning to speak, and by having the frænum linguæ larger than its moderate size, and that without any previous ulceration. When the complaint is occasioned by a cicatrix it is easily recognised. Wherefore the patient is to be placed on a proper seat, the tongue raised to the roof of the mouth, and the membranous frænum cut transversely. But if the curvature is occasioned by a cicatrix, we transfix the callus with a hook and draw it upwards, and making a cross incision free the bent part, taking care not to make deep incisions of the parts; for hemorrhages which have been found difficult to stop have thereby been occasioned. After the operation the part is to be washed with cold water or oxycrate; and after all these things the cure is to be completed with relaxing and incarnative applications.

Commentary. Celsus thus describes the treatment in congenital affections: "Horum extrema lingua vulsellâ prehendenda est, sub eâque membrana incidenda, magnâ curâ habitâ, ne venæ quæ juxta sunt, violentur et profusione sanguinis noceant." (vii, 12, 4.)

Aëtius's plan of treatment is quite similar to our author's. (viii, 38.)

Albucasis gives a similar account of the operation. He cautions against opening the artery below the tongue, for fear of hemorrhage. Should this accident occur he directs the surgeon to use the actual cautery. (Chirurg. ii, 34.)

Rhases recommends when the frænum extends to the tip of the tongue that it be divided, so as to allow freedom of motion. However, one of the authorities quoted by him directs us to pass through the frænum a needle armed with a thread, which is to be tightened so as to divide the intermediate space. He recommends this method in order to obviate the fear of hemorrhage from the incision. Rhases himself states that a dangerous hemorrhage will result from opening the green veins below the tongue. (Cont. vii, 1.)

Avicenna also recommends the operation with the ligature. (iii, vi, 11.)

Haly Abbas describes very distinctly the operation of dividing the frænum. (Pract. ix, 35.)

Alsaharavius mentions that the operation is sometimes necessary. (Pract. ix, 35.)

XXX—ON ANTIADES, OR INDURATED TONSILS

As indurated glands are called strumæ, so the almonds of the ears when inflamed, swelled, and as it were, dried, occasioning difficulty of deglutition and of breathing, are called antiades, from their being placed opposite one another. When therefore they are inflamed we must not meddle with them; but when the inflammation is considerably abated, we may operate, more especially upon such as are white, contracted, and have a narrow base.

But those which are spongy, red, and have a broad base, are apt to bleed. Wherefore, seating the person in the light of the sun, and directing him to open his mouth, while one assistant holds his head, and another presses down the tongue to the lower jaw with a tongue spatula, we take a hook (tenaculum) and perforate the tonsil with it, and drag it outwards as much as we can without drawing its membranes along with it; and then we cut it out by the root with the scalpel suited to that hand, called ancylotomus, for there are two such instruments, having opposite curvatures. After the incision of one we may operate upon the other inversely in the same manner. After the operation the patient must gargle with cold water or oxycrate; and if any hemorrhage come on he may use a tepid decoction of brambles, roses, and myrtle-leaves; or if the blood flows copiously we must give for a gargle the juice of plantain and comfrey, and the trochisk from amber and the Lemnian earth, dissolved in oxycrate. When the hemorrhage stops, the parts on the next day may be anointed with the flower of roses, saffron, and starch with milk, or with water, the white of an egg, or hydrorosatum. When sordes collect about the ulcers, we may use injections and linctuses made from honey.

Commentary. Celsus directs us when the tonsils are indurated to scrape the membrane with the finger, and tear it out; or, if this does not succeed, to seize the tumour with a hook or tenaculum, and cut it out; then the wound is to be washed with vinegar, and a styptic medicine applied to it. (vii, 12.)

Aëtius directs us to seize the tonsil with a hook and cut it out at the middle. When cut out at the base, he remarks there is danger of hemorrhage. (viii, 57.)

Albucasis directs us to make the patient sit with his head on the operator's bosom, and, while an assistant presses down his tongue, the operator is to seize the indurated tonsil with a hook, and drawing it out, to cut it off with a sharp instrument resembling a forceps, or, in other words, with a pair of scissors. He likewise gives a drawing of another instrument which consists of a lunated piece of iron fixed to a handle. He relates an interesting case in which he performed the operation. (ii, 36.)

Rhases, upon the authority of a surgeon called Ancilisius, in the barbarous translation of his works, which probably is a corruption of Antyllus, briefly describes this operation. He directs us to open the mouth and take hold of the tonsils, the fourth part of which may be cut off. He recommends us to make the patient gargle with vinegar. He forbids the operation when the tonsils are enlarged and red. (Contin. vii, 2.)

Haly Abbas (Pract. ix, 36,) and Mesue (de Ægr. Gutturis, 4,) describe the operation, but not so minutely as Albucasis.

Guido de Cauliaco copies the descriptions of Albucasis and Haly Abbas. (c. vi, 2.)

XXXI—ON THE UVA

The uvula being, as it were, the quill or plectrum of the organ of speech is often the seat of defluxion from the head, and becoming preternaturally enlarged, of a lengthened form and slender shape, it is called columella; but when thick below and round it is named uva, from its resemblance to a grape, as the other is so called from its resemblance to a column. If, therefore, it cannot be made to yield to general treatment,—I mean evacuations by bleeding and purging,—nor to topical, such as astringents, repellents, and discutients,—we must proceed to the operation, lest, by its constant irritation, it bring on coughs, sleeplessness, and even suffocation. Such, therefore, as are contracted, round, not of a lengthened shape, bloody, or somewhat black, we must decline operating upon; but those that are slender, long, small at the extremity, loose, not very bloody, but whitish, we must operate upon; for the inflammation of them soon subsides. We must only take away as much of the uva as exceeded its natural size; for the complete extirpation of it proves greatly injurious to the parts about the chest, and occasions the loss of voice. Wherefore, having placed the patient on a seat in the rays of the sun, and directed him to gape wide, we seize with the forceps adapted for this purpose, or a common tenaculum, upon the redundant part and drag it downward, and cut it out with the instrument called staphylotomus, or the scalpel used in the operation for the suture of the upper eyelid. After the operation the same things are to be done as are recommended for angiology. But since often, from the timidity of the patient, or the fear of the hemorrhage, or the success attending the treatment by medicines, he declines the operation by instruments, we may rather consume it by means of a caustic medicine. Wherefore, taking the caustic used for burning the eyelids, or some such, we are to fill with it the hollows of the instrument called staphylocaustos, and directing the patient to gape wide, and getting the tongue pressed down with a tongue spatula, we open the instrument sufficiently and grasp with it as much of the uva as we cut off in the other operation. The medicine must neither be of too liquid a consistence, lest it run down from the uva improperly, and burn the adjoining parts (and, therefore, we direct the patient not to swallow during the whole operation of burning), nor very hard, that it may soon act upon the uva. And if from one application the extremity of the uva become black, this will be sufficient, but if not we must use it again. During the whole time of its action the patient must sit with his head bent forwards, in order that the saliva which is melted down with the portions of the medicine may flow from the mouth. The part becomes dead in one hour, and falls off about the third or fourth day. After the burning, having wrapped the index-finger round with soft wool or tow, we wipe the parts about the uvula, or direct the patient to gargle with water. But after this operation, and also that on the tonsils, soothing fomentations from the oil of camomile are to be applied around the neck, and in like manner we may use gargles and liniments.

Commentary. It appears from the Hippocratic treatises that excision of the uvula was sometimes performed in early times. (Prognost. de Morbis, ii; De affect.)

Celsus recommends us not to meddle with the operation when the uvula is red and enlarged, for fear of hemorrhage; but when it is slender, sharp, and white, or when it is pale and thick below, but slender above, it may be extirpated without danger. For this purpose he merely directs us to seize upon it with a forceps and cut it out. (vii, 12.)

Galen describes fully the operation by medicines, but says nothing of excision. (De Med. sec. loc. vi.) Aëtius describes the operation in nearly the same terms as our author. He directs us to grasp the enlarged uvula with a forceps and cut it off, using afterwards some astringent gargle. (viii, 44.) Oribasius briefly mentions the operation, which he directs to be performed with extreme circumspection. (Med. Collect. xxiv, 10.)

Albucasis describes the operation similarly to the Greeks. He directs the operator to get the patient's tongue pressed down by an assistant; when the operator is to seize upon the uvula and cut off as much as is proper of it. He gives a drawing of an instrument for the operation with caustic medicines. (Chirurg. ii, 37.)

Avicenna's description is to the same effect, but not so circumstantial. (iii, 9, 15.) Mesue directs us to perform the operation with a heated scalpel of gold. (De Ægr. Gutturis, 3.)

Rhases states that when the uvula is enlarged, but is not red, the operation may be performed without danger. He mentions that some preferred the actual or potential cautery, but that he preferred excision. He describes, but not distinctly, an instrument for applying the caustic medicines. He states that loss of the entire uvula impairs the voice and exposes the lungs to danger from cold. (Contin. vii; and Divis. i, 49.)

XXXII—ON THORNY SUBSTANCES FIXED IN THE PHARYNX

Thorns, or the bones of fishes, or other substances, are often swallowed in eating, and fix in different places. Wherefore, such as can be seen we are to extract with the forceps for that purpose; but those which are lower down in the gullet we must manage differently. Some are of opinion that the patient ought to be made to swallow large morsels, such as the stalk of lettuces, or pieces of bread; but others direct us to bind a thread about a small piece of clean soft sponge and give it to the patient to swallow, and then taking hold of the thread to draw it up, and to do this frequently in order that the thorn may get fixed in the sponge and be brought up. Leonidas orders suppurative cataplasms to be applied, such as those from raw barley-flour, in order that the part may be converted into pus and the thorn fall out of its own accord. If we see the patient at the time of swallowing, before digestion has taken place in the stomach, and cannot perceive the substance which is fixed, we may order him to vomit by pushing the fingers or feathers down the throat, for sometimes the thing which is fixed will be brought up with the matters that are vomited.

Commentary. Our author's directions are mostly taken from Aëtius. (viii, 50.)

Albucasis repeats our author's directions, and further recommends us, when they fail, to introduce an instrument made of lead, which he gives a drawing of, and either to extract the substance or push it downwards. (Chirurg. ii, 38.) A similar plan of treatment is recommended by Mesue (de Ægr. Gutturis); by Avicenna (iii, 9, 43); and by Alsaharavius (Pract. xii.) When a morsel of food sticks to the œsophagus, Alsaharavius directs that the person should be struck on the back, which will facilitate the descent of it. (6.)

XXXIII—ON LARYNGOTOMY

The most famous surgeons have also described this operation. Antyllus, therefore, says, "In cases of cynanche (as we will explain under the head of Dietetics) we entirely disapprove of this operation, because the incision is utterly unavailing when all the arteries (the whole of the trachea?) and the lungs are affected; but in inflammations about the mouth and palate, and in cases of indurated tonsils which obstruct the mouth of the windpipe as the trachea is unaffected, it will be proper to have recourse to pharyngotomy, in order to avoid the risk of suffocation. When, therefore, we engage in the operation we slit open a part of the arteria aspera (for it is dangerous to divide the whole) below the top of the windpipe, about the third or fourth ring. For this is a convenient situation, as being free of flesh, and because the vessels are placed at a distance from the part which is divided. Wherefore, bending the patient's head backwards, so as to bring the windpipe better into view, we are to make a transverse incision between two of the rings, so as that it may not be the cartilage which is divided, but the membrane connecting the cartilages. If one be more timid in operating, one may first stretch the skin with a hook and divide it, and then, removing the vessels aside, if they come in the way, make the incision." These are the words of Antyllus. We judge that the windpipe has been opened from the air rushing through it with a whizzing noise, and from the voice being lost. After the urgency of the suffocation has passed over, we pare the lips of the incision so as to make them raw surfaces again, and then have recourse to sutures, but sew the skin only, without the cartilage. Then we use the applications proper for bloody or fresh wounds, but if it does not unite we must treat it with incarnants. We must follow the same plan of treatment if we should meet with the case of a person who had cut his own throat from a wish to commit suicide.

Commentary. Aretæus makes mention of this operation in such terms as proves that it must have been practised occasionally in his time. He, however, does not approve of it, at least in cases of angina. (De Curat. Morb. Acut. i, 7.)

Cælius Aurelianus says that Asclepiades performed the operation in cases of cynanche; but he himself disapproves of it. (De Morb. Acut. i, 7.) We may mention further in this place that Avicenna, Avenzoar, Haly Abbas, Mesue, and Rhases express themselves rather favorably of the operation in urgent cases of cynanche. From the circumstance mentioned by Pollux of cynanche, that it mostly attacks children, we are inclined to think that the ancients meant the *croup* by it.

None of the Greek authorities, except our author, have left a description of the operation. Psellus, however, mentions it in such a manner as would lead us to infer that the operation had not been lost sight of in his time, i. e. "Laryngotomy is a certain surgical operation."

Avicenna and Albucasis merely copy our author's description, and appear to have never seen the operation performed. To show, however, that the windpipe may be opened without occasioning death, Albucasis relates the case of a female who cut her trachea while attempting to commit suicide; in which case, by sewing up the wound, he effected a cure without difficulty. (Chirurg. ii, 13.)

Rhases mentions that, in cases of cynanche which threaten instant death, a certain physician, Ancilisius (Antyllus?) recommends the surgeon to open the windpipe. His description of the operation is as follows: The patient's head being kept back the skin is to be divided, and the sides of it separated by means of threads, so as to expose the windpipe, which is to be opened by making an incision in the membrane which connects two of the rings together. After the abcess bursts the wound is to be sewed up. (Cont. vii, 2.)

Haly Abbas likewise describes the operation accurately. He directs us to make an incision in the skin, and to separate the edges with hooks so as to expose the windpipe, which is to be opened between two cartilages. (Pract. ix, 38.)

The modern history of the operation is given in Van Sweiten's Comment. (814); Mémoires de l'Acad. Royale (ii); and Cooper's Surgical Dictionary. See a complete history of the operation by Sprengel. (Hist. de la Méd. 18, 6.) He says, that Anthony Benivieni, a surgeon of Florence, is the first after Antyllus who is known for certain to have performed the operation.

XXXIV—ON ABSCESS

That the abscess is a corruption and transmutation of the flesh or fleshy parts, and what are its modes of formation, and how many kinds of abcesses there are, we have sufficiently explained in the Fourth Book. Now we have only to treat of the operation upon it. If it be completely changed to pus, which we ascertain from the pains, fever (if any was formerly present), redness, pulsation, and the other symptoms of inflammation being diminished, from the swelling assuming a sharp point, and from pus being felt under the fingers upon pressure, more especially if the abscess be superficial, in that case we may proceed to the operation. But if it is not felt to the touch, nor is elevated to a point, owing to its being deep-seated, we must attend to the other symptoms before operating. It is to be understood, however, that before the conversion to pus is completed, we sometimes open abscesses when they are unripe, on account of their being near joints or vital parts, lest, by their continued putrefaction, a ligament or some necessary part should be corrupted by it. And Hippocrates directs us to open abscesses about the anus before they are completely ripened, for fear of their perforating the intestine. In opening them we must not, in all cases, make the incisions in the same manner, but observe the natural lines—as on the face; and the growth of the hairs—as on the head, and taking as much care as possible not to occasion deformity. Straight incisions are to be made in the legs, as in the muscles and tendons; and nerves, arteries, and vital parts are to be avoided, taking care of their safety by sometimes making a straight incision and sometimes a transverse one into the abscess, according to the circumstances of each case. When the abscesses are small we make one incision, but when they are larger we make more, always dividing the thinner parts, and those which are most convenient for the escape of the matter. When the swelling is much raised up to a point, unconcocted, thin, and devoid of vitality, we must cut out a piece either like a triangle, or like a myrtle leaf, or of some other angular figure, because the circular is unfavorable to cicatrization. Those which are not pointed we open by a simple incision, and when we find a sinus, if the part is fleshy and the skin proper for uniting, we only make such incisions into the part as will allow the matter to be discharged; but if it be thin and very devoid of flesh we make a simple incision along its whole length; and after this simple incision, if the parts on each side appear thin and not fleshy we must pare them off. After the operation, having first sponged the part, if the abscess be small, and if only one incision has been made, we may use a simple pledget, but if it be large, and there be many incisions, we draw through them a fillet which can be easily extracted; and when the part has been cut out we fill it in like manner with lint. If a hemorrhage take place we must use cold water or oxycrate, and if the bleeding continue we may sprinkle upon the part finely powdered chalcitis, which we may also have recourse to often when the part is gangrenous and flaccid. In winter, and when the parts are nervous, we may soak oblong pledgets in wine and oil and apply them; and in summer, when the parts are fleshy, we may soak these applications in water and oil, or in the same cold wine and oil, and binding them, on the following day we may bathe with the same fluids; but on the third day, having loosed the dressings and sponged the parts, we may use the application called tetrapharmacon on a pledget, and if there be no inflammation present we may apply the same wash for the preservation of the pledget; but if there be inflammation, we must apply a digestive cataplasm, having first poured water on the parts. When the inflammation abates we may effect the cure by promoting suppuration and incarnation. Sinuses are to be cured by agglutinative remedies, as has been said, in the Fourth Book, on sinuses.

Commentary. All the authors quoted under this head in the Fourth Book may be consulted.

Celsus is more than usually prolix in laying down the rules for the surgical treatment of abcesses. Before the abscess harden, he directs us to make incisions in the skin, and apply a cupping instrument, in order to remove any symptoms of inflammation which may have been present, or, in other words, to procure resolution. Sometimes, however, as he explains, the matter is collected in a cyst (tunica), in which case it is not to be supposed that the contents of the abscess can be removed by a cupping instrument. When the pus ripens it is seldom proper to let it out if seated in the armpits, or groins; nor when the collection is superficial, or in the flesh; and it is better, as he prudently directs, to apply cataplasms until the pus make an opening for itself. When it is judged necessary to open an abscess, he recommends us, if not seated in a nervous part, to perform the operation with a red-hot iron, because a small opening made in this manner will remain longer open. Abscesses in nervous parts are to be opened with a scalpel. In making an incision, the form and size of it are to be considered. In general the openings are to be made as small as possible; but large sinuses require larger incisions, and sometimes two or three are necessary: when the skin is livid or diseased it sometimes must be cut off to further the cure. In this case an opening is to be made of the shape of a myrtle-leaf. When the pus is evacuated, if in the armpit or groins, no pledget is to be used, but a sponge out of wine is to be applied. In other places, a little honey is first to be used; then agglutinative medicines; and above these likewise, if necessary, a sponge squeezed out of wine. (vii, 2.)

The treatment of abscesses is fully explained by Galen. (Therap. ad Glauc. ii.) He directs us, when an abscess is slow of ripening, to make superficial scarifications in it, and afterwards to apply a cataplasm of barley-meal.

Aëtius's directions are, upon the whole, similar to our author's, but not quite so minute and precise. Like our author, he directs us to make the incision long and narrow, like a myrtle-leaf. The ancients were well aware that circular sores are slow of healing; and the causes of this fact are fully explained by Cassius and Alexander Aphrodisiensis.

Little additional information is to be obtained from the other authorities. Albucasis directs us, when the abscess is large, not to evacuate all its contents at once, lest it produce dangerous prostration, especially if the patient be weak; for, he remarks, the animal spirits will escape along with the pus. Like our author, he forbids us to open abscesses until they are ripe, unless seated near the anus, or some vital part. (Chirurg. ii, 40.)

Haly Abbas justly remarks that if an abscess be opened prematurely, the lips of it remain in an indurated state, and prevent the sore from healing. But when seated near nerves or ligaments, he advises not to wait until it is ripe. His treatment upon the whole does not differ from our author's. (Pract. ix, 8.)

The method of opening abscesses, by means of caustic applications, is described in the Fourth Book, 18.

XXXV—ON STRUMÆ, OR SCROFULOUS GLANDS

The chœras, or scrofula, is an indurated gland, mostly forming in the neck, armpits, and groins, deriving its name either from a Greek word, signifying a species of rock, or from swine, because they are fruitful animals, or because swine have swellings of the neck. The strumæ are formed either on the anterior part of the neck, or on either side of it, or on both, and they consist of one, two, or more, all contained in their proper membranes, like the steatoma, atheroma, and meliceris. Those, therefore, which are painful to the touch, and on the application of medicine, are of a malignant nature, are to be considered as carcinomatous and it is obvious that they do not readily yield to a surgical operation. But such as are mild to the touch and the seasonable application of medicines, may be operated upon in this manner. To such as are superficial and incline towards the skin we use a simple section, and free them from the surrounding bodies, and stretching the skin with hooks we flay the lips of the incision, as we said in describing the operation of angiology, and by degrees remove them entirely. But such as are larger, having transfixed them with hooks, we raise up, and dissecting away the skin from them in like manner, we must free them entirely from the surrounding bodies, avoiding in particular the carotid arteries and recurrent nerves. If any divided vessel obscure the operation, we may include it in a ligature, or cut it asunder, if not large. And when the base of the scrofulous tumour runs out into a narrow point, we may cut it away readily, and introducing the index finger search if there be any other strumæ lying there, and remove them in the same manner. But if we suspect that a large vessel or vessels are situated at the bottom of the scrofulous tumour, we need not cut it out from the base, but include it in a ligature, so that it may fall off spontaneously in pieces without danger, when we may effect the cure by the application of lint; but if cut away at once we may unite the lips of the incisions. The incisions are to be made direct, and if there be nothing redundant we may immediately sew them up. But, if owing to the size of the scrofulous swelling there be a redundancy of skin, having cut away a part of it like a myrtle-leaf, we may have recourse to sutures, and use the applications for recent wounds.

Commentary. See all the authors referred to in the 34th section of the Fourth Book.

Galen briefly recommends incision or septic applications. He relates an unfortunate case in which an ignorant surgeon, by cutting the recurrent nerve, occasioned loss of speech. (See Meth. Méd. xvi; and Loc. Affect. i, 6.)

Aëtius gives a long extract from Leonidas on the treatment of scrofula. His directions for dissecting out the tumours in the neck are such as experience alone could have dictated. In operating on the neck, he cautions us to avoid the jugular veins, carotid arteries, and the nerves of speech, and with this intention he recommends us rather to make the incisions longitudinal than transverse. When the tumour is small a simple incision, he says, will be sufficient; but if large, the skin is to be cut in the form of a myrtle-leaf, and the lips of the incision being stretched with hooks, the skin is to be separated from the struma with the fingers and a scalpel; but the base of the tumour is to be cut with great caution. He does not, like our author, make any mention of the ligature. When there is a discharge of blood he recommends styptics. (xv, 5.)

Celsus says nothing of the treatment by a surgical operation, (v, 28.)

Haly Abbas, Avicenna, and most of the Arabian authorities approve of excision, and describe the operation in much the same terms as our author. Albucasis directs us when there is a large vein at the bottom of the tumour to apply a ligature round its root, and allow it to drop out by putrefaction. When the contents of the tumour are fluid, he recommends us to open it, and apply an ointment to consume the corrupted flesh; after which incarnants and detergents are to be used. When scrofulous tumours resist, the ordinary treatment, he directs us to burn them with a red-hot iron.

XXXVI—ON STEATOMA, ATHEROMA, AND MELICERIS

These also belong to the class of abscesses, but differ from them in this respect, that those which are properly called abscesses are of an inflammatory nature, painful, and contain an acrid and corroding fluid; neither are they surrounded by a proper membrane or tunic. They differ from one another, in as much as that which is contained in the steatoma is, as its name implies, like suet; that which is in the atheroma is like pap made from corn; while the fluid in the meliceris is like honey. You may distinguish them from one another thus. The steatoma is harder than the others, is unyielding to the touch, and has a narrower base. The meliceris conveys to the touch the sensation of a soft body, is slowly diffused, and soon returns again to its shape. We operate upon them as upon scrofulous tumours, by incision, dissection, sutures, and the rest of the treatment, only avoiding to wound the membrane, lest its fluid contents be poured out and obstruct the operation, and lest a part of it should be left behind, which often occasions a renewal of the complaint at the wrists, ankles, and the moveable parts about joints, as a scrofulous tumour does in like manner, if the whole or a part of it be left behind. If any such thing be left it will be better not to sew up the wound, but to consume the remainder with septic applications.

Commentary. We have given an explanation of the nature of these tumours in the Fourth Book.

Galen states that the indications of cure in all these cases are to discuss their contents, produce putrefaction of them, or to cut them out. The steatoma, he remarks, being of a solid nature, can be remedied only by an operation. (Meth. Méd. xiv.)

Celsus directs us, in extirpating steatomatous tumours, to open the cyst and evacuate its contents; but recommends not to wound the cyst of the others. Should the whole or part of the cyst be unavoidably left behind, he directs suppurative applications to be used. After the operation he directs us to unite the lips of the wound by a clasp (fibula) and an agglutinative medicine. (vii, 6.)

The surgical treatment of these tumours is very fully laid down by Aëtius, in an extract from Leonidas; but his description is so long that we cannot do justice to it within our narrow limits. Like Celsus, he directs us to avoid wounding the tunics which surround the atheroma and meliceris; but states that this may be done in the case of the steatoma. He judiciously directs the skin to be cut in the form of a myrtle-leaf. (xv, 7, 8.)

Albucasis directs us, in the first place, to prick the tumour, in order to ascertain the nature of its contents. When they are found to be fatty, he recommends us to cut it out by making a crucial incision, and removing it with its cyst if possible. When the cyst is wounded he directs us to dissect it out in pieces, and to endeavour to leave no part of it behind. He gives drawings of various instruments, namely, scalpels, tenacula, and perforators, for dissecting out these tumours. (ii, 45, 46.)

Rhases and Avicenna give very judicious directions for the treatment of these tumours, but they scarcely differ at all from those of Aëtius and our author. They recommend us to avoid opening the cysts of the atheroma and meliceris, if possible; but if any part remain they direct us to destroy it by septics. (Contin. xxvii.)

XXXVII—ON ANEURISM

Aneurism is a tumour soft to the touch and yielding to the fingers, having its origin from blood and spirits. Galen says "an artery having become anastomosed (i. e. dilated) the affection is called an aneurism; it arises also from a wound of the same, when the skin that lies over it is cicatrized, but the wound in the artery remains, and neither unites nor is blocked up by flesh. Such affections are recognised by the pulsation of arteries; but, if compressed, the tumour disappears in so far, the substance which forms it returning back into the arteries." Thus Galen.—But we distinguish them from one another in this way: That formed from anastomosis of an artery appears longer, is deep seated, and when pressed upon by the fingers, a sort of sound is heard; whereas no noise is heard in the cases arising from rupture, and these, moreover, are more rounded, and feel superficial. Those therefore which form in the armpits, groin, and neck, and those in other parts of the body, which are very large, we must decline operating upon, on account of the largeness of the vessels. But those which occur in the extremities, the limbs, or the head, we operate upon thus. We make a straight longitudinal incision in the skin, and then having separated the lips with hooks, as we mentioned in the operation of angiology, and having dissected away the skin, and separated it with the instruments used for operations on membranes, we lay bare the artery, and passing a needle under it, and tying it with two ligatures, and having first divided the intermediate part of the artery with a lancet used for bleeding, and evacuated its contents, we have recourse to the suppurative treatment until the falling off of the ligatures. If the aneurism be occasioned by rupture of the artery, we must seize in the fingers along with the skin as much as possible of the aneurism, and then below what we hold in our hand we push a needle having a double thread, and after it has passed through we cut the double, and thus with the two threads we bind the tumour on this side and on that, as we mentioned for staphyloma. If any apprehension be entertained from the falling off of the ligatures, we must push another needle entirely through, in the course of the first, having in like manner a double thread, and, cutting the noose into four pieces, we may bind the tumour. Or, having opened the tumour in the middle, after the evacuation of its contents, we cut away what is redundant of the skin, leaving what is secured with the ligatures, and applying an oblong compress soaked in wine and oil, we have recourse to the treatment by lint.

Commentary. Galen, we believe, is the first author who treats of aneurism. He states that he had known cases in which an aneurism had been occasioned by a wound of the artery at the bend of the arm in performing venesection. He relates the case of a cure having been accomplished by the application of a sponge with bandages. (Meth. Med. v, 7.) The passage quoted by our author is from his work De Tumoribus (11.)

Aëtius gives a most interesting account of aneurism. He states that it arises most frequently in women during labour, owing to the breath being violently retained, but that it may take place in any part of the body from a wound, as when an unskilful surgeon in opening a vein at the bend of the arm, opens an artery at the same time. It proceeds, he says, either from rupture or dilatation, and its contents are blood and spirits. The symptoms of an aneurism are a swelling of a smaller or larger size, without change of colour, free from pain, of a spongy softness, disappearing upon the pressure with the fingers, and returning again when they are removed; this last symptom being particularly characteristic of aneurism from dilatation. But when it arises from a wound the tumour is not equally soft, as the blood becomes coagulated. With regard to the treatment, he declares that aneurisms in the neck and head ought not to be interfered with; but when the disease arises at the bend of the arm he directs us to proceed in the following manner. In the first place having marked the course of the artery from the armpit to the fore-arm, we are to make a simple incision, three or four fingers' breadth below the armpit along the inside of the arm, where the artery is most superficial; and having laid it bare and separated it from the surrounding parts, to seize the artery with a blunt hook and bind it with two ligatures; after which it is to be divided between them, and the wound filled with fine frankincense, and a suitable pledget of lint bound over it. The swelling at the bend of the arm may then be opened without any fear of hemorrhage. When the coagula have been cleared away the artery from which the blood was discharged is to be seized with a hook, secured and divided like the former; after which the wound is to be filled with fine frankincense, and suppuration promoted. (xv, 10.)

Albucasis treats of aneurism in the following terms. When an artery is divided, and the skin heals over it, a tumour frequently is the consequence, and the same thing sometimes happens from the wound of a vein. Aneurism of an artery is characterized by a deep-seated tumour in the situation of an artery, the swelling subsiding when pressed upon by the fingers, and being attended with a hissing sound. When it arises from the wound of a vein it is round and exposed. He adds, to open such tumours, especially if seated in the armpits, groins, and neck would be a fatal mistake. When the aneurism arises from dilatation of the artery, we are to make a longitudinal incision, and having dissected away the artery from the surrounding parts, to pass below it a needle armed with a double thread, and to tie the threads in two places as recommended in angiology. The part between the two ligatures is then to be divided and the blood evacuated. Suppurative applications are then to be made, until the ligatures fall out; after which suitable ointments are to be applied. If the disease arise from the opening of a vein, we are to grasp as much as possible of the tumour in the hand, to push a needle through it armed with a double thread, when the aneurism is to be firmly bound with the threads in the manner described in the operation for staphyloma. When danger is apprehended from the falling out of the threads, we are to introduce another needle armed with another thread under the whole tumour at the opening made by the first needle, and to tie the threads in four places. The aneurism is then to be cut in its middle, and its contents evacuated, when the superfluous skin is to be removed, and a compress dipped in wine and oil applied. (Chirurg. ii, 49.) The threads which he speaks of are meant to decussate one another like the letter X. This part of his description is somewhat obscure.

We need scarcely remark that the operation of Albucasis is exactly the same as our author's.

Rhases borrows his account of aneurism from Antyllus and Paulus. The operation of Antyllus consisted of tying the artery above and below the tumour, and then evacuating its contents. (xiii, 7.) He states that when the disease occurs in the hams, groins, or neck, it is dangerous to meddle with it, but that when seated in the extremities it is easily cured. All the cases in which he had known the artery to be opened during the performance of venesection had terminated in aneurism, except one in which a cure was effected by compression. (Cont. xxviii.)

Haly Abbas directs us when an artery has been wounded in bleeding, to dissect away the parts about it, and having applied a silk thread on each side of the wound, to divide the artery in the middle. When an aneurism takes place he recommends a plan of treatment similar to that recommended by Albucasis. (Pract. ix, 45.)

Avicenna and Alsaharavius do not describe the operation. Alsaharavius directs us when an artery has been opened in bleeding at the arm, to attempt a cure by means of compresses and tight bandages. (Pract. xxix, 11.)

It will be perceived from the foregoing account of the practice recommended by Aëtius, that the ancient surgeons were aware of the advantages of securing the artery above the seat of the aneurism, as practised by the late Mr. John Hunter, and that they actually had recourse to two ligatures in the manner directed by Mr. Abernethy; but that they afterwards opened the tumour and evacuated its contents, not having yet learned from experience to trust to the absorbent powers of the system. It will likewise be remarked that carotid, axillary, and inguinal aneurisms were in ancient times abandoned as incurable; so that modern surgery may undoubtedly boast of having so far improved upon the practice of the Greeks and Arabians.

Sprengel gives an interesting history of the operation for aneurism. (Hist. de la Méd. xviii, 3.) According to him, John de Vigo was the first who conceived the idea of curing aneurism by compresses and styptics. This, however, is not exactly true, for, as mentioned above, Galen, Rhases, and Alsaharavius recommended compresses and bandages to prevent aneurism after the accident which most commonly gives rise to it.

XXXVIII—ON BRONCHOCELE

A large round tumour forms on the neck from the inner parts, whence it obtains the appellation of bronchocele, of which there are two varieties, the steatomatous and the aneurismatical. The aneurismatical we judge of from the symptoms of aneurism, and abandon as hopeless, like all other aneurisms which it is dangerous to meddle with, as is the case most especially with those of the neck, owing to the size of the arteries.

The steatomatous we operate upon like steatomes in general, distinguishing and avoiding the vessels, in the same manner as we described for strumæ.

Commentary. The surgical operation for bronchocele is described by Celsus. He says that its contents may be evacuated by caustics, but that the knife is a more expeditious process of cure. For this purpose he directs us to make a single incision down to the cyst, and to dissect it from the surrounding parts with the fingers. When its cyst cannot be removed he recommends us to destroy it with caustic medicines. (vii, 13.)

Aëtius and Albucasis give exactly the same account of bronchocele as our author.

The poet Juvenal alludes to the prevalence of bronchocele among the people at the foot of the Alps. (Sat. xiii, 162.)

Pliny attributes it to the corruption of the water. (xi, 37.)

Rolandus, Guy of Cauliac, and other of the earlier modern authorities, direct us to remove the tumour by means of two cross setons.

XXXIX—ON GANGLION

A ganglion is a round tumour of a tendon, arising from a blow or violent exercise, being formed most frequently about the wrists, ankles, and the parts about a joint which are much moved, but likewise in the other parts. It is attended with a swelling, which is free from discoloration, unyielding, and without pain, but if strongly pressed upon it has a dull feeling. It is not deep-seated, but takes its origin under the skin, and may be moved laterally, but cannot by any means be forced forwards or backwards. Those then which form in the legs, arms, and extremities it is not safe to cut out, for there is danger lest the part be mutilated. But those about the head or forehead we operate upon by dividing the skin with a scalpel, and if the tumours be small, seizing them with a flesh forceps and cutting them out by the roots. But if they are larger, we transfix them with hooks, and remove them by dissecting them from the skin, and uniting the lips with sutures, complete the cure by the treatment applicable to fresh wounds.

Commentary. We have treated of ganglion in the Fourth Book, and mentioned the principal authorities on the subject. Hippocrates and most of the others forbid ganglia to be opened. The hard tumour on the head, to which likewise he applies the name, may safely be removed in the manner described by our author. Albucasis repeats his directions. (Chirurg. ii, 50.)

Haly Abbas recommends discutients at first, and if these have not the desired effect we are to strike the tumour with a hard body so as to break its cyst. (ix, 10.)

Rhases recommends striking the tumour with a hammer, binding a piece of lead on it, and excision. When excision is practised he directs us to take pains to extirpate the cyst or tunic which surrounds it. (Cont. xxviii.)

XL—ON VENESECTION

Although the mode of performing venesection be known to everybody, yet, in order that no part of surgery may be omitted, and for the sake of its technical distinctions, it must not be overlooked by us. The first object then in venesection is the evacuation of a fulness of blood. It has been shown that fulness of blood is of a twofold nature: first, with regard to the strength, although the veins do not appear full, in which case those affected soon become weak and enervated, nature not being able to support, as it were, the load; and second, with regard to the containing vessels, as is seen in the parenchymatous parts, in which case, although the strength seems able to support the fulness without stress, the vessels sometimes burst, and a spitting of blood or some other discharge takes place. Plethora then as regards the strength may be ascertained from the heaviness upon the body; and plethora of the veins from their distension and from their appearing full. In both cases evacuation is indicated; and, therefore, if necessity require, you must bleed on the first attack of the disease, waiting only for the digestion of the food in the stomach, or the complete sanguification thereof in the liver. But if on any account venesection has not been had recourse to in the beginning, and has been postponed until after the seventh day, there will be no impropriety of bleeding even then when necessity requires it, and the strength does not contra-indicate. But when about to let blood it is necessary to ascertain that there be not a great obstruction of fæces in the intestines, and, if there be, the bowels ought first to be evacuated by an emollient clyster, lest the veins of the intestines suck in the putrid matter of the excrements. Those requiring the abstraction of blood from the presence of a disease we may bleed at any season, avoiding only the acme of particular paroxysms in fevers. But if it be a continual fever, the morning is by all means the fittest season for the operation. Those who require the evacuation of blood, not from the presence of any disease, but as a preventive, will find the spring the fittest season of the year. With regard to age, bleeding must not be practised before the fourteenth, nor after the seventieth year, unless some urgent necessity compel us. And upon the whole we must avoid bleeding those persons whose strength is reduced. In recent inflammations we must make the evacuation from the opposite parts, but in chronic from the adjoining. We abstract blood from many parts of the body, but more especially from the inner part of the elbow. But it is to be recollected that in general the artery lies below the inner vein called the alar; that below the middle one (median) there is a nerve; whereas the upper one, called also the humeral, is free from all risk. In diseases of the head we open the humeral, but in those below the neck, the alar. The median is applicable in both cases. Wherefore we must tie a narrow band around some muscular part of the arm, and having by friction of the hands upon one another produced the necessary fulness of the vein, we divide it transversely, but only along its breadth; for larger incisions than this are difficult to heal, whilst those which are very narrow occasion inflammations by obstructing the passage of the thicker fluids. When we expect to have to abstract blood again on the second, third, and sometimes the fourth day, we must divide the vein more obliquely, in order that by bending the arm the incision may be kept open and not heal speedily. Such is the opinion of Antyllus. The quantity of the evacuation must be determined by the strength of the patient and the magnitude of the disease. When, therefore, there is a humeral plethora, and the matter is in a state of inflammation, we are to make our evacuations to deliquium animi, provided the strength be firm, and the patient does not swoon from an overflow of the humour upon the stomach. Wherefore many at the commencement fall into deliquium animi before a sufficient evacuation has taken place, and, therefore, the deliquium must be judged of from the measure of the evacuation. If there is a necessity for much evacuation, and the strength is weak, we must husband the evacuation, and making the first abstraction in small quantity, bleed again, or even a third time, if required. We have recourse to general evacuation not only when the body is in a plethoric state (as Galen says), but on account of the magnitude of the affection, when the general system is in a moderate state with regard to the humours, as we do also in hemorrhage from the nose or elsewhere, when although the discharge do not proceed from plethora, we bleed from the opposite parts in order to produce revulsion; and so also in violent inflammations, as in colics and affections of the kidneys from calculi, ophthalmies, and other such acute and urgent attacks; for the heat and pain of the inflamed parts occasion a defluxion upon it, although the general system be free from superfluities. In such cases we must bleed more sparingly, proportioning the evacuation particularly to the age and constitution of the patient, and also taking into account the season, country, and habits of the person affected. When there is a strong inflammation near the vein which is opened, as in pleurisy and hepatitis, it will be most proper to wait the change of the blood in colour and consistence. Blood in inflammation is different from the natural, since being excessively heated, if it was formerly crude, it becomes ruddier and brighter; or if it was such before, it turns black from being over-heated. Yet we must not in every case wait for the change, but sometimes give over before this takes place; for two reasons, either from the weakness of the patient's powers, which you may ascertain to have sunk by feeling the pulse (for you will find it either unequal as to strength and magnitude, or indistinct, the stream of the blood failing also indicates that the strength is sunk), or from the malignity of the inflammation; for sometimes it will not remit, but the constriction continues strong. But if none of these circumstances contra-indicate, and if the patient be in the vigour of age, we may wait until a change takes place, especially if the atmosphere be mild. But if the flow of blood stop before a sufficient evacuation has taken place (this happens from fear, deliquium animi, and coagulum, or too tight an application of the bandage), we must attend to each of these causes, rousing from deliquium with strong-scented things, slackening the bandage when too tight, and a coagulum may be dissolved by pouring in oil, or by rubbing it with the fingers. The rest of the apparatus for phlebotomy is known to everybody. But these things apply to venesection at the bend of the arm. When we would abstract blood from the forehead as for headache, having first used fomentations, we apply a bandage round the neck, placing a finger over the windpipe to prevent suffocation, and when the frontal vein is properly filled we divide it with the point of a lancet or scalpel. In the same manner we may open the external jugulars for chronic ophthalmy, producing a discharge of blood with the concave part of the scalpel. The vessels also below the tongue we open transversely for angina, but without the application of any bandage. Some also open in like manner the veins which appear in the great canthi, as for chronic affections of the head or eyes, in which cases they also sometimes rupture the vessels within the nostrils either by rubbing them with the extremity of a specillum, or by tickling them with rough substances. They also open those behind the ears for the affections about the head; and those about the top of the thighs, as in affections of the kidneys; and those in the extremities they also open, after by the application of the ligatures to the parts above, by friction in the case of the hands, and walking in that of the feet, the vessels having become distended with blood; in affections of the spleen opening the vessel in particular between the small and middle finger of the left hand, and in affections of the liver those of the right hand; for the evacuation of the extremities, being from a distance, occasions a more powerful revulsion. In ischiatic diseases, and those of the uterus, they open the vein in the foot above the inner toe.

Commentary. We have to regret that our limits prevent us from doing more ample justice to the sound and enlarged views of the ancient physicians on this subject, and we must be content with making a few desultory observations and giving a few extracts.

We have had occasion frequently to remark that Hippocrates practised venesection freely in various diseases. He has left no treatise, however, expressly on the subject.

Celsus says, that to let blood was no new discovery in his day; but that blood might be let with advantage in almost every disease was a discovery. He states it also as a recent discovery that children, old men, and pregnant women might be safely bled, the operation having been anciently proscribed in all these cases. Yet, notwithstanding the authority of Celsus, the prejudice against bleeding young and old persons seems to have generally prevailed, for it will be perceived, that our author, copying from Galen, forbids persons to be bled before fourteen and after seventy, except in urgent cases. However, Averrhoes mentions that his countryman Avenzoar had bled a child only three years old with great success; and relates further that he had known certain persons who had been bled at the age of eighty. Celsus properly directs us to judge of a patient's ability to endure venesection from his strength, and not from his tender or advanced age. He also acutely remarks that there is a difference between a strong body and a fat, and between a lean and a weak; for that a lean body contains most blood, and a fat most flesh. (See also Arist. H. A. iii, 19.) Those, therefore, who are lean bear depletion best, and the corpulent suffer most from it. The strength of the body, therefore, is to be estimated from the veins rather than from the general appearance. When the nature of the disease indicates evacuation, and the strength appears ill fitted to bear it, he advises us first to give warning of the danger, and then to abstract blood; for, he adds, "satius est remedium anceps experiri quam nullum." In general he forbids venesection when the stomach is loaded with impurities; and upon this rule of practice all the ancient authorities, we believe, agree with him. Thus, to give an example from the Arabians, Averrhoes says, our famous physician, Abumeron Avenzoar, states that venesection ought not to be had recourse to until the body is purged, for the veins being emptied of blood attract the crude superfluities. (Collig. vii, 1.) This rule of practice is now too little attended to. In general Celsus holds that the second or third day of a disease is the fittest time for abstracting blood. He forbids bleeding upon the very onset of a fever, which he says is enough to kill a man outright. Upon the whole he approves of letting blood as near as possible to the affected part. He admits, however, that venesection may sometimes act by producing revulsion. The operation, he remarks, although easy to a skilful person may prove dangerous when performed by an unskilful one, as a nerve or artery may be wounded. In securing the arm after the operation he directs us to bind on the wound a compress soaked in cold water. (ii, 10.)

Galen wrote three treatises on venesection, to which operation he was very partial. They are: *De venesectione adversus Erasistratum; de venesectione adversus Erasistrateos in Româ*; and *de curatione per venæ sectionem*. These works are deserving of great attention as containing many judicious observations and rules of practice, but which are delivered at so great length that we can scarcely venture even upon an abstract of them. His principles of treatment, however, are nearly the same as those of our author. He appears to have abstracted blood in great quantities. Thus he mentions having seen six lib. taken away in the course of a fever, and six heminæ at once in a case of hæmoptysis. Now the hemina being somewhat more than a half a pint, the quantity abstracted must have exceeded three pints. He strenuously inculcates that venesection proves useful by occasioning revulsion, and as a proof of this he instances the beneficial effects produced by opening a vein of the arm in cases of epistaxis. He practised bloodletting occasionally in cases of dropsy, as we have mentioned under that head. Bleeding from the arm he thinks prejudicial in cases of amenorrhœa, as it causes a determination of blood to the upper parts of the body, and, therefore, he directs us rather to bleed at the ankle. He agrees with Celsus that lean persons bear depletion better than such as are fat; and that venesection is not to be performed when there are undigested matters in the stomach. He states that persons in extreme heat or cold do not bear bleeding. He mentions that in bleeding from the basilic vein there is danger of wounding the artery, that a nerve lies under the median; but that the cephalic may be opened without danger.

Oribasius gives an interesting dissertation on venesection, principally condensed from the works of Herodotus, Antyllus, and Galen. (Med. Collect. vii.) Antyllus directs us when going to bleed at the elbow to apply a ligature two fingers broad round the arm, so as to produce a swelling of the veins; and remarks that they are mistaken who affirm that the same effect may be produced by applying the ligature below, for that the veins will not then swell, even when the arm is fomented. When going to bleed at the ankle he directs us to apply the ligature above the knee; to put the limb into hot water, and make the person walk about. When the blood does not flow readily, he advises us to slacken the bandage if too tight; or if the opening in the vein be covered with the skin, to turn the arm into all positions until the opening of the vein and of the skin correspond; and if it be too small, to enlarge it. When fear retards the flow of the blood it will be of advantage, he says, not to allow the patient to hear the sound of it. When it stops from deliquium animi he advises us to lay the patient in a reclining posture on a couch; to promote vomiting, and to rouse by tight ligatures to the extremities, and by aromatics. When a clot of blood obstructs the vein he directs us to squeeze it out, or to dissolve it with oil or vinegar. When coldness of the body, occasioned whether by the temperature of the air, or the nature of the disease, prevents the flow of blood, he recommends fomentations and frictions. When a piece of fat or flesh blocks up the opening of the vein, he says there is no remedy for it but to cut it out or push it aside. When the object is to produce a sudden depletion he directs us to make a large incision in the vein, but a small one when it is intended to procure revulsion.

According to Drs. Freind and Milward, Alexander Trallian is the first authority who recommends bleeding by opening the jugulars. As far as we know this statement is correct.

Aëtius's account of this subject is similar to our author's, but less copious. (iii, 10.)

Actuarius in like manner has many judicious remarks on venesection, which our limits prevent us from giving to the reader. He forbids venesection when any natural secretion is increased, and this is in general a very proper rule, although, as Galen and Avicenna remark, profuse sweatings are sometimes remedied by bleeding. Bloodletting, he says, is contra-indicated by crudities in the stomach, and a loose state of the bowels. (Meth. Med. iii, 1.)

Little additional information is to be gleaned from the Arabians. We have mentioned, however, that Averrhoes and Avenzoar approved of venesection at a later and earlier period of life than the Greeks permitted it.

Avicenna with his customary accuracy collects everything of importance which had previously been written on the subject, but makes hardly any addition to the ancient stock of information. We can scarcely venture upon an abstract of his important chapter on phlebotomy. We may just mention that as a general rule he approves of bleeding after any accident. He disapproves of bleeding both at the onset and the crisis of a disease. In constitutions requiring bloodletting he holds that spring is the best season for it. Even in cases in which there is a deficiency of blood, but there is congestion in some particular part, he permits blood to be abstracted, in order to produce revulsion, the patient's strength being recruited afterwards by a nourishing diet. When the colour of the blood is dark, and it is thick in consistence, a larger amount is to be abstracted than when it is thin and of a light colour. He makes the important remark, that bleeding sometimes kindles up a fever. He forbids the bath immediately before the operation, and food or exercise immediately afterwards. When a piece of fat obstructs the flow of blood, he directs that it should be gently pushed aside, but not cut out. (i, 4, 20.)

No author, ancient or modern, has described the modes of performing venesection in all parts of the body more accurately than Albucasis. Bleeding from the jugular vein he describes in much the same way that it is now practised by veterinary surgeons, namely, by placing a sort of scalpel, bent at the point, which he calls fossorium, upon the vein, and striking the instrument with a hammer, or some such body. He gives drawings of variously-shaped lancets for opening the veins of the arm. (Chirurg. ii, 97.)

The reader is also referred to Haly Abbas for a copious account of the operation, and the circumstances under which it may be performed. It is contra-indicated, he says, when the bowels are loaded with vitiated fæces. He allows it to be performed even after seventy years of age, provided the patient be of a vigorous constitution. (Pract. ix, 2.)

Rhases, with admirable judgment, condenses all the information supplied by preceding authorities, and mixes it up with his own personal observations. He forbids us to give food immediately after bleeding, as the empty veins will absorb the chyle before it is properly digested, which will prove a pabulum of disease. For the same reason, he, like the others, forbids bleeding when the stomach is loaded with crudities, lest they should be absorbed, and carried over the system. In retention of the menses he directs us to open the saphena, or to apply a cupping instrument to the ankle. When the disease is an acute attack of inflammation, he recommends us to abstract blood fully from an opposite part, so as to procure revulsion; but when it is a chronic affection, he advises to take it from the part affected. (Contin. xxviii.) He enjoins, as a prudent precaution in bleeding a person who is intoxicated, to apply two bandages about the arm, and to have proper attendants to restrain the bleeding, which is often difficult to stop in such cases. (Ad Mansor. vii, 21.)

The veterinary surgeons practised bleeding freely in the treatment of the diseases of cattle. Vegetius, the great authority on this subject, mentions that many persons bled their cattle every year, in the spring. He adds, however, that the ancient and more prudent authorities disapproved of indiscriminate depletion. (Mulom. i, 22.)

XLI—ON CUPPING

We must not have recourse to cupping at the commencement of complaints, nor when the body is in a plethoric state, but when the general system has been evacuated, and when there is no defluxion any longer to the part, and especially when there is a necessity of removing, dislodging, and determining something outwardly. Dry cupping then dissipates flatulence, stops defluxions to the stomach, attracts blood to a part, and stops it again, when determined to a part, if applied to the opposite parts; and it also occasions a translation from the deep-seated parts to the surface, and on the whole produces a metastasis of the fluids, and an evacuation of the spirits. But cupping with scarifications facilitates the evacuation of the offending causes, which it manifestly brings from the deep-seated parts; for it produces the discharge not only of blood but of the other humours, and especially if applied with much heat. And if we wish to make the abstraction from parts that are fleshy, we must first scarify and then apply the cupping instrument;

but if the part is not fleshy, we must first have recourse to dry cupping, and when the parts becomes swelled up, we scarify and apply the cupping instrument again. If we wish to make but a small evacuation we must be satisfied with one incision, but if we wish much we must make several. And if we apprehend that the contained blood is of a thinner consistence we will make superficial scarifications, but if of a thicker, deep-seated. When we wish to evacuate coagulated blood, occasioned by a blow, we must be regulated as to the depth of the incisions by the thickness of the skin above. Some have devised an instrument for this purpose, by joining three equal lancets together, so that by one application it may produce three incisions, but we consider it inconvenient, and use a simple lancet. Others have used cupping instruments of glass, in order that the quantity of blood which is evacuated may be seen; but those made of copper have a more powerful attraction, as being able to endure a stronger fire, whereas those of glass are apt to break. But such as draw out the blood by sucking with the mouth through horns, evacuate less, but do not dry, like those applied with fire. If necessary, when we are about to apply the cupping instrument, having placed the limb in an erect posture, we fasten it to the side; for if we apply the lamp above when lying, the wick falling upon the skin with the flame burns in a painful manner, whereas there is no necessity for this. Sometimes the size of the instrument is proportioned to the part on which it is applied; and on that account there is a great variety of cupping instruments with regard to smallness and greatness of size. For the same reason, those which are made with longer necks and broader bellies are possessed of a stronger power of attraction. We must avoid applying the cupping instrument near the breasts, for sometimes they fall into it, and swelling greatly, render the removal difficult, and in that case sponges out of hot water are to be applied round the cupping instrument, which make it relax. But if even with this it do not fall off we must perforate it.

Commentary. On this mode of abstracting blood, and of altering its determination, the records of ancient surgery are so full of information that our only difficulty lies in selection.

It appears that the father of medicine and his successors practised cupping. (De Articulis, 49, and de Medico, 6.)

Celsus mentions two kinds of cupping instruments, the one being made of horn, and the other of copper. Those of copper were open at one end and shut at the other. Those of horn had a larger opening at one end and a smaller at the other. A piece of cloth was set on fire and thrown into the copper one, and its mouth was then fitted to the body and pressed on until it fastened. In applying the one made of horn, the air was exhausted by sucking at the smaller end, which was then covered up with wax, and in this state it would fasten to the part. He remarks that when the part to which the instrument is applied had been previously scarified, blood is discharged, but otherwise nothing but spirits. He states that the principal use of the cupping instrument is to remove any local affection when the general constitution is sound. Upon the whole, he considers it to be a safer but less efficacious remedy than venesection. Cupping, he adds, is to be had recourse to in chronic diseases, in order to remove any corrupted matter which may be seated in a part; and in acute, when the strength will not allow of venesection. (ii, 11.)

According to Galen, cupping is useful after evacuation, but does not answer when there is plethora. In inflammation of the brain and its membranes, therefore, he forbids cupping at the commencement, and also in inflammation of other parts, until the defluxion is stopped and the general system has been evacuated; and states that the object of cupping in such diseases is to move and determine the inflammatory particles outwards. In general, he advises us not to apply the instrument to the part affected, but to the adjacent part, with the view of producing revulsion, *de hirud. revuls. cucurb.*, &c. He likewise gives an interesting account of leeches. He recommends their tails to be clipped off when it is wished to abstract much blood by means of a few leeches. (Ibid.)

Oribasius is the ancient author who discusses this subject at the greatest length, and to him Paulus is principally indebted. He mentions that cupping instruments are made of glass, horn, or copper. Those of silver, he says, are to be rejected; those of copper are in most general use; those of glass answer best when we wish to see the quantity of blood that flows into the instrument; and those of horn are to be applied to the head because copper ones are difficult to remove; and besides, timid persons are afraid of the flame in such cases. Those which are made deep attract more strongly than such as are shallow; instruments of the latter description are to be applied to the head. Before using them he recommends us to warm the part with fomentations and cataplasms. Upon the authority of Herodotus he enumerates the beneficial effects which may be derived from cupping; such as evacuating the matters fixed in the part, diminishing inflammation, recalling the appetite, strengthening the stomach, determining to the surface, provoking menstruation, and so forth. (Med. Coll. vii.)

Aëtius gives a similar but less copious account of this subject. (iii.)

Actuarius forbids us to apply cupping instruments until after general evacuation, when, he says, they will be useful by producing revulsion of the noxious humours. He also approves of cupping for strengthening the stomach when it has lost its tone, and to discuss flatulence in the bowels. (Meth. Med. iii, 4.)

Albucasis gives a most circumstantial and interesting account of the methods of cupping every part of the body. He particularly recommends cupping the nape of the neck in affections of the brain and eyes. He gives a full account of dry cupping. He recommends it to be applied when the disease is seated in places which do not bear cupping with scarifications, such as the region of the liver and spleen, the kidneys, the bowels, and the joints affected with gout. In applying the instrument he directs us either to create a flame in it, or to fill it with hot water. He gives drawings of various instruments for cupping. (Chirurg. ii, 98.) He also treats fully of leeching, which, however, he recommends only in cases in which the cupping instrument cannot be applied. When the bleeding continues longer than is desired, he directs a piece of cloth soaked in cold water to be applied to the place, or if that does not prove effectual, styptics, such as galls, beans without their skins, and the like. When the leeches will not take, the place is to be smeared with fresh blood. When it is desired to make them drop off, powdered aloes, salts, or ashes are to be sprinkled upon them. (ii. 99.)

Haly Abbas gives an ample enumeration of the cases in which cupping is applicable. He recommends it particularly in such cases as do not admit of general bleeding, for ophthalmies, cynanche, and in an especial manner for amenorrhœa, when it is applied to the breasts.

The other Arabians, although some of them treat fully of this subject, especially Avicenna and Rhases, yet give little additional information. Rhases speaks of applying a glass or a cupping instrument to draw off the blood after leeching. He gives a full account of the different kinds of leeches. Before applying them, some, he says, smear the part with blood and some with milk. When they are too long of falling off he directs us to sprinkle salt upon their mouths. He recommends them to be kept in a vessel containing water herbs. (Cont. xxviii.) When it is wished to abstract more blood after the leeches have fallen off, Albucasis directs us to foment the part with hot water, to rub it, and apply a cupping instrument to it. When, on the contrary, it is wished to stop the discharge, Avicenna recommends us to apply galls, lime, or other astringents, to the part. For this purpose Albucasis likewise directs us to apply a mass of beans deprived of their skins.

XLII—ON BURNING THE ARMPIT

In dislocation at the joint of the shoulder, it sometimes happens that the head of the arm falls out over and over again, either from the prevalence of too much humidity, or because the way is paved to it by its frequent occurrence. In this case then we have recourse to burning. Wherefore, the patient being laid on his back, or on the sound side, the skin at the inner part of the armpit, where the dislocation mostly takes place, is to be stretched between two fingers of the left hand, or with hooks, and burnt with heated cauteries, of a slender and oblong shape, until the cautery, being pushed through to the other side, occasion the formation of two eschars at one application. And if the distance between them is considerable, having passed the head of a specillum through them, we make another eschar in the middle by burning down until the cautery reach the specillum. And Hippocrates wishes two other eschars to be formed on each side of the middle one at the same distance as they, so as to form a quadrangular figure. We must not burn deeper than the skin, because nerves, glands, and other substances, which may give rise to inflammation and disturbance, lie below. The treatment may be conducted by means of leeks applied with pounded salts, and the rest of the treatment of eschars. Afterwards we may use the hand cautiously.

Commentary. Hippocrates (as stated by our author) recommends this operation for preventing the recurrence of dislocation at the shoulder-joint: it is minutely described by him. (De Artic. xi.) Albucasis describes the operation, but it will be readily understood from our author's account of it. (Chirurg. i. 27.) It is described in like manner by Haly Abbas. (Pract. ix. 73.)

XLIII—ON PRETERNATURAL FINGERS, AND ON PERSONS HAVING SIX FINGERS

Preternatural fingers are formed in the hand sometimes near the thumbs, and sometimes near the little finger, but rarely beside any of the others. Of preternatural fingers, some are wholly fleshy, and others have bones in them, and sometimes they have likewise nails. Of those having bones, some derive their origin from a joint, having a common articulation with some other finger; and some arise from the phalanx, and these have no motion. The others sometimes have motion. Now the excision of those which are fleshy is easy, for we cut with a scalpel the preternatural finger all through. But on those which have their origin from a joint the attempt is more difficult. Of those which arise from the phalanx we must first cut away the flesh all around to the bone, and as to the bone itself we either chop it through with a chisel, or remove it by sawing; and in the treatment we scrape and cicatrize them as mentioned by us with regard to the wounds of bones.

Commentary. Galen (de Diff. Morb. 4,) and Avicenna (Cant. i, 2,) allude to the preternatural growth of fingers.

Haly Abbas describes the operation in the same terms as our author. (Pract. ix, 39.) Rhases repeats our author's description of the method of treatment, and also mentions that of Antyllus, which, however, is little or nothing different from our author's. Thus, he directs us first to make an incision of the soft parts down to the bone, which is to be sawn across; the skin is then to be united, and the part treated with agglutinants. When the supernumerary finger grows from a joint he directs us to make the separation cautiously; and if it grows between two fingers, or contains a bone, he forbids it to be amputated. (Cont. xxiv.)

Albucasis's account of preternatural fingers is evidently taken from our author. (Chirurg. ii, 91.) When there is a preternatural adhesion of two fingers to one another, he directs us to divide it with a scalpel, and introduce a pledget wetted in the oil of roses, or a thin plate of lead between them, until the parts heal. (Ibid.)

XLIV—ON THE OPERATION OF BURNING FOR EMPYEMA

The most effectual remedy which has been discovered for empyema is burning. Wherefore, the parts are to be burnt by applying the root of the long birthwort soaked in oil, so as to form eschars, one of which we must make between the junction of the clavicles, having stretched the skin upwards; and two small ones a little distance from the chin and remote from the carotids; two of considerable size below the mammæ, between the third and fourth ribs; two others between the fifth and sixth, inclining a little backwards; another at the middle of the sternum, and another above the mouth of the stomach, and three behind, one at the middle of the back, and two on each side of the spine, higher up than the eschar in the back, and not very superficial. Others, as Leonidas says, having passed a knobbed cautery, heated in the fire, through the interstice between the ribs to the abscess, have carried the burning down to the pus. Some have dared to operate upon them by making a transverse incision, or one a little obliquely in the skin, between the fifth and sixth ribs, then perforating with a knife the membrane lining the ribs, and thus evacuating the pus; but they and those who burn with iron to a considerable depth either occasion immediate death, the vital spirit being evacuated with the pus, or occasion incurable fistulæ.

Commentary. Galen mentions the operation of burning the chest for phthisis. (De Morb. Vulg.)

In phthisical complaints, which do not yield to ordinary treatment, Celsus recommends the cautery to be applied in this manner: One eschar is to be burnt with a red-hot iron under the chin, another on the throat, two upon each breast, and two under the scapulæ. They are to be kept open until the cough is removed. (iii, 22.)

Aëtius directs us to burn the chest and neck much in the same manner as recommended by our author. (viii, 73.)

This operation is described by Albucasis, who gives a drawing of an instrument for performing it expeditiously. (Chirurg. i, 26.) See also Rhases (Cont. ix.)

Haly Abbas recommends such an operation as that described by Celsus and our author. He directs us to do it, not with iron, but with the root of the long birthwort smeared with oil. (Pract. ix, 74.) The use of the root of the birthwort (aristolochia) as a cautery is also mentioned by Aëtius. (xii, 3.) Cornarius, by the way, seems not to have been aware of this circumstance, which has led him into a mistake in translating the sentence where it is mentioned.

The practice of burning the chest in chronic diseases of the lungs is strongly advocated by Caillot. (Elemens de Physiologie, i.) It was tried by Dr. Mudge in his own person with great success. (See Dr. M. Good's 'Study of Medicine,' ii, 786.)

Our author, it will be remarked, disapproves of paracentesis thoracis. This operation is recommended and described in one of the Hippocratic treatises. (De Morbis, i, and ii.) It is also mentioned in the 'Isagoge' of Galen. Rhases likewise mentions it in brief terms. (Cont. iv, 3, and x.) Rhases directs us to open the chest by a small orifice, that the matter may be slowly evacuated. He mentions that Galen recommends burning the chest, and also the operation of paracentesis in such cases.

XLV—ON CANCER

Cancer is an uneven swelling, rough, unseemly, darkish, painful, and sometimes without ulceration (which Hippocrates called also concealed cancer), and if operated upon, it becomes worse, and sometimes with ulceration, for it derives its origin from black bile, and spreads by erosion; forming in most parts of the body, but more especially in the female uterus and breasts. It has the veins stretched on all sides as the animal the crab (cancer) has its feet, whence it derives its name. Wherefore, the treatment of it by medicine has been sufficiently delivered by us in the Fourth Book; and cancer of the womb has been treated of in the Third. But since putrid parts and such as are simply altered from their natural state require amputation, cancers in the womb, indeed, it is neither possible nor expedient to operate upon; but of those of the external parts, and especially of the breasts, we have now to explain the surgical treatment. Some, then, have consumed the whole redundant matter by cauteries; but others first make an excision of the whole breast, and then burn the place. But Galen approves only of the excision, writing thus of the operation: "If ever you attempt to cure cancer by an operation, begin your evacuations by purging the melancholic humour, and having cut away the whole affected part, so that not a root of it be left, permit the blood to be discharged, and do not speedily restrain it, but squeeze the surrounding veins so as to force out the thick part of the blood, and then cure the wound like other ulcers." Such are the words of Galen. And other malignant and putrid ulcers, such as phagedæna, gangrene, and the like, must be treated in the same manner.

Commentary. Hippocrates forbids the surgeon from interfering with occult cancers, that is to say, with such as have not ulcerated, remarking that if healed the patient soon dies, whereas, if let alone, he may live a long time. (Aph. vi, 38.) Upon this his commentator, Theophilus, remarks that even if the disease is eradicated by cutting or burning, many untoward symptoms follow, and the strength of the patient does not stand out. (Ed. Dietz. ii, 506.)

Celsus describes, we fear but too truly, the general result of every known method of treating cancer. He says, some use corrosive applications, some burning irons, and others cut it out with the scalpel; but medicines are of no avail, burning only exasperates the disease, and excision only removes the part affected, for the disease immediately returns, (v, 28.)

Galen's sentiments are partly explained by our author. He states, that the disease is curable only at its commencement. When it has attained any considerable magnitude, he says, it admits of no remedy without a surgical operation; and when the tumour is cut out all around there is danger of hemorrhage, which, if restrained by ligatures, may give rise to the disease in the neighbouring parts, whereas, if cauteries be used to burn the roots of the vessels no inconsiderable danger may result from their application so near to the vital parts. (Therap. ad Glauc. ii; Meth. Med. xiv; Isagoge.)

Aëtius gives from Leonidas the following description of the operation on cancerous mammæ. Laying the patient in a supine position, he says, I make an incision into the mammæ above the cancer, and immediately apply a cautery until an eschar be produced to stop the bleeding. I then make another incision deep into the substance of the mamma, and again burn the parts, and so proceed—first cutting and then burning alternately, in order to restrain the bleeding. In this way there is no danger of hemorrhage. After the amputation is completed I again burn the parts until they are quite dry. The first burnings are for the sake of the bleedings, and the last with the intention of eradicating the disease. (xvi, 45.) This operation, described in nearly the same words, occurs in Soranus. (61.) He says, when the disease is scrofulous the burning may be omitted. (Ibid.)

Avicenna mentions that after the excision of a cancerous part the actual cautery may be required. And yet, he adds, there may be danger from the burning provided the part affected be near any vital organ. (iv, 3, 2.)

Rhases says, that they who make an incision into a cancerous part merely produce ulceration thereof, unless it be so seated that the disease can be completely removed and the parts afterwards burned. (Ad Mansor. vii, 9.) In another work he expresses himself rather favorably of excision and burning. (Contin. xiii.)

Haly Abbas approves of the operation when the cancer is seated in the mammæ or extremities. He recommends us to allow the part to bleed until all the melancholic humour is evacuated, and says nothing of the cautery or ligature. (Pract. ix, 12.)

Albucasis says that he never saw a case of cancer cured unless the tumour was small and recently formed. He directs us, when the operation is attempted, to cut out the tumour by the roots, and if the hemorrhage from any vein be profuse to stop it by the cautery. (Chirurg. ii, 53.)

Serapion expresses himself rather diffidently of excision. (v, 24.)

Soranus gives a full account of scirrhous breast distinct from the cancerous. He states that when the whole breast is scirrhous and adheres to the chest, the excision of the sound parts from the diseased ought not to be attempted; but when only the extremity of the breast, or only the half of it is hardened, he approves of amputation without burning, there being no danger of bleeding in this case as in cancer. (66.)

XLVI—ON MALE BREASTS RESEMBLING THE FEMALE

As at the season of puberty the breasts of females swell up, so in like manner those of the males also swell to a certain extent; but for the most part they subside again. In some cases, however, having acquired a beginning they go on increasing, owing to the formation of fat below. Wherefore, as this deformity has the reproach of effeminacy, it is proper to operate upon it. Having, therefore, made a lunated incision below the breast, and dissected away the skin, we unite the parts by sutures. But if, as in women, the breast incline downward, owing perhaps to its magnitude, we make in it two lunated incisions, meeting together at the extremities, so that the smaller may be comprehended by the larger, and dissecting away the intermediate skin, and removing the fat, we use sutures in like manner. But if, through mistake, we should cut away too little, we must again remove what is redundant, and apply the remedies for fresh wounds.

Commentary. The description given by Albucasis is so like our author's that there can be no doubt of its being borrowed from him. When there is a great redundance of fat and flesh, he directs us to make two lunated incisions, the larger comprehending the smaller, and having dissected away the intermediate skin to unite the edges by sutures. (Chirurg. ii, 47.)

Haly Abbas repeats the same description in almost the same words. (Pract. ix, 40.)

Rhases recommends the operation upon the authority of Antyllus and our author. (Contin. xiv.)

XLVII—ON BURNING OVER THE LIVER

If the pain be attended with weight in those who have abscess in the liver, it is an indication that the fleshy part of the liver is affected; but if the pain be acute the matter is rather in the coats, and we must burn the part thus:—Having strongly heated slender, knobbed cauteries, we apply them a little above the loins at the extremity of the liver, making an eschar. But having burnt the whole skin and reached the coat we must evacuate the pus: after the discharge of which, having used lentils and honey, with the applications from honied water, and things of an incarnative nature, we have afterwards recourse to epulotics.

Commentary. In cases of hepatitis, which do not yield to the usual remedies, the author of one of the Hippocratic treatises advises us to burn the side with spindles of boxwood dipped in oil, or with fungi. (De Morbis Internis.)

Aretæus directs us to open abscesses of the liver with red-hot irons. (Morb. Chron. i, 13.) Celsus mentions that some open abscesses of the liver with a scalpel, and some burn the vomica. (iv, 8.) Cælius Aurelianus, however, disapproves of this practice. (Pass. Tard. iii, 4.)

Albucasis describes the operation like our author, and gives a drawing of a spear-shaped instrument for opening the vomica. (Chirurg. ii, 30.) Haly's description is quite similar. (Pract. ix, 75.)

XLVIII—ON BURNING OVER THE SPLEEN

Having stretched the skin which lies over the spleen with hooks, we burn it through by one application of a long ignited cautery so as to form two eschars; and this we do three times so that there may be six eschars formed altogether. But Marcellus by using a trident or trident-shaped cautery formed six eschars at one application.

Commentary. In cases of diseased spleen the Coan surgeons burned eschars on the side affected. (Hippocr. de Affect. intern. and de Affect. 5.)

Aëtius directs us to burn the eschar either with the actual cautery or with caustics. (x, 12.) The ancients used an issue paste, very like the modern, prepared from potass. See above (s. 9.)

Avicenna recommends the same practice as the Greeks (iii, 15, 1); and so in like manner Haly Abbas (Pract. ix, 76); Albucasis (Chirurg. i, 32); and Rhases (Contin. xx.)

Guido de Cauliaco repeats Albucasis's description of the process of burning the side in cases of scirrhous spleen. (ii, 2.)

XLIX—ON BURNING OVER THE STOMACH

In chronic defluxions of the stomach the moderns have recourse to burning,—some with knobbed cauteries, forming three eschars, one at the ensiform cartilage, and the other two below, so as to make a triangle, the depth of the burning being the thickness of the skin. Some form only one large eschar at the mouth of the stomach. But others do not burn with iron but with the substances called iscæ. The iscæ are spongy bodies forming on oaks and walnuts, being mostly in use with the barbarians. They allow the ulcers to remain for some time without cicatrizing, and rather stimulate them in order that by the great diaphoresis thereby occasioned, the mouth of the stomach may be freed from the defluxions.

Commentary. Hippocrates, Galen, and Celsus say nothing about burning over the stomach in affections of it. Aëtius's account is similar to our author's. He calls the iscæ the medullary part of the wood of walnuts. (vii, 91.) They are mentioned likewise by Haly Abbas, who says they are called *ducanum* in the Persian language. (Pract. ix, 77.) Albucasis directs us to burn with iron. (Chirurg. i, 28.)

L—ON DROPSIES

The formation of dropsical swellings, their varieties and causes, how they are to be distinguished from one another, and their treatment by medicine, having been explained in the Third Book, and it having been there shown that ascites alone falls under the province of surgery, we are now going to give an account of it. Wherefore we must make the patient stand erect; or if that cannot be done, we must cause him to be seated; or if he be so weak that this cannot be done, we must abandon the operation entirely. If then the man be standing erect we give orders to the assistants standing behind to press with their hands and push downwards the swelling to the pubes. Then taking a sharp-pointed knife or lancet, if the dropsy is among the intestines, in the perpendicular line of the navel, and about three fingers' breadth distance from it we divide the hypogastrium as far as the peritoneum. But if the liver be primarily affected we must make our incision on the left side of the navel; or if the spleen, on the right, for we must not make an incision in that part on which the patient is disposed to lie. And having dissected with the point of the instrument the skin that lies over it, we divide the peritoneum a little above the first incision until the instrument comes to an empty space. After this we introduce through the incision of the abdomen and peritoneum a copper tube, having an opening like those of writing-pens, and by this we must abstract the fluid in proportion to the strength; feeling the pulse, and then removing the tube, we stop the flow of the fluid, (for it will stop immediately from the alteration of the incision,) and, for the sake of security, we introduce a twisted tent into the incision of the abdominal parietes alone; and having placed the man in a recumbent posture and recruited him, we may next day again evacuate through the tube a small quantity of fluid proportionate to his strength; and thus, in like manner, until very little be left, avoiding, by all means, a sudden evacuation. For some ignorant persons having evacuated the vital spirit with the fluid have immediately killed the patient. Some for the sake of greater security having evacuated a small quantity of the fluid by the operation so as to relieve the powers of the system from its great load, procure the discharge of the remainder by hydragogue medicines, by burying the patient in heated sand, by insolation, abstinence from liquids, giving desiccative food; and they have recourse likewise to burning over the stomach, liver, spleen, and hypogastrium; and make five eschars about the navel, some by slender cauteries of iron, and others by those substances called iscæ, or some other such like material. And many have been rather cured by this method alone, sometimes without paracentesis having been had recourse to at all.

Commentary. Hippocrates declares in one of his Aphorisms, that the sudden evacuation of the matter in empyema, or of the water in dropsy, proves fatal. He speaks of evacuating the fluid with an instrument called τρυπαντρωγλητήριον, which Camper thinks must have been a kind of trochar.

Galen, in his Commentary on the Aphorisms of Hippocrates, (vi, 7) remarks, that in his time the operation of paracentesis was in general use, instead of burning. He states, however, that he had seldom seen recovery take place after the operation. (See in particular Meth. Med. xiv.)

Aristotle alludes to paracentesis near the conclusion of his work on the 'Generation of Animals.'

Cælius Aurelianus mentions that Erasistratus, Evenor, and Thessalus were advocates for paracentesis, but that Asclepiades, Themison, and Soranus disapproved of it. He himself approves very much of the operation, and answers all the objections which had been made to it. He says, it relieves the fulness and difficulty of breathing, and prepares the parts for the action of the remedies. He agrees, however, with the other authorities, that a sudden evacuation of the water is attended with danger. (Pass. Tard. iii, 8.)

Celsus gives a good description of the operation. Some, he says, perform it at a spot four fingers' breadth below the navel in the left side; some do it at the navel; and some burn the skin and then perforate the abdominal parietes. He directs the operator to be careful not to wound a vessel. The size of the point of the perforator, he says, should be the third part of a finger's breadth. After the perforation has been made, a tube (canula) of lead or copper is to be introduced and the water drawn off gradually. The whole is not to be removed at one time, but a tent is to be introduced into the opening, unless it was made with fire, to prevent it from healing too soon. He speaks favorably of the operation, unless the patient be much debilitated. (vii, 15; also ii, 10.)

Aëtius and most of the medical authors subsequent to Galen, mention the operation of paracentesis, and approve of it.

Vegetius, the veterinary surgeon, recommends paracentesis for the dropsy of cattle, when the swelling is not removed by purging. (Mulom. iii, 25.)

Avicenna expresses himself rather unfavorably of paracentesis. He says, it ought never to be attempted until every other remedy has proved ineffectual, and unless the strength of the patient be good, and he can endure exercise, abstinence from drink, and restricted diet. His description of the operation is taken from Paulus. (iii, 14; iv, 13.)

Serapion mentions the operation in very brief terms. (iv, 7.)

Albucasis's description is very minute; but, upon the whole, little different from our author's as to the place of the incision or the instruments with which it is to be performed. After the perforation has been made in the manner directed by our author, he recommends the introduction of a canula made of silver, copper, or brass, and having a small hole at the bottom and three in its sides; he advises us to evacuate only half the water at first. He adds, that when the canula is removed the skin will cover the opening in the abdominal muscles, and thereby stop the discharge. The remaining part of the water is to be removed afterwards, according to the strength of the patient. (Chirurg. ii, 54.)

Haly Abbas does not in general approve of the operation. He mentions, that he never saw it performed but once, and then it did not save the patient. He adds, that Galen relates that he only knew of one case in which it had proved successful. He directs the incision to be made three fingers' breadth, straight below the navel, that is to say, in the linea alba; but if the liver is diseased he recommends it to be made in the left side, or if the spleen, in the right. (Pract. ix, 41).

Rhases gives Antyllus's description of the operation, which, however, is scarcely at all different from that of our author. He directs us to make the assistants stand behind and compress the sides of the abdomen, and, if possible, recommends to make the patient sit on a bench. He directs us to make the incision with a large needle below the navel, when the collection is connected with disease of the intestines; but if from the liver, on the left side; or if from the spleen, on the right. Like the other authorities noticed above, he directs us to make the opening of the peritoneum higher up than that of the skin. A canula, made of copper, is then to be introduced into the opening. If the pulse sink during the operation he advises us to stop the discharge of the water. (Cont. xix.)

We have mentioned in our notes on Book Third, section 48, that Hippocrates and Aëtius approved of scarifications at the ankles. It appears that Archigenes also was an advocate for this practice in dropsical cases.

Dropsy of the womb and hydatids thereof are correctly described by Soranus. It seems to be now agreed that the dropsy in this case is a species of large hydatid. (120.)

LI—ON EXOMPHALOS, OR PROLAPSUS OF THE NAVEL

Protrusion of the navel takes place when the peritoneum there is ruptured and prolapsed; or from the omentum, intestine, and sometimes an inert fluid falling down upon the navel, sometimes from hypertrophy of the flesh, and sometimes from a collection of blood there, proceeding from the rupture of a vein or artery, as in aneurisms; and sometimes the collection consists not of blood, but of spirits only. If, then, the omentum be protruded, there appears a swelling at the navel, which is free from discoloration, soft to the touch, without pain, and uneven; but if it is intestine in addition to the afore-mentioned symptoms, there is greater inequality,—the tumour, when pressed by the fingers, disappears, sometimes with borborygmi; and it is increased by baths and straining. If its contents be a fluid, the tumour is equally soft, not yielding to pressure, and is neither diminished nor increased by it. If it consist of blood, in addition to the afore-mentioned symptoms, the swelling is more livid; but if it arise from hypertrophy of flesh, the tumour will be harder, elastic, and will continue of the same size. Those occasioned by flatulence are attended with softness, a certain sound when tapped, and disappearance upon pressure. We must operate then in this manner. Having placed the man in an erect posture, we order him to press down at the same time that he retains his breath; then, having marked the whole prominence of the navel with black ink, we are to lay him on his back, and dissect around the tumour with a scalpel, agreeably to the marking; then, stretching the middle with a hook, we must apply a thread or string around the part which is dissected, for thus it will be prevented from falling down, when secured with a knot. Then, at the top, having opened the constricted tumour, we must introduce the index-finger, and search carefully lest any fold of the intestine, or part of the omentum, be included in the ligature; and if intestine be included, we must loosen the fold of the thread, and push it inwards, but if it is omentum we may draw it out, and cut off what is redundant of it, securing, as is proper, with a thread, any vessel that may come in the way; and then taking two needles, containing a plain thread, we pass them through the scarified part in the form of the Greek letter X, and cutting the doubles of the threads, as we mentioned for aneurism, we make constriction with the four heads. After the bodies secured by the ligatures have become putrid and dropped off, we complete the cure by dressing the part with pledgets, and strive to make the cicatrix particularly hollow. Such is the operation when the part concerned is the intestine or omentum. But if flesh, or fluid, or blood occasions the complaint, having divided the middle of the tumour circularly, and then removed whatever lies external to the peritoneum at the navel, we perform the cure by incarnative applications. But exomphalos arising from aneurism, or the presence of flatus, we must abandon as hopeless, like other cases of aneurism.

Commentary. Celsus gives an interesting abstract of the ancient opinions upon this subject, but as it differs but little from our author's description, we shall not dwell very particularly upon it. He directs us to cure the disease either by passing through the tumour a needle armed with two threads, in the manner described for staphyloma, or to produce mortification of the part by pressure between two rules. Some, he says, first make an incision in the tumour, so as to be enabled to remove with the greater facility whatever is protruded, but this he thinks unnecessary, as it will be sufficient merely to return the prolapsed substance, and apply a ligature round its base; after which the outer part is to be destroyed by medicines or the cautery. This operation, he adds, will be sufficient, whether the contents of the hernial tumour be intestine, omentum, or water. He intimates, however, that the operation is attended with some danger, and that it is only to be performed between the ages of seven and fourteen, and when the body is in a healthy state. He forbids to interfere with scirrhous tumours. (vii, 14.)

The description of the operation given by Albucasis is very minute, but is to the same effect as our author's. (Chirurg. ii, 52.) Rhases, in like manner, recommends us to pass a needle, armed with two threads, through the tumour, and to secure it by a crucial knot. He, Avicenna, and Haly Abbas evidently copy our author's description.

The operation with the ligature, as first described by Celsus, was revived, with very slight modifications, by the celebrated Desault, of Paris, but is now seldom practised.

LII—ON WOUNDS OF THE PERITONEUM, AND ON FALLING DOWN OF THE INTESTINE OR OMENTUM, WHERE GASTRORAPHÉ ALSO IS DESCRIBED: FROM THE WORKS OF GALEN

How wounds of the peritoneum are to be treated is next to be considered. If then the wound be small, so that the prolapsed intestine being distended with air, cannot be restored to its place, it will be necessary either to evacuate the flatus or enlarge the wound. The former measure is the better, provided one can accomplish it. But how may this be most probably done? By removing the cause which occasions the inflation of the intestine. But what is this? Congelation of the surrounding air; so that the cure is to be performed by heating. Wherefore, having soaked a soft sponge in hot water, and then squeezed it out, foment the intestine therewith. In the meantime let hot austere wine be prepared, for it is more heating than water, and communicates strength to the intestine. If, after having had recourse to all these things, the intestine remain inflated, we must divide as much of the peritoneum as the prolapsed intestine requires. The straight instruments called syringotoma, used for operating upon fistulæ, are very proper for this incision. A recumbent position of the patient is the best when the wound is in the lower part; and when in the right side, he may lie on the left, and when in the left, on the right; and this is common both to great and small wounds. But the replacement of the intestine into its proper place when the wound is large, requires a skilful assistant. For he must take hold of the wound externally with his hands, and contract and compress it a little, so as to expose always a small portion to the sewer, and also must compress moderately what is sewed until the whole is sewed. What is the most proper mode of performing the operation called gastroraphé, we must next explain. Since the abdomen must be united with the peritoneum, we have to begin by passing a needle through the skin from without inwards; but when it has transfixed the skin and the whole rectus muscle, passing by the adjacent peritoneum, we must push the needle from within through the other part of the peritoneum, and so hence from within outwards, through the rest of the abdomen; and when it has passed out we must push the needle again from without inwards through this part of the abdomen, and, passing by the adjacent portion of the peritoneum, and beginning again from the opposite side of this membrane, perforate it from within outwards, and at the same time all the other parts of the abdomen; then beginning again from this, sew it with the opposite membrane, and afterwards transmit it from the neighbouring skin outwards; and do this repeatedly until the whole wound be sewed up. The space between the sutures required to keep the under parts together must be very small, but the interval between those required to keep the skin from falling asunder need not be so small. Excess in either respects must be avoided, and a medium chosen between the two extremes. And a medium is likewise to be observed as to the consistence of the thread, for that which is too hard breaks the soft skin, and what is too soft is itself first broken. In the same manner, passing the needle too near the lips of the wound, occasions often a rupture of the remainder which is too narrow. But if too much is taken in, much of the skin remains ununited. These observations apply to the treatment of all ulcers, but are more especially to be observed in gastroraphé; and, as aforesaid, we must act, forming a conjecture as to the adhesion of the peritoneum with the abdomen, from the circumstance that the latter being membraneous seldom adheres; or, as some do, by bringing together the parts of the same kind; that is to say, peritoneum to peritoneum, and abdomen to abdomen. Or, it may be done thus: in the same manner as above, we must pass a needle from the side of the abdomen nearest us, from without inwards, and through it above; then passing both lips of the peritoneum, we must again turn the needle from without inwards through both lips of the peritoneum, and again turning it from within outwards, pass it through the opposite part of the abdomen. This mode differs from the common and vulgar one, inasmuch as the needle is passed through the four lips at one perforation, and exactly conceals the peritoneum within the abdomen. The proper applications are those formed of the same materials as the applications for recent wounds; but in order that no vital part may be affected sympathetically, some tender wool is to be dipped in moderately hot oil, and the whole space between the groins and armpits wrapped in it. It will be better, also, to evacuate the bowels by a clyster of warm oil. But if any of the intestines be wounded, dark austere wine, in a tepid state, should be injected, more especially if it be perforated quite through. The large intestines are easily cured, but the small ones with difficulty, and the jejunum is utterly incurable, from the multitude of its convolutions and the magnitude of its vessels, and owing to its coats being thin and nervous; besides, it receives all the bile in an undiluted state, and is nearest to the liver. The under and fleshy parts of the stomach we may attempt to cure, for we may succeed, not only because these parts are thicker, but because curative medicines are more readily applied to them, owing to their situation. The parts, however, about the mouth of the stomach and œsophagus are affected by the medicines only in passing down; and the exquisite sensibility of the mouth of the stomach is an obstacle to the cure of wounds of it. When, from a rupture of the peritoneum, the omentum is prolapsed, and either becomes livid or black, the part anterior to the black portion may be included in a ligature, for fear of hemorrhage, and then the part behind the ligature is to be cut off, and the extremities of the ligature allowed to hang from the under part of the sewed wound of the abdomen, in order that they may readily escape when cast off by the suppuration of the wound.

Commentary. The description of gastroraphé here given will be sufficiently intelligible upon an attentive perusal. It is taken from Galen. (Meth. Med. vi, 4.) By abdomen, in this place, is to be understood the abdominal parietes, namely, the skin and muscles. Galen explains that ἐπιγάστριον is used in this sense.

Celsus gives a long description of a somewhat different method of performing gastroraphé. He uses two needles. (vii, 16.)

Several modes of performing the operation are minutely described by Albucasis. He relates the history of a case in which he practised gastroraphé. (ii, 87.)

Haly Abbas recommends the warm bath, to facilitate reduction. The method of performing gastroraphé which he directs, is similar to the suture now practised upon dead bodies after dissections. (Pract. ix, 43.)

Rhases describes various modes of gastroraphé. He speaks of performing the operation with the string of a harp. (Cont. xxviii.) That the strings of the ancient harp were made of the guts of a sheep is clearly proved from the following passage in the Odyssey of Homer:

> ὡς ὅτ' ἀνὴρ φορμίγγος ἐπιστάμενος καὶ ἀοιδῆς
>
> ῥηϊδίως ἐτάνυσσε νέῳ ἐπὶ κόλλοπι χορδὴν,
>
> ἅψας ἀμφοτέρωθεν ἐυστρεφὲς ἔντερον οἰὸς.

Οδυσ. φ.

The modes of gastroraphé described by Galen and Celsus are explained and commented upon by Van Swieten (Comment. cccxi), and by Fabricius ab Aquapendente. (Œuv. Chir. ii, 53.) A complete history of the operation is given by Sprengel. (Hist. de la Méd. xviii, 21.) Ambrose Paré performed the operation exactly like Galen.

LIII—ON DEFICIENCY OF THE PREPUCE

When there is a small deficiency in the skin of the penis, some, in order to repair the deformity, have attempted a double surgical operation; sometimes cutting the skin all round above at the commencement of the penis, in order that by this solution of continuity the skin may be drawn downwards until the glans (as it is called) be covered; and sometimes with a scalpel dissecting its inner surface from the root of the glans, and then drawing it downwards, and surrounding the glans with a soft ligature; but a piece of cloth must be interposed at the incision, in order to prevent an adhesion of the prepuce to the glans. Antyllus approves most of this method, of which he gives a full description, but we have been content with a brief outline, because it is rare that this surgical operation is required, as the complaint neither occasions any defect of the functional office, nor such deformity that one would choose to submit to the hazard of an operation on account of it.

Commentary. Celsus describes the operation as follows: "Cutis circa glandem prehenditur et extenditur, donec illam ipsam condat; ibique deligatur: deinde, juxta pubem, in orbem tergus inciditur, donec coles nudatur; magnâque curâ cavetur, ne vel urinæ iter, vel venæ quæ ibi sunt, incidantur. Eo facto, cutis ad vinculum inclinatur, nudaturque circa pubem velut circulus; eoque linamenta dantur, ut caro increscat, et id impleat: satisque velamenti supra latitudo plagæ præstat. Sed, donec cicatrix sit, cinctum esse id debet: in medio tantum relicto exiguo urinæ itinere." (vii, 25.)

Rhases directs us to put a proper piece of lead upon the glans, then to draw the prepuce over it, and secure it with a ligature, having previously dissected it from the parts below, if necessary. (Cont. xiv.) This is much the same as our author's operation for phimosis. See section lv.

The reader will find the ancient operation described by Fabricius ab Aquapendente. (Œuv. Chirurg. ii, 61.)

LIV—ON HYPOSPADIÆUM, OR IMPERFORATE GLANS PENIS

In many children the glans is not perforated at birth, but the meatus is situated under the part called canis, at the termination of the glans. Hence they can neither make water forwards unless they draw up the member to the pubes, nor procreate, as the semen cannot be injected direct into the uterus. In addition to these defects, the complaint occasions no ordinary deformity. Wherefore, the simplest and least dangerous mode of operation is that by amputation. Having then placed the patient in a supine posture, we have to stretch the glans forcibly with the fingers of the left hand, and then with the point of a scalpel we are to amputate the glans at the corona, not making the amputation obliquely, but carving it, as it were, all round, so that an eminence may appear in the middle resembling the glans. And since a hemorrhage frequently takes place, we may stop it by styptics if possible, but if not, we must have recourse to burning with slender cauteries.

Commentary. Galen makes mention of this deformity. (De usu Partium.) See also Theophilus. (De Fab. Hom. v, 22.)

Albucasis evidently transcribes our author's description. The part named *canis* (κυὼν) by our author is called *finis capitis virgæ* in the translation of Albucasis, and *finis coronæ* in the translation of Haly Abbas. (Pract. ix. 44.) We do not remember to have seen the term κυὼν applied by any other medical author to a part of membrum virile. Perhaps the proper word is ἶς *gent.* ἰνὸς which is applied by Galen to a part of the genital member. (Meth. Med. xiv. 16.)

Guido de Cauliaco directs us to make an opening with a suitable instrument and introduce a canula of lead or wood. (iv, 2.)

LV—ON PHIMUS, OR PHIMOSIS

There are two causes of phimosis; for sometimes the prepuce so covers the glans that it cannot be retracted; and sometimes when drawn behind, it cannot be brought forward, which last species is properly called paraphimosis. The first variety is occasioned either from a cicatrix formed in the prepuce, or from an adhesion by flesh. But the second variety takes place in inflammations of the genital organs when the skin being brought back, the glans swells, and it cannot longer allow of being drawn forward. If it is the first species of phimosis we may operate upon it in this manner. After having placed the patient properly, and drawn the prepuce forwards, and having fastened three or four hooks into its extremity and giving them to assistants to hold, we direct them to stretch and open it; and then if the external adhesion be from a cicatrix, we divide the prepuce from the internal parts with a lancet or sharp knife in three or four places, making the divisions at the inner parts direct and equally distant from one another. The prepuce at the glans is double, wherefore we divide the mouth of the inner part; for having thus opened the contraction formed by the cicatrix, we are enabled to retract the prepuce. But if a preternatural adhesion of the flesh of the internal parts occasion the phimosis we may make scarifications in all the flesh, drawing back the prepuce and scraping away the fleshy prominences between the incisions, and afterwards apply a tube of lead to the whole glans, having wrapped it in dried paper (papyrus), the tube having its opening the same everywhere; for thus, by the application of the tube, the prepuce, when brought forwards again, is prevented from forming adhesions, being kept separate by the lead and the paper wrapped round it; for by getting swelled with the moisture it separates the skin still more. This we may do whether we operate upon a phimosis occasioned by a cicatrix, or one from a preternatural adhesion of flesh. But if the complaint called paraphimosis take place, and become chronic, adhesions take place, and the complaint is incurable, unless one choose to submit to the operation for deficiency of prepuce. But if it has not yet formed adhesions, we may make three, four, or more direct incisions circularly, and having bathed with much tepid oil, draw the prepuce outwards.

Commentary. Celsus describes the operation as follows: "Subter a summâ orâ, cutis inciditur recta linea usque ad frænum; atque ita superius tergus relaxatum, cedere retro potest. Quod si parum sic profectum est, aut propter angustias, aut propter duritiem tergoris, protinus triangula forma cutis ab inferiore parte excidenda est, sic ut vertex ejus ad frænum, basis in tergo extremo sit. Tum superdanda linamenta sunt alia que medicamenta quæ ad sanitatem perducant. Necessarium autem est, donec cicatrix sit, conquiescere: nam ambulatio, atterendo ulcus sordidum reddit." (vii, 25.)

Our author's description of the operation for keeping the prepuce separated from the glans, by means of a leaden tube, is mostly taken from Galen. (Meth. Med. xiv, 16.)

LVI—ON ADHESION OF THE PREPUCE TO THE GLANS

When there has been a previous ulceration about the glans, or prepuce, an adhesion of the one part to the other takes place. We must, therefore, dissect around, as far as may be, endeavouring to separate the adhesion with the point of a scalpel, or of a polypus knife, and more especially to free the glans completely from the prepuce, to which it adheres; but, if this be found difficult, we must rather add of the glans to the prepuce with which it is united, than contrariwise; for the prepuce, being thin, is readily perforated. After the disengagement of the adhesion, a thin cloth, dipped in cold water, is to be placed between the glans and the prepuce, that no adhesion may again take place, and the parts are to be healed with some astringent wine.

Commentary. Albucasis describes the operation in exactly the same terms. (Chirurg. ii, 56.)

LVII—ON CIRCUMCISION

We do not treat at present of those who are circumcised in conformity to a heathen rite, but of those in whom the prepuce has become black from some affection of the privy part. In such cases, it becomes necessary to cut off the blackened portion all around; and afterwards we must have recourse to the squama æris, with honey, or to pomegranate-rind and tare, in the form of those applications which are made upon a pledget. And if there be a hemorrhage, we must use lunated cauteries, which contribute to two good purposes: I mean the stoppage of the bleeding and of the spreading sore. But if the whole glans be consumed, having introduced a leaden tube into the urethra, we direct the patients to make water through it.

Commentary. See a similar description in Albucasis. (Chirurg. ii, 57.) Albucasis describes the mode of performing the operation on boys, as a rite of the Jewish religion. He directs the prepuce to be cut with a pair of scissors, and the part allowed to bleed freely. From the manner in which he expresses himself respecting the operation, there can be no doubt that he was a Jew, and it is equally clear that our author was a Pagan.

Fabricius ab Aquapendente describes a similar operation. (Œuv. Chirurg. ii, 64.) Guido de Cauliaco directs us to draw the prepuce forwards, and cut it off; after which the bleeding is to be stopped with powders, or the cautery. (vi, 2.)

LVIII—OF THYMI ON THE PENIS

Thymi are fleshy excrescences, forming sometimes upon the glans, and sometimes upon the prepuce; and some of them are malignant, and some are not. Those which are of a mild nature it will be proper to pare away with the edge of a scalpel, and sprinkle the part with chalcitis; but when malignant, the part must be burned after they are removed. If there be thymi on both sides of the prepuce, some internal and others external, we must not attempt all at the same time, lest by mistake we should cut off the prepuce, which is thin; but we must first cut off the internal, and, when they are healed, we may next attempt the external. Some of the moderns effect a cure by cutting them off with a pair of scissors, and by binding them with a horse-hair; as, in like manner, some burn them with the cold cautery.

Commentary. Albucasis copies our author's description. (Chirurg. ii, 56.) When the tumour is of a malignant nature, he particularly approves of using the actual cautery. These intractable tumours on the genital member are now frequently met with.

LIX—ON CATHETERISM, AND INJECTION OF THE BLADDER

When the urine is suppressed in the bladder, owing to some obstruction, such as a coagulum, or stones, or from any other cause, we have recourse to catheterism for the removal of it. Wherefore, taking a catheter proportionate to the age and sex we prepare the instrument for use. The mode of preparation is this: having bound a little wool round with a thread, and introduced the thread with a sharp rush into the pipe of the catheter, we adapt the wool to the opening at the head of the catheter, and having cut off the projecting parts of the wool with a pair of scissors, we put the catheter into oil. Having then placed the patient on a convenient seat, and used fomentations, if nothing prohibit, we take the catheter and introduce it at first direct down to the base of the penis, then we must draw the privy parts upwards to the umbilicus, (for at this place there is a curvature of the passage,) and thus push the instrument forwards. When in the perineum it approaches the anus, we must bend the member with the instrument in it down to its natural position, for from the perineum to the bladder the passage is upwards; and we must push the instrument forwards until it reach the cavity of the bladder. We afterwards take out the thread fastened into the opening of the catheter, in order that the urine being attracted by the wool may follow, as happens in syphons. Such is the method of introducing the catheter. But since we have often occasion to wash an ulcerated bladder, if an ear-syringe be sufficient to throw in the injection it may be used, and is to be introduced in the manner described above. But if we cannot succeed with it we may fix a skin or the bladder of an ox to the catheter, and throw in the injection through its opening.

Commentary. Although we have treated succinctly of strangury and retention of urine in the Third Book, it may be proper, before explaining the ancient methods of introducing the catheter, to give some further account of the causes of these complaints, and the opinions entertained by the physiologists with regard to the functional offices of the urinary organs. Galen states that the bladder is possessed of two faculties, a retentive and an expulsive, both of which arise from muscular power; that the retentive resides in the neck of the bladder, and is of the voluntary kind of powers; but that the expulsive belongs to the class of natural or involuntary powers, being of the same kind as the peristaltic faculty of the intestines. When a person, then, makes water voluntarily, it is by suspending the voluntary action of the sphincter vesicæ, that is to say, of the retentive faculty of the bladder, whereby the expulsive or peristaltic powers are brought into action, and the contents of the bladder are thereby evacuated. He properly adds, however, that this involuntary or expulsive faculty may be assisted by the action of the voluntary muscles which surround the bladder, especially the recti muscles of the abdomen. Retention of urine, therefore, may arise from the loss of either of these faculties. The expulsive faculty is most commonly lost, either from over-distension of the bladder, as when its contents have been allowed to accumulate too far, or from injury of the spinal marrow which supplies it with nerves. Rhases remarks that when retention of urine proceeds from debility of the expulsive faculty, the bladder may be evacuated by merely making pressure above the pubes.

According to Rhases, retention of urine arising from derangement of the retentive faculty, that is to say, from its no longer being under the control of the will, may be occasioned by inflammation, by some swelling, such as a fleshy tumour forming in the meatus urinarius, or by the presence of some foreign body, such as a stone, a clot of blood, or the like. He alludes several times to this fleshy tumour in the passage, by which he probably means either an enlargement of the prostate gland, or stricture of the urethra. He calls it a very intractable case. For a fuller exposition of the ingenious speculations and opinions stated above, see Galen (De Locis Affectis, iv, 4); Rhases (Contin. i and xxiii.)

Celsus describes very accurately the operation of catheterism. The tube or catheter, he says, should be made of copper, and the male catheter ought to be somewhat bent, smooth, and neither too large nor too small for the passage. The length of the largest male catheter should be 15 inches, of the middle-sized 12, and of the smallest 9; the largest female catheter should he 9, and the smallest 6 inches. The patient is to be laid on his back, and the surgeon standing by his right side, and holding the penis in his left hand, is to introduce with his right the catheter into the urinary passage; and when it reaches the neck of the bladder, the instrument along with the penis is to be bent downwards and introduced into the bladder. When the water is evacuated the catheter is to be extracted. The female passage, he remarks, is shorter, and is discovered by a sort of mammary protuberance above the vagina, by which he evidently means to describe the clitoris. The operation, he adds, in this case is less difficult. (vii, 26.)

The operation is mentioned by Aëtius and other of the Greek authorities, but none of them describe it fully but Paulus.

Albucasis recommends a catheter made of silver. His account of the operation is evidently borrowed from our author. He describes and gives a drawing of an instrument for throwing injections of oil and water into the bladder when inflamed. It is a tube of silver or copper having the bladder of a ram attached to it. (Chirurg. ii, 59.)

Avicenna and Serapion mention the operation but do not describe it minutely. Haly Abbas directs us to make the patient sit and to pour warm water and oil upon the penis. This is evidently recommended with a view of producing relaxation. The ordinary steps of the operation are very properly described by him. (Pract. ix, 45.)

Rhases gives a fuller account of catheterism, and all the circumstances connected therewith, than any other ancient author. He very properly forbids the catheter to be introduced when the retention arises from inflammation at the neck of the bladder. (Ad Mansor. ix, 73.) He first gives Antyllus's description of the operation, which is very accurate, but similar to our author's. He recommends us, before attempting the introduction of the instrument, to put the patient into a warm bath, or to apply hot fomentations to the parts. He then directs us to lubricate the instrument with oil or thick mucilage, and to introduce it into the passage until it arrives at the under extremity of the penis, when it is to be gently pushed upwards in the direction of the navel, turning it to one side or another according as it encounters obstruction. He states that it is best to have the openings of the catheter in its sides as they are less likely to be obstructed by clots than when in the extremity. He also mentions that he was sometimes in the practice of using a ductile instrument of lead which accommodated itself to the passage.

Both Serapion and Rhases mention the operation of puncturing the bladder. Rhases says that when there is retention of the urine and the bladder is inflamed, if the case be urgent, and there be reason to apprehend that the introduction of the catheter would aggravate the symptoms, it may be proper to make an incision in the perineum into the side of the bladder, and to draw off the urine with a canula. Both add, however, that there is danger of the wound not closing. (Cont. xxiii, 2.)

The ancients seem to have fancied that it was necessary to fill up the internal cavity of the catheter with wool, or some such substance, in order to produce a vacuum when drawn out, believing that the catheter in this case acted upon the principle of the syphon. See Alexander Aphrodisiensis (Prob. ii, 59.) It is singular that they should have fallen into this mistake, when Galen, as we have mentioned above, had so clearly explained that the evacuation of the bladder is accomplished by the action of its expulsive powers whenever its retentive faculty is suspended or overcome. The earlier writers on surgery likewise adopt the notion that the cavity of the instrument requires to be filled up with wool. See Guido de Cauliaco (vi, 2.) They describe stricture of the urethra under the names of *hypersarcosis* and *caruncula in meatu urinario*. See Henricus Regius (An. Med. 44.)

LX—ON CALCULUS

The cause of the formation of stones, and that in children they are formed most readily in the bladder, and in adults in the kidneys,—all this having been explained in another place, we now proceed to the method of performing lithotomy, but shall first give the symptoms of stones lodged in the bladder. The patients then void urine of a watery consistence with a sandy sediment; and from constant itching the member is now relaxed and again stretched in an uncommon degree, because, owing to the irritation, they are perpetually handling it, more especially in the case of children. When the stone falls into the neck of the bladder a sudden retention of urine takes place. Of those cut for the stone, children to the age of fourteen are the best subjects for the operation, on account of the softness of their bodies: old men are difficult to cure because ulcers of their bodies do not readily heal; and the intermediate ages have an intermediate chance of recovery. And again, those who have larger stones recover best because they have become habituated to the inflammation, whereas those who have smaller recover with difficulty for the opposite cause. These things being so, when we proceed to the operation, we first have recourse to shaking the patient, sometimes by means of assistants, and sometimes by making him jump from a height, in order that the stone may be forced down to the neck of the bladder. We have then to place him sitting in an erect posture, with his hands under his thighs, in order that the bladder may be forced down into a small space. If then we ascertain by feeling externally that the stone with the shaking has fallen down to the perineum, we proceed immediately to the operation; but if it has not descended, we must introduce the index finger of the left hand well oiled, or, if an adult, the middle also, into the anus, and with the fingers in a supine direction we search with them for the stone, and, bringing it down gradually to the neck of the bladder, we fix it there, pushing it out with the finger or fingers when so fixed; and having given directions to the assistant to press down the bladder with his hands, and ordering another assistant to raise the testicles in his right hand, and with the other to stretch the perineum to the other side from that upon which the incision is to be made, we take the instrument called a lithotome, and between the anus and the testicles, not, however, in the middle of the perineum, but on one side, towards the left buttock, we make an oblique incision, cutting down direct upon the stone where it protrudes, so that the external incision may be wider, but the internal not larger than just to allow the stone to fall through it. Sometimes, from the pressure of the finger or fingers at the anus, the stone starts out readily at the same time that the incision is made, without requiring extraction; but if it does not start out of itself we must extract it with the forceps called the stone-extractor. After the removal of the stone, having stopped the bleeding by manna of frankincense and aloes, comfrey, misy, and such like styptic powders, and having dipped wool or compresses in wine and oil, we apply them; and also apply the bandages for calculous diseases, namely, that having six legs. But if there be any apprehension of hemorrhage we must apply a compress which had been soaked in oxycrate, or water and rose-oil, and placing the patient in a reclining posture, bathe the parts frequently. After the third day, having loosed the bandages, and poured much water and oil into the wound, we may dress it with the ointment called tetrapharmacon (basilicon) on a pledget, removing them and dressing often on account of the acrimony of the urine. If inflammation come on, we must have recourse to the cataplasms and fomentations proper for it. And we may also inject into the bladder oil of roses, oil of camomile, or butter, unless some inflammation prevent. In like manner, if the sore become spreading, or otherwise malignant, we must suit the applications to the state of it. When the ulcer is freed from inflammation we may loose the dressings, and use diachylon plaster to the groins and bottom of the belly. During the whole time of the treatment, the thighs must be bound together, which contributes to the cure with the other remedies. If the stone, being small, fall into the penis, and cannot be voided with the urine, we may draw the prepuce strongly forwards, and bind it at the extremity of the glans. We must next apply another ligature round the penis behind the member, making the constriction at its extremity next the bladder, and then make an incision down upon the stone, and bending the penis we eject the stone, and undoing the ligatures we clear away the coagula from the wound. The posterior ligature is applied lest the calculus should retreat backwards, and the anterior, in order that, when untied, after the extraction of the stone, the skin of the prepuce may slide backwards and cover the incision.

Commentary. We will now attempt to explain all the ancient descriptions of lithotomy.

Hippocrates in his *Oath* binds his pupils not to perform this operation, but to leave it to those who made it their business. It appears then that in his days lithotomy was a separate branch of the profession. Celsus is the earliest author who describes lithotomy, although it is probable that he merely explained the method of operating in Alexandria, the surgeons of which city had acquired great celebrity in performing this operation. He forbids the operation, except after every other remedy had failed; and in children between the ages of nine and fourteen, and in the season of spring. The patient is to be kept upon a spare diet beforehand; and when the operation is about to be performed, he is to be directed to walk, so as to bring down the stone to the neck of the bladder, which is to be ascertained by introducing a finger into the anus. Then a strong and experienced person, sitting on a high seat, is to take the patient and hold him secure, his buttocks being placed upon the assistant's knee, and his legs being drawn in and his hands placed on them and held there. But if the patient be strong he is to be held by two assistants, one on each side, upon two seats placed beside one another, and they are to be directed to press upon his shoulders with their breasts, so as to force down the bladder. Two other assistants are to be at hand, to prevent any risk of the former two losing their hold. The surgeon having pared his nails, is to introduce gently first the index and then the middle finger into the anus, whilst with the right he makes pressure upon the abdomen, and in this way the stone is to be secured at the neck of the bladder. The shape of the stone is to be considered, and it is to be pressed down so as to favour its exit. These matters being properly arranged, a lunated incision is to be made over the neck of the bladder near the anus down to the neck of the bladder, the horns of the incision inclining a little towards the (left?) buttock; then at that part where the incision is bent round (at the curvature of the incision?) even under the skin, another transverse incision is to be made, by which the neck is to be opened, and the urinary passage dilated, the opening being somewhat larger than the stone. When the stone is small it may be propelled and drawn out by the fingers; but if large, it is to be extracted by a hook or crotchet made for that purpose. This hook is of a semi-circular form, smooth externally, and rough on the inside. By the help of it the stone is to be taken out dexterously, attention being paid to the shape of it. He mentions that Ammonius the lithotomist was in the practice of breaking down the stone into pieces when it was so large that it could not be extracted without tearing the neck of the bladder. He states that the operation is seldom required in the case of females, but that if the stone be large it may sometimes be necessary. The fingers are to be introduced into the vagina, as they are into the rectum of males, and then, if the patient be a girl, an incision is to be made under the left edge (of the labia pudendi?); but if in an adult female, a transverse incision is to be made on both sides between the urethra and os pubis.

The above is but an abridgment of the Celsian description, which, it must be admitted, is attended with considerable difficulties. We shall give the passage in which he describes the form and place of the incisions. "Incidi super vesicæ cervicem juxta anum cutis plaga lunata usque ad cervicem vesicæ debet, cornibus ad *coxas* spectantibus paulum: deinde eâ parte, qua resima plaga est, etiamnum sub cute altera transversa plaga facienda est, qua cervix aperiatur; donec urinæ iter pateat, sic, ut plaga paulo major, quam calculus sit." Sprengel renders the words "cornibus ad coxas spectantibus paulum" by "dont les angles regardant les aines;"

but *coxæ* signifies properly not the groins, but the *nates*, viz., the buttocks, or perhaps the hips. (Celsus viii, 1.) In the English translation of M. Foubert's paper on Lithotomy, in the 'Memoirs of the French Academy of Surgery,' these words are more correctly rendered, "the extremities of which incision must be in some measure directed towards the thighs." Dr. Milligan, however, in his edition of Celsus, proposes to read *coxam*, by which he supposes that Celsus understood the *coxa sinistra*. He adds: "hinc liquet, cornua plagæ Celsianæ, ut hodiernæ, coxam sinistram respexisse." We are inclined to adopt this conjecture, as it makes the Celsian description agree with that of our author and his Arabian copyists, all of whom direct the first incision to be made towards the left *nates*. The words "qua resima plaga est," must signify, we suppose, the curvature in the middle of the incision where the two horns unite. M. Foubert reads "qua strictior ima plaga est," but we suspect without any proper authority from MSS.

We may be permitted to remark that the advantages of the semi-lunar incision are pointed out by Bromfield, and the Celsian operation was generally practised by the late Baron Dupuytren of Paris.

Aëtius and other of the Greek authorities allude frequently to the operation, but none of them describe it minutely except Paulus. Our author's statement, that there is less danger from the extraction of large than of small stones, is at variance, we believe, with modern experience. Aretæus states that small stones are most easily extracted. He was, however, no advocate for the operation at all, except in extreme cases. He speaks of cutting "the neck of the bladder." (Morb. Acut. Curat, ii, 9.) Does he not allude to attempts at lithotrity in the following passage?—ὄυτε γὰρ (λίθος μέγας) θρύπτεται, ἣ πόσι, ἤ φαρμάκῳ, ἣ αμφιθρυπτοιτο, ὂυτε ἀσινέως τέμνεται. (Morb. Chron. ii, 4.) Which passage may be thus translated: "when the stone is large neither lithotrity, or lithotripsy, nor lithotomy, can be practised safely." Theophilus, in his 'Commentary on the Aphorisms of Hippocrates,' states that in lithotomy it is not the bladder, properly speaking, but the neck of the bladder, which is muscular, that is cut.

We now proceed to the Arabians. Albucasis, after detailing the symptoms in much the same terms as our author, goes on to describe the operation as follows. Having cleared out the bowels with a clyster, the patient is to be shaken so as to make the stone descend, and he is then to be secured in the arms of an assistant, with his hands under his *nates*. The surgeon is then to press upon the perineum, and, if the stone be felt, the operation is to be proceeded with; but otherwise, the index finger of the left hand, if the patient be a child, and the middle if an adult, is to be introduced into the anus, and the stone is thereby to be gradually brought down to the neck of the bladder. Having pushed it outwards to the place where you mean to make your incision, an assistant is to be directed to press down the bladder from above the pubes, while another draws up the testicles with the one hand, and with the other stretches the skin under them. Then with a proper scalpel the operator is to make an incision between the anus and the testicles, not in the middle, but towards the left *nates*, straight upon the stone which is to be pressed out by the finger. Let the incision be transverse (oblique?), large externally, but internally of the size of the stone. If the stone does not then start out, the operator must seize upon it with a forceps, or a hook having a lunated extremity. If there be more than one stone, the largest is to be extracted first, and then the others may be easily removed. When the stone is large he directs us to break it down with a forceps. His directions respecting the treatment afterwards are similar to those of Paulus. When the stone sticks in the urethra he recommends us to cut down upon it. His description of the operation on women is likewise similar to our author's, but more circumstantial. Having got a dexterous midwife, or some proper person to introduce her finger into the rectum or vagina, and press the stone down to the left hip, the operator is to make first a small incision over it, and afterwards, by the help of a sound or specillum, it is to be enlarged so as to allow a passage for the stone. (Chirurg. ii, 60, 61.)

Avicenna's description is nearly the same as that of Albucasis, but not so minute. He directs the surgeon to introduce a finger into the anus, if the patient be a male, but into the vagina if a woman who is not a virgin, and to push the stone outwards, so as to make it protrude. He is then to cut down upon it, making an incision proportionate to the size of the stone; but if the stone be very large, the incision must not be made of the same size, but it is to be grasped in a forceps and broken into pieces. If inflammation come on after the operation, he recommends him to have recourse to clysters, the warm bath, and venesection, and a piece of cloth dipped in oil of roses and some vinegar is to be applied to the part. The bad symptoms after the operation are said to be violent pain in the part and under the navel, coldness of the extremities, prostration of strength, loss of appetite, and, at last, singultus and involuntary discharges from the bowels. (iii, xix, 1, 7.)

The description given by Haly Abbas being nearly the same as that of Albucasis, need not be noticed here but very briefly. He prefers performing the operation in infancy, but permits it to be done at all ages. For the reason assigned by our author he states that recovery is most likely to take place when the stone is large. Like the others, he directs the surgeon to introduce either the fore-finger alone, or it and the middle finger into the anus, behind the stone, and to push it outwards, and then the operator is to cut down upon it, making the incision between the testes and the anus, yet not in the middle, but towards the left side. When the incision is carried down to the stone it will sometimes start out from the pressure of the fingers in the anus; but otherwise, it is to be seized upon with a forceps and extracted. If inflammation come on he recommends us to apply a cataplasm, and to throw into the bladder an injection consisting of oil of roses and of camomile, or of melted butter. (Practic. ix, 46.)

Rhases gives from preceding authors several descriptions of lithotomy, but as they closely resemble our author's, we shall treat of them only in a cursory manner. In his first description he directs the surgeon to place the patient with his hands fastened to his ankles so as to press down the bladder. When the stone does not descend properly, so as to be felt externally, he recommends him to introduce one or more fingers into the rectum and push it outwards; and then while an assistant draws up the testicles the operator is to make a transverse (oblique?) incision, larger externally, but internally only of such a size as to allow the stone to pass out. If the stone does not come out readily it is to be extracted with an instrument, and the hemorrhage checked with a composition of aloes, frankincense, and vitriol. When the patient is a child he recommends the operator to place him upon the knees of an assistant, and to make pressure on the abdomen so as to force down the bladder. He forbids the operation when the stone cannot be brought down to the neck of the bladder. When the stone is large he directs it to be broken into pieces before extraction. His next description is taken from the celebrated Antyllus, but as it scarcely differs at all from the preceding one, we shall merely select a few remarks. When the stone is smooth, round, and small, he directs the surgeon to push it down to the neck of the bladder by means of a finger introduced into the rectum, and to make an incision down upon it; after which the stone is to be forced out. When pain supervenes after the operation, he recommends him to place the patient in a bath medicated with camomile, linseed, mallows, &c.; or if it be summer, and there be any disposition to hemorrhage, to place him in a vessel filled with strong vinegar. When it is ascertained that there are clots of blood in the bladder obstructing the urine, he directs the surgeon to introduce a finger by the incision, and extract them gradually. His next description is from an author named Sarad, whom he frequently quotes in other parts of his works. He directs the operator to introduce a finger into the rectum and push the stone outwards to the left side of the perineum, removed about the size of a grain of barley from the raphe (*daram*), and then to make an incision into the neck of the bladder. He afterwards gives a very circumstantial account of the operation from another author called Athuriscus. He particularly directs the operator to make an incision in the left side of the perineum and to open the neck of the bladder, as a wound of the body of the bladder seldom unites. When the stone is large he recommends him to seize it with strong pincers and break it into pieces. When a stone sticks in the urethra he directs him to tie one ligature behind it and to secure the prepuce before the glans with another, and then to cut down upon the stone. He gives very minute directions about the after treatment, recommending especially the removal of any clots which obstruct the passage. (Cont. xxiii.)

The practice of lithotomy appears to have been reckoned a disreputable occupation among the Arabians, for Avenzoar mentions it as an operation which an upright and respectable man would not witness, far less perform. (ii, 2, 7.)

As there are some doubts regarding the form of the incisions in the ancient methods of performing lithotomy, we will now give the words of some of the Arabian translators. Stephanus Antiochensis, the translator of Haly Abbas, has the following words: "Inter testes anumque finde et non in mediâ viâ sed in sinistri lateris parte ab intestinis, sitque *perallela* fissura, et ab exterioribus larga, ab interioribus non." The translator of Albucasis expresses himself thus: "Finde in eo quod est inter anum et testiculos et non in medio, ad latus natis sinistræ: fiat sectio *transversa*." The following are the words of Avicenna's translator: "Cave ne scindas super commissuram quum sit malum, commissura enim secundum veritatem est locus mortalis. Amplius fac super ipsum (lapidem?) scissuram tendentem ad *transversum*, studendo ut cadat scissura in collo vesicæ." The translator of Rhases expresses himself in the following terms: "Scinde super lapidem cum instrumento *camadan*; et scissura debet fieri *transversa*, et sit exterior caro larga et in interiori vesicæ stricta."

Yet notwithstanding all this we are inclined to think that the incision was *oblique* and not *transverse*; for our author, whom they all follow, directs us to make the incision oblique (λοξὸς), and it is further clear that a transverse one would not answer the purpose so well. No dependence can be put in the accuracy of these barbarous translations. The language of Stephanus Antiochensis is particularly obscure. Casiri justly characterizes the translations of the Arabian authors as being "*perversiones* potius quam *versiones*." (Bibl. Hisp. Arab, i, 266.)

The ancient operation, with scarcely any alterations, is described by the earlier modern writers on surgery. See Brunus (Chirurg. Magna. ii, 17); and Guido de Cauliaco (Chir. vi, 2.) They direct us to introduce a finger into the rectum and push the stone outwards; then to make an incision down upon it on the left side of the raphe. Brunus recommends a longitudinal incision.

It appears that the ancient operation of lithotomy is still practised with great success by the native doctors of Hindostan. See 'Transactions of the Medical and Physical Society of Calcutta,' vol. iv. An interesting case in point, related in the 'Medical Gazette' for Feb. 7, 1845, forms a valuable commentary on the Celsian description of lithotomy. In the year 1827 Mr. Madden the traveller saw it performed in Tyre by an old pilot on a boy of thirteen years of age. The case did well.

LXI—ON THE PARTS ABOUT THE TESTICLES

As contributing to the understanding of the operations on herniæ, we shall premise a description of the parts about the testicles. The testicle itself is a glandular and friable substance, formed for the production of semen. The substances called parastatæ and cremasteres, are processes from the membrane of the spinal marrow, descending along with the arterial vessels in the testicles, by which the semen is injected into the pudendum; the spermatic vessels are veins from the vena cava passing to the testicles in a convoluted manner, and by them the testicles are nourished. The tunica vaginalis (erythroides or elytroides?) is of a nervous nature; at the convex and anterior part not adhering, but at the concave and posterior parts united to the testicle, deriving its origin from the peritoneal coat. This part, where it is united to the testicle, they call the posterior adhesion. The darti are membranes connecting the external skin to the tunica vaginalis, being united to it at the part where it is united behind to the testicle. But that wrinkled skin which forms an external covering to the testicles is called the scrotum.

Commentary. Celsus gives a similar description of the parts connected with the testicles. The testicles themselves, he says, consist of medullary matter and possess no sensibility of their own, but experience violent pains and inflammations from the membrane which surrounds them. They hang from the groins by nerves called cremasters by the Greeks, with each of which descend two veins and arteries. These are covered by a thin nervous white coat, without blood, called elytroides by the Greeks. (This must be the tunica vaginalis of modern anatomists.) Above it is a stronger tunic which adheres strongly to the inner at its lower part, and is called dartos by the Greeks. (This appears to be the cremaster muscle of modern anatomists.) The veins, arteries, and nerves are surrounded by many small membranes. (By these he seems to have meant the fasciæ from the aponeurosis of the external oblique muscle.) All these parts are covered by an external investment called the scrotum. (vii, 18.)

Ruffus Ephesius says that the scrotum is a loose substance in which the testicles are placed, being in particular fleshy externally; that it consists of two tunics, the external being corrugated and called dartos, and the internal being called erythroides (elytroides?). The dartos and scrotum connect the testicles to the parts above, but the erythroides (vaginalis?) is united to and surrounds the testicle itself. (De Corporis Humani partium appellationibus, ii.)

Oribasius describes the cremasters as being two muscles which descend from the groins and surround the tunica vaginalis. (Anatomica ex Galeno.) (This is very similar to Cloquet's description of them.)

Theophilus's description unfortunately has come down to us very incomplete. (De Fabricâ Hominis, v, ad finem.)

LXII—ON HYDROCELE

An inert fluid, collected about the parts which are enveloped by the scrotum, and occasioning a marked swelling there, has obtained this appellation. The fluid is, for the most part, collected in the tunica vaginalis around the testicle, at its anterior part; but the affection is sometimes, though rarely, formed externally to the tunica vaginalis. Often, however, it is collected in the proper tunic of the testicles, and surgeons call this affection hydrocele of the tunica adnata. If the complaint is formed from some preceding cause, such as weakness of the parts, the blood brought there for the purpose of nourishment is converted into an inert watery or serous substance. But if it is occasioned by a blow, a sanguineous or feculent substance constitutes its contents. The common symptom is a permanent swelling without pain about the scrotum, not disappearing under any circumstances, yet somewhat compressible when the collection is small, but not at all compressible when it is large. When the fluid is collected in the tunica vaginalis the swelling is globular, but somewhat oblong like an egg; and in these cases the testicle is not to be felt as being everywhere surrounded with the fluid. But that which is collected externally to the tunica vaginalis, is felt as through a small intervening substance. When it is formed in the adnata, being everywhere circumscribed and globular, the swelling has the appearance of another testicle. If the fluid be watery, the swelling is of one colour and transparent; but if it be feculent and bloody, it appears red or livid; and if these symptoms appear in both parts of the scrotum, you may be sure that there is a double hernia. We operate upon it in this manner. Having shaven the pubes and scrotum, unless the patient be a boy, we lay him in a supine posture upon a bench, and apply to his buttocks a cloth several times folded, and to the scrotum a sponge of considerable magnitude, and sitting at the left side of the patient, we give directions to an assistant sitting at his right side to draw the genital organs to the other side, and to draw up the skin of the scrotum to the abdomen. Then taking a scalpel we divide the scrotum longitudinally from its middle to near the pubes, making the incision straight and parallel to the raphe which divides the scrotum into two parts, and extending the incision down to the vaginalis. When the fluid is in the adnata, we make the incision where the apex of the tunica adnata makes its appearance, and separating the lips of the incision with a hook, and having dissected the darti with a knife for hydrocele and a scalpel, and laid bare the tunica vaginalis, we divide it through the middle with a lancet for bleeding, more especially in that part where it is separated from the testicle; and having discharged into some vessel the whole or most of the fluid, we cut away the vaginalis, especially its thinnest parts, with hooks. Afterwards, Antyllus uses sutures and the treatment for recent wounds; but the moderns have recourse to what is called the incarnative mode of treatment. If the testicle is found in a state of putrefaction, or otherwise diseased, the vessels which pass along with the cremaster are to be separately inclosed in a ligature, the cremaster cut, and the testicle removed. And when there are two hernias we may operate in the same manner twice, directing the incisions on both sides at the parts of the scrotum about the loins. After these things, having introduced the head of a probe through the incision below at the extremity of the scrotum, and elevating the scrotum upon it, we make an incision with a sharp-pointed scalpel in a convenient situation for the discharge of the coagulated blood and pus. By means then of the head of the probe we introduce an oblong pledget into the upper incision, and having sponged away the clotted blood, we introduce wool dipped in oil through the incision down to the testicle; and externally we may apply other pieces of wool dipped in wine and oil to the scrotum, hypogastrium, groins, perineum, and loins; and applying a compress three times folded upon them, and binding them with a six-legged bandage, and other proper bandages, we place the man in a reclining posture, putting wool under the scrotum for the sake of ease, and spreading the soft skin under him to receive the embrocations. We bathe with warm oil until the third day, after which having loosed the bandages we must use the ointment tetrapharmacon on a pledget, having changed the oblong one. Afterwards we may again apply the embrocations proper for inflammation until the seventh day, after which we have recourse to the medicine called motophylacion. After the ulcer has been cleaned and moderately incarnated, and the parts have been bathed, we must remove the oblong pledget, and have recourse to the subsequent treatment as formerly described. But if inflammation, hemorrhage, or any such disagreeable consequence come on, we must, in a word, treat each of these in a suitable manner, that I may not have occasion to make repetitions. But if we would rather have recourse to the cautery in cases of hydrocele (as is the practice of the moderns), we must follow all the directions given as to what is to be done before and after the operation, and also those given with regard to the operation itself, omitting only the incision with a scalpel, and the division for allowing the discharge of its contents. Wherefore having heated ten or twelve cauteries, shaped like the Greek letter Γ, and two sword-shaped ones, we must first burn the scrotum through the middle with the gamma-shaped, and having dissected away the membranes with a scalpel or blunt hook, we must burn with the sword-shaped as if cutting. Having laid bare the tunica vaginalis (which is easily recognized by its whiteness and density) with the extremity of a gamma-shaped cautery, we evacuate the fluid. Afterwards, when the whole is laid bare, we stretch it with hooks and remove it with a sword-shaped cautery.

Commentary. Celsus directs the surgeon, when water is contained in a hernial tumour, to make an incision in the groin, if the patient be a child, unless the largeness of the collection prevent; but in adults, and when the swelling is great, he recommends him to make it in the scrotum. Then if the incision be in the groin, the coats are to be drawn up there and the water discharged; but if in the scrotum, and if the disease be seated there, nothing more is to be done but to evacuate the fluid, and remove any membranes which may happen to contain it; after which the parts are to be washed with a solution of salt or soda. When the fluid is situated under the middle or inner coat (the tunica vaginalis and tunica albuginea?), all these tunics are to be removed without the scrotum and cut out. (vii, 21.) Celsus, as well as our author, describes the hæmatocele or bloody tumour, the existence of which is affirmed by Heister. (ii, 5, 123.)

Galen alludes incidentally to the evacuation of the fluid in hydrocele. (Meth. Med. xiv.) Sprengel and Guy de Cauliac affirm that he makes mention of the seton as a mode of cure; but if this assertion be correct we have not been able to find out the passage in which he does so.

Aëtius gives a very distinct account of the nature of hydrocele, but his description of the operation is by no means so accurate as our author's. He trusts mostly to astringent and desiccative applications. (xiv, 22.)

Albucasis describes the operation in nearly the same terms as Paulus. His operation consisted of making an incision in the swelling and dissecting out the coats of the testicles. The dressings which he recommends are similar to those mentioned by our author. He also describes the operation by the cautery in nearly the same terms as Paulus. He adds, that if the patient be timid and do not choose to submit to these operations, the surgeon may let out the water either with a scalpel or the instrument used for tapping in dropsy. He states, however, that after this operation the water will collect again. (Chirurg. ii, 62.)

Avicenna briefly describes the operation of opening the tumour, and applying cauteries or strong medicines to the membranes. (iii, xxii, i, 6.)

Haly Abbas directs us to open the tumour, and cut out its tunics, and then to apply incarnative dressings. This treatment, he adds, the moderns prefer to the escharotic applications used by the ancients. (Pract. ix, 47.) He also describes the process of burning. (Pract. ix, 79.)

Rhases describes the operation of puncturing the scrotum for hydrocele. He also speaks of burning the part with a slender rod of iron, and of cutting out its tunics. (Cont. xxiv.)

The membrane called tunica adnata in our translation is the "ima tunica" of Celsus, and the "panniculus proprius" of the Arabian translation of Albucasis, and seems to be the same as the tunica albuginea of modern anatomists.

Sprengel gives an excellent history of the operation of hydrocele. (Hist. de la Méd. 18, 8.)

LXIII—ON SARCOCELE AND TOPHI OF THE TESTICLES

When flesh is formed in any part of the bodies which are connected by the scrotum, it gives rise to the disease called sarcocele. This arises either from some obscure cause, the testicle being attacked with a defluxion and becoming indurated, or from a blow, or from unskilful treatment after the operation for hernia. Its consequences are, a swelling of the same colour, with hardness; when the swelling is of a scirrhous nature, it is devoid of colour and sensibility; and when it is malignant there are sharp pains. When going to operate we place the patient as in the former case, and make the incisions in like manner; and if the complaint is occasioned by the growth of a fleshy tumour to the testicle, we divide the dartos and tunica vaginalis in like manner; then stretching the testicle and bringing it to the outside of the vaginalis, we separate the cremaster from the vessels, tie a ligature round the vessels, and cut the cremaster; then we remove the testicle affected with the fleshy tumour as a foreign body. But if the fleshy tumour be formed about any of the coats of the testicle or its vessels, having divided the scrotum and the membranes lying under the flesh, we must dissect out the whole fleshy tumour. But if the posterior process ("epididymis"?) be affected with sarcocele, having dissected all the surrounding parts, we remove the testicle along with it; for it is impossible for the testicle to continue without it. If tophi be formed about the testicle and the tunica vaginalis, they may be distinguished from sarcocele and hydrocele by their resistance, hardness, and inequality, and are to be operated upon as sarcocele.

Commentary. Celsus describes and recommends the same operations. He directs us to divide the nerve by which the testicle is suspended (the cremaster?), then to tie the veins and arteries at the groin with a thread, and cut them below the ligature. When a fleshy tumour is formed between the coats he recommends us to cut it out. (vii, 22, 23.) When the parts are indurated he forbids us to meddle with them.

Albucasis directs us to separate the cremaster from the vessels, to tie the vessels, and then remove the testicle from the surrounding parts. When the disease consists of a fleshy tumour which adheres to the testicle he directs us to cut it out. After the operation the wound is to be filled with rose-oil and wine. (Chirurg. ii, 63.) The other Arabians treat of the operation less minutely, with the exception of Haly Abbas, who describes it exactly as Albucasis. (Pract. ix, 48.)

LXIV—ON CIRSOCELE AND PNEUMATOCELE

When the vessels about the scrotum or darti are in a varicose condition, they are called simply varices, but if the nutrient vessels of the testicles be in a varicose state, the affection is named cirsocele. The symptoms of it are obvious. There is a collection attended with swelling, and somewhat curved, of a botryoidal shape, and accompanied with relaxation of the testicle. It also occasions certain inconveniences, especially in running, exercising, and walking. We may operate upon it thus. After putting the patient in a convenient posture, we must lay hold of the scrotum and push the cremaster to the under part; it is easily distinguished from the vessels, being more slender, firmer, and elastic, as being strong and firm; the patient also feels pain upon pressure, and moreover it is connected with the penis. Having secured the vessels in the scrotum by our own fingers and those of our assistant, and stretching them strongly, we press obliquely the point of a scalpel direct upon the vessels; then having transfixed the parts with hooks and dissected what lie under the skin, and having exposed the vessels, as mentioned in the operation of angiology and that for aneurism, and pushing through them a needle having a double thread, and cutting the loop of the thread, we tie the ligatures round the vessels where the varices arise and where they terminate, and make a straight incision in the intermediate space. Having evacuated the blood collected in the tumour, we apply the treatment for suppurations until the ligatures with the vessels themselves fall out of their own accord. Leonides says, that when a few of the vessels which nourish the testicles are in a varicose state this operation should be performed, but that when all are affected, the testicle should be cut out along with them, lest being deprived of its nutrient vessels it should decay. Pneumatocele being a species of aneurism, Leonides forbids us to operate upon it for fear of a hemorrhage, which cannot be restrained from taking place at the time; but, there being two kinds of it, the one occasioned by the four vessels which nourish the testicle, and the other by the arteries of the darti and scrotum being affected, the moderns refrain from meddling with the latter, but operate upon the former. We distinguish them from one another, inasmuch as that which arises from the arteries is easily made to disappear upon pressure with the fingers, whereas that from the nutrient vessels of the testicles, not at all or with much trouble. We operate upon it as for cirsocele, taking up each of the veins and securing it with a thread.

Commentary. Celsus thus describes the cirsocele: "Venæ intumescunt; eæque intortæ conglomeratæque a superiore parte, vel ipsum scrotum implent, vel mediam tunicam vel imam: interdum etiam sub imâ tunicâ, circa testiculum nervumque ejus, increscunt." (vii, 18.) He describes the operation at great length afterwards. If the varicose tumour is upon the scrotum he directs us to burn it with slender and sharp irons, which are to be applied to the veins themselves, but in such a manner as to burn them alone. Then suitable dressings are to be applied for producing cicatrization. When the varicose veins are situated above the middle tunic, an incision is to be made in the groin, the tunic drawn out, and the veins separated from it with a finger or the handle of a scalpel. The veins are afterwards to be tied with a thread above and below; then they are to be cut below, and the testicle restored to its place. When the disease is situated above the third tunic (tunica albuginea?) the middle one must be cut out. Then if only two or three veins are in a varicose state they may be tied, as above directed, at the groin and where they join the testicle and cut out. When the disease is situated between the internal coat and the testicle, he says, there is no other remedy but the removal of the testicle. For this purpose he directs us to secure the arteries and veins with a thread, divide them, and then to cut the nerve by which the testicle is suspended (the cremaster?). (vii, 19 and 22.) He does not treat of pneumatocele. It must be obvious that the pneumatocele of our author was an aneurismal varix or erectile tissue. We see no good reason, therefore, for the animadversions which Heister makes upon his account of it. (See Surgery.)

This operation is briefly noticed in the 'Isagoge' of Galen, and 'Meth. Med.' (xiv.)

Albucasis considers it a dangerous operation, but says he will describe it as it was performed by the ancients. He accordingly gives our author's account of it, directing us to dissect the congeries of vessels from the surrounding parts, to pass a needle, armed with a double thread, under them, and to tie them above and below; then to make a longitudinal incision in them, and to evacuate the feculent fluids which they contain. The wound is afterwards to be dressed with incarnants. If all the vessels are involved in the disease, he directs us to remove the testicle altogether. (Chirurg. ii, 64.)

He says he never saw the operation performed for pneumatocele; but that the ancients operated for it in the same manner as for cirsocele. (66.)

Avicenna and Rhases treat of the pneumatocele, and recommend carminative applications to it; but they do not describe the surgical operation.

Haly Abbas borrows the description of Paulus. (Pract. ix, 49.)

LXV—ON ENTEROCELE, OR INTESTINAL HERNIA

Enterocele is a descent of the intestine into the scrotum, and is occasioned either from rupture of the peritoneum which takes place in the groin, or from stretching of the peritoneum. Both these, I mean rupture and stretching, are occasioned by previous violence, such as a blow, a leap, or loud crying, but that from stretching in particular is connected with relaxation and other weaknesses of the body. The common symptoms of both are a marked swelling in the scrotum, which is increased by exercise, heat, retention of the breath, and other exertions; and its symptoms are, that it goes up slowly upon pressure, and quickly falls down again, and that while the person affected with it lies in a recumbent posture it remains in its proper place until he stands again erect. The retention of fæces in the region of the scrotum often brings on dangerous symptoms; for it is attended with pain, and sometimes with rumbling of wind upon pressure. The peculiar symptoms of hernia from distension are, that it does not occur suddenly, but gradually; that it falls down occasionally from any ordinary causes; that the swelling appears equable and deep-seated, the protruded intestine being surrounded by the peritoneum. In those from rupture the descent at first is sudden, and happens only from violence; the swelling is very large, and appears seated superficially immediately under the skin, owing to the intestines having burst through the peritoneum. If the omentum alone falls down to the scrotum in rupture of the peritoneum the affection is called epiplocele, but if intestine descend along with it, it is named epiploenterocele; and if water be contained in the tunica vaginalis it receives an appellation compounded from all the three. But neither these nor the intestinal hernia from rupture of the peritoneum are proper subjects for surgery, but we operate upon enterocele alone from distension, in the following manner: after placing the patient in a recumbent posture, and getting the skin in the groin stretched by an assistant, we make a transverse incision, cutting as in the operation of angiology (but some make the incision not transverse but longitudinal), then having transfixed it with hooks we stretch out the incision to such a degree as to afford room for the testicle to pass through; then passing through the inner skin a number of hooks proportionate to the size of the wound, and dissecting the membranes and fat with a blind hook or scalpel we cut them across. When the peritoneum is everywhere laid bare, introducing the index-finger at the back part of the scrotum between the darti and peritoneum, we free the posterior process (epididymis?); and then with the right hand doubling its extremity to the inside of the scrotum, and at the same time stretching the peritoneum in the left hand, we bring the testicle with the vaginalis tunica to the incision, and give directions to one assistant to stretch the testicle, whilst we, having completely cleared the posterior process, ascertain by the fingers whether a fold of intestine be comprehended in the tunica vaginalis, and if so we must press it down to the belly; then we take a large-sized needle containing a doubled thread of ten pieces, and we pass it through the middle at the extremity of the peritoneum close to the incision; and cutting the double we make four pieces of them, and laying them over one another in the form of the Greek letter X, we bind the peritoneum securely, and again twisting round the pieces we secure it so that none of the nutrient vessels may have a free passage to it lest any inflammation be occasioned, and we apply another ligature farther out, less than two fingers' breadth distant from the former. After making these ligatures we leave about the size of a finger of the peritoneum, and cut off the whole all round, removing at the same time the testicle, then making an incision at the lower part of the scrotum to favour the discharge, we introduce an oblong pledget, and apply embrocations of oil and bandages as for hydrocele. We must also make the other applications as there laid down. I have known some not unskilful surgeons who after the incision into the tunica vaginalis burnt the extremity of it with heated cauteries for fear of hemorrhage, as would appear. These after the operation straightway bathed their patients in a long wooden trough containing hot water, until the seventh day, repeating this as often as five times during the period of a day and a night, more especially with children; and it succeeded wonderfully, for they remained free from inflammation, and the ligatures fell out speedily along with the parts. In the intervals between the bathings the afore-mentioned embrocations were applied. Another surgeon, in addition to the means already mentioned, rubbed into their back at the time pepper triturated with oil.

Commentary. Celsus recommends us, if the patient be a child, to make an attempt, in the first place, to effect a cure with bandages. In more advanced ages, if a large portion of intestine has fallen down, and if attended with pain and vomiting, which symptoms generally arise from retention of the fæces, it is clear, he says, that the knife is not applicable, and that the case is to be remedied by other means. He recommends venesection in the arm, the tepid bath, warm cataplasms, and spare diet; but he disapproves of purgatives. This is his treatment of strangulated hernia. When an operation with the scalpel is resolved upon, an incision having been made in the groin down to the middle tunic (tunica vaginalis?), the lips of it are to be separated with the assistance of hooks, while the surgeon frees the tunic from all the small membranes (external fascia?). When this tunic is removed, an incision is to be made from the groin down to the testicle, which is to be carefully cut out. This process, however, is only applicable when the patient is of a tender age, and the mischief is moderate. When the patient is a strong man and the disease greater, the testicle is not to be removed, but is to be allowed to remain in its place. It is accomplished in this manner: the groin being opened with a scalpel, in the same manner, down to the middle tunic, it is to be seized with two hooks, so that an assistant may prevent the testicle from falling out at the wound; then that tunic is to be cut downwards with a scalpel, and under it the index-finger of the left hand is to be pushed down to the bottom of the testicle so as to force it up to the wound: then the thumb and index-finger of the right hand separate the vein, artery, nerve, and their tunic, from the upper tunic. But if any small membranes (fasciæ?) come in the way, they are to be cut out with a scalpel, until the whole tunic be exposed. Having cut out what is proper, and replaced the testicle, a somewhat broader thong of skin is to be removed from the lips of the wound in the groin, in order to enlarge the wound, and thereby occasion a greater formation of new flesh. The object of this operation, it will be remarked, is to produce a firm cicatrix at the external abdominal ring. In cases of epiplocele, he recommends us either to replace the omentum, or to cause the death of it by septic medicines, cauteries, or the ligature; or to cut it out with a pair of scissors, but of this proceeding he does not much approve, as it may occasion dangerous hemorrhage. (vii, 20, 21.)

Galen briefly states that intestinal and omental herniæ are to be cured by pressing up the intestine or omentum, removing as much as possible of the spermatic vessels; or otherwise drawing out the peritoneum, fomenting it, and then cutting it off. (Isagoge.) He mentions that it was customary to bleed the patient before the operation when he was plethoric. (De Opt. sec.)

Aëtius speaks of the operation as being highly dangerous. He forbids attempts at reduction while the prolapsed parts are affected with inflammation, tormina, and flatus. (xiv, 23.)

Albucasis's account of the treatment is quite similar to our author's. He states that the disease is occasioned by the descent of a portion of intestine to the testicle, owing to rupture or distension of the peritoneum. Sometimes, he says, fæces get into the prolapsed bowels, and being retained give rise to violent and sometimes fatal symptoms. When going to operate he directs us, in the first place, to make the patient reduce the intestine if reducible. Then an incision is to be made along the whole skin of the testicle, and hooks are to be fixed in the lips of the wound so as to enlarge it, and allow a passage for the testicle. The membranes, then, below the skin, are to be dissected, so as to expose completely the tunica vaginalis (*sifac album.*) The index-finger is then to be introduced between the tunica vaginalis and the second coat (tunica albuginea?) so as to free the adhesions at the back part of the testicle. The operator is afterwards to separate the testicle from all its adhesions and raise it up to the external wound. He must now examine whether any portion of intestine remain protruded, and if so, it must be replaced. The operator is then to take a large needle armed with a cord of ten threads, and having introduced it behind the tunic under the skin of the testicle (tunica vaginalis?) its extremities are to be cut, and the threads arranged into four pieces. With them the peritoneum is to be tightly bound in a crucial form, so as that the nutrient vessels may not be able to reach it, which will obviate inflammation. Another ligature is to be applied afterwards at the distance of less than two fingers' breadth from the former. After applying these two ligatures, about a finger's breadth of the peritoneum is to be left, and the rest is then to be cut all around, and the testicle removed along with it. An incision is then to be made at the lower part so as to allow an outlet for the blood and matter. Wool dipped in oil is to be applied afterwards, and bound as formerly described. Sometimes, he adds, the cautery is applied to the tunica vaginalis after the incision for fear of hemorrhage. (Chirurg. ii, 65.) He describes minutely the treatment by burning in another place. (i, 47.)

Avicenna recommends the cautery, but does not describe the other operation. Haly's description is evidently taken from our author. (Pract. ix, 50.)

Rhases states correctly that hernia generally arises from dilatation of the passage which leads from the cavity of the abdomen to the testicle. In ordinary cases, he says, there is no rupture of the peritoneum. He states that the contents of the hernial tumour are either intestines or omentum. The omentum, he adds, is the intestine most commonly found in ruptures. He says the peritoneum (*sifac*) lines the whole intestines and surrounds the testicles. Antyllus, from whom he gives a subsequent extract, states in like manner that the peritoneum descends to the testicles and forms the tunica elytroides, i. e. vaginalis. Antyllus also affirms that hernia arises from relaxation of the passage between the cavity of the abdomen and the testicles. This opinion regarding ruptures is maintained by several of the authorities quoted by Rhases. (Contin. xxiv.)

Sprengel says of Rhases: "Sa théorie des hernies proprement dites est infiniment préférable à celle des Grecs." (Hist. de la Méd.) The account which Rhases gives of ruptures is, no doubt, very correct; but there is every reason to suppose that it was entirely taken from the works of the Greek surgeons.

The operations practised by the ancients for the radical cure of hernia cannot but appear to us extremely cruel and hazardous; and yet the danger attending them must have been less than is generally supposed, otherwise they could not have been so frequently performed as they were about two centuries ago. Fabricius ab Aquapendente mentions that a celebrated rupture doctor of his time informed him that he used to operate upon 200 patients at an average every year. Fabricius, however, prudently recommends us not to perform the operation except in extreme cases, and to be content in general with supporting the parts by means of a truss.

The ancients never operated to relieve strangulated hernia.

LXVI—ON BUBONOCELE, OR INGUINAL HERNIA

Enterocele arising from distension commences as bubonocele; for at first the peritoneum being stretched the relaxed intestine is protruded as far as the groin, and forms this disease, which the ancients operated upon in this manner. After making the incision to the extent of three fingers' breadth transversely across the tumour in the groin, and removing the membranes and fat, and the peritoneum being exposed in the middle where it is raised up to a point, let the knob of a probe be applied, by which the intestines will be pressed deep down. The prominences, then, of the peritoneum formed on each side of the knob of the probe are to be united to one another by sutures, and then we extract the probe, neither cutting the peritoneum nor removing the testicle, nor anything else, but curing it with the applications for fresh wounds. But since burning in cases of bubonocele is preferred by most of the moderns it will be right for us to give an account of this operation. After the man has undergone moderate exercise, let him cough violently and strain to keep in his breath; and when the swelling appears at the groin we mark with black ink or collyrium the place that is to be burned in a triangular figure, making its transverse line above in the situation of the groin, and we also make a mark in the middle of the triangle. Having laid the patient in a recumbent posture we first apply to the mark in the middle nail-shaped cauteries heated in the fire, afterwards burn the sides of the triangle with gamma-shaped (Γ) cauteries, and afterward level the triangle with cauteries shaped like tiles or lentils, an assistant during the whole process of burning wiping away the ichorous discharges with a rag; and in those who are of a moderate habit of body the burning should be carried to such a depth as to touch the fat. But in those who are lean we must not attend to this mark lest by mistake we should burn the peritoneum; nor again in those who are grosser and fatter, for in them the fat appears before a sufficient burning has taken place. We must, therefore, be rather guided as to its extent by a skilful conjecture. After the burning, having triturated salts with leeks we apply them to the eschar, and use the inguinal bandage shaped like the Greek letter X. On the following days we complete the cure with the dressings fitting for eschars, such as lentils with honey, and the like.

Commentary. Celsus directs us, when the inguinal tumour is moderate in size, to make one incision; but if larger, he recommends two lines to be made, so that the middle may be cut out; then, without extracting the testicle, as advised in certain cases of prolapsed intestines, the veins are to be bound together and tied where they adhere to the tunics, and afterwards cut below the knots. (vii, 24.)

Avicenna speaks of astringent applications and the actual cautery, but disapproves of the incision and suture. (iii, 22, 1.)

The operations of the suture and burning are described by Albucasis (Chirurg. ii, 67, and i, 47); by Rhases (Cont. xxiv); and by Haly Abbas (Pract. ix, 52, and ix, 80.) They all evidently copy from our author.

Garengoit affirms that Paulus has made mention of crural hernia, but we agree with Heister that this is a mistake.

LXVII—ON RHACOSIS, OR RELAXATION OF THE SCROTUM

When the skin about the scrotum is relaxed without the bodies within being affected, rhacosis is formed, being a most unseemly complaint. Wherefore Leonides, having placed the man in a recumbent posture, cut off the redundant skin with a scalpel direct upon some board or some hard skin, and united the lips of the wound with sutures. But Antyllus, having first transfixed the redundant skin with three or four ligatures, cut off what was external to them with a sharp-pointed pair of scissors or scalpel, and having secured the parts with sutures, effected the cure by the treatment for recent wounds.

Commentary. Our author's description of the two modes of performing the operation is copied by Albucasis. (Chirurg. ii, 68); and by Haly Abbas (Pract. ix, 53.)

LXVIII—ON CASTRATION

The object of our art being to restore those parts which are in a preternatural state to their natural, the operation of castration professes just the reverse. But since we are sometimes compelled against our will by persons of high rank to perform the operation, we shall briefly describe the mode of doing it. There are two ways of performing it, the one by compression, and the other by excision. That by compression is thus performed: children, still of a tender age, are placed in a vessel of hot water, and then when the parts are softened in the bath, the testicles are to be squeezed with the fingers until they disappear, and, being dissolved, can no longer be felt. The method by excision is as follows: let the person to be castrated be placed upon a bench, and the scrotum with the testicles grasped by the fingers of the left hand, and stretched; two straight incisions are then to be made with a scalpel, one in each testicle; and when the testicles start up they are to be dissected around and cut out, having merely left the very thin bond of connexion between the vessels in their natural state. This method is preferred to that by compression; for those who have had them squeezed sometimes have venereal desires, a certain part, as it would appear, of the testicles having escaped the compression.

Commentary. We have given Celsus's description of the operation in the 64th section of this Book. Albucasis describes the operations by compression and by excision. In the former the testicle is squeezed by the operator while the patient is seated in hot water. In the other the spermatic cord is to be first secured with a ligature and then the testicle cut out. (Chirurg. ii, 69.)

They are likewise described in nearly the same terms by Haly Abbas. (Pract. ix, 54.) The castration of the inferior animals is mentioned by Aristotle (Hist. Animal. ix, 50); by Varro (De Re Rustica, iii, 9); by Columella (De R. R. vi, 26); and by Palladius (De R. R. vi, 7.) Varro informs us that it was customary to make capons by burning the testicles of cocks with a red-hot iron. It appears from Juvenal that the surgeons in his time were often called upon to perform castration. (Sat. vi, l. 370.) Abulpharagius likewise mentions that the performance of this operation constituted at one time an important part of the surgical practice in Bagdad. (Dynast. ix.) But the Emperor Justinian condemned the operation as being dangerous and often fatal.

Sprengel gives an interesting history of castration. One of the most important points in this operation is the mode of tying the cord. Some modern authorities affirm that no bad effects result from putting a ligature round the whole cord, but others condemn this practice as bringing on convulsions and tetanus. All admit the difficulty of securing the artery separately.

LXIX—ON HERMAPHRODITES

This affection derives its name from a combination of the names Hermes and Aphrodite (Mercury and Venus,) and occasions great deformity to both sexes. There being four varieties of it, according to Leonides; three of them occur in men and one in women. In men, sometimes about the perineum and sometimes about the middle of the scrotum, there is the appearance of a female pudendum with hair; and in addition to these there is a third variety, in which the discharge of urine takes place at the scrotum as from a female pudendum. In women there is often found above the pudendum and in the situation of the pubes the appearance of a man's privy parts, there being three bodies projecting there, one like a penis, and two like testicles. The third of the male varieties in which the urine is voided through the scrotum is incurable; but the other three may be cured by removing the supernumerary bodies and treating the part like sores.

Commentary. This section of our author is copied by Albucasis (Chirurg. ii, 70); and by Haly Abbas (Pract. ix, 55.) Avicenna briefly mentions this monstrosity. (iii, 20, 2, 43.)

Guy of Cauliac and Brunus describe it in the same terms as the Arabians.

LXX—ON EXTIRPATION OF THE NYMPHA AND CAUDA PUDENDI

In certain women the nympha (clitoris?) is excessively large and presents a shameful deformity, insomuch that, as has been related, some women have had erections of this part like men, and also venereal desires of a like kind. Wherefore, having placed the woman in a supine posture, and seizing the redundant portion of the nympha in a forceps we cut it out with a scalpel, taking care not to cut too deep lest we occasion the complaint called rhœas. The cauda is a fleshy excrescence arising from the mouth of the womb, and filling the female pudendum, sometimes even projecting externally like a tail; and it may be removed in the same manner as the nympha.

Commentary. That the nympha and clitoris were used anciently as synonymous terms is evident from Ruffus Ephesius (De Partibus Hominis); Soranus (c. 6); and Pollux (Onomasticon, ii.) Martial, in more than one place, makes allusion to unnatural practices connected with an enlarged clitoris. Aëtius says that it is a small muscular substance situated at the commissure of the alæ pudendi above the meatus urinarius. He adds, that when preternaturally enlarged it is to be amputated. Like our author, he directs us to take hold of the tumour with a forceps and cut off the protuberance, taking care not to carry the excision too far. He recommends us to apply a sponge squeezed out of an astringent wine or cold water, with suitable dressings. He gives the same account of the cauda as our author. (xvi, 103 and 104.) It was a tumour arising from the uterus itself. Albucasis merely transcribes our author's account of these operations. (Chirurg. ii, 71.) Avicenna briefly recommends us to remove the enlarged nympha by medicines or the knife.

(iii, 22; i, 24.) It would appear that this operation, like circumcision, is still often practised in the East.

The chapters of Soranus, in which these operations were treated of, are unfortunately wanting.

On extirpation of the enlarged clitoris see Heister's Surgery (ii, 5, 147). The *cauda pudendi* was probably the cauliflower excrescence of the os uteri described by late authorities on midwifery.

LXXI—ON THYMI, CONDYLOMATA, AND HEMORRHOIDS ABOUT THE FEMALE PARTS OF GENERATION

The thymus is an excrescence sometimes red, but sometimes white, for the most part without pain, and resembling the clusters of thyme. The condylomata are rugose protuberances; and the hemorrhoids resemble those about the anus, and, like them, sometimes pour forth blood. Such excrescences in women, when brought into view and exposed, are to be seized with a forceps and cut out with the point of a half-spatula. And we are then to use pounded galls, or fissile alum. For the more distinguished surgeons do not approve of ligatures in these cases.

Commentary. Aëtius gives a fuller account of these tubercles. He recommends us to seize them with a forceps and cut them out by the roots. He directs us not to interfere with such hemorrhoids of the womb as are varicose and malignant. Those which are hard and do not bleed are to be cut out at once, but such as are disposed to bleed are to be seized with a forceps and a ligature put round them before they are cut. Moschion, however, condemns this practice as being highly dangerous.

Albucasis evidently copies from our author. (Chirurg. ii, 73.)

Haly Abbas briefly directs us to seize these tubercles with a forceps and cut them out with a pair of scissors. (Pract. ix, 65.)

Rhases, treating of diseases of the uterus, says, "if there be a red piece of flesh in the mouth of the womb, if situated at its anterior part, and if it be round, or long, and not attended with pain, some surgeons cut it off, but I prefer tying it." (Cont. xxii.) This description seems to apply to polypus of the womb.

See a full account of the condylomata and hemorrhoids of the womb, by Lodovicus Mercatus (in the Gynæcia, p. 962.) He remarks that Celsus and Aëtius call any tubercle arising from inflammation by the name of condyloma, whereas Paulus applies the term only to callous tubercles of the uterus. He approves of seizing them with a forceps and cutting them out.

LXXII—ON IMPERFORATE PUDENDUM AND PHIMUS

Some women have the genital parts imperforate, sometimes naturally, and sometimes owing to some previous disease. And sometimes it is deep-seated, sometimes in the alæ pudendi, or in the intermediate places, and is sometimes occasioned by an adhesion of the parts, and sometimes by obstruction. The obstructing substance is either flesh or membrane. The disease occasions great impediment sometimes in coition, sometimes in conception, or in parturition, and occasionally during the menstrual purgation, provided the membrane or flesh occasion a complete obstruction; for in certain cases there is a perforation in the middle. Having ascertained the cause, either from its being obvious to the sight, or by introducing the speculum, if it be a simple adhesion only, it may be separated by a straight incision, made with a scalpel, for operating upon fistulæ. But if it is an obstruction, having transfixed the connecting body, whether it be membrane or flesh, with hooks, we stretch it and divide with a scalpel for fistulæ; and having stopped the hemorrhage with such applications as are desiccative without being stimulant, we have then recourse to such medicines as promote cicatrization, applying a priapus-shaped tent covered with some epulotic medicine, in those cases especially in which the operation is performed upon a part not very deep-seated, in order that the parts may not unite again. And the phimus which is formed at the mouth of the uterus is operated upon in the same manner.

Commentary. Aristotle makes mention of imperforate vagina. (De Generat. Animal. iv, 4.) Aëtius treats of these diseases at considerably greater length than our author, but his practice is nearly the same. Upon the whole the amount of his directions respecting the treatment is, that when the obstruction is occasioned by a membrane, it is to be divided and the lips of the incision prevented from adhering by the introduction of suitable tents; or, if it is a fleshy body, it is to be dissected out, and the parts separated by a piece of sponge or tents. (xvi, 96.) The same operation is described by Soranus. (219.)

The same method of treatment, however, had been previously recommended by Celsus. Thus, when the obstruction is occasioned by a simple membrane, he recommends us to divide it by two transverse incisions like the letter X, taking great care not to wound the urinary passage, and then the membrane is to be cut out. When the obstruction is produced by a fleshy tumour, he directs us to expose it by making a straight incision; then, having seized it with a forceps or hook, to dissect it out, and introduce an oblong tent (λημνίσκος) soaked in vinegar, and apply externally wool moistened with vinegar. The dressings are to be removed on the third day, and the sore treated upon general principles. When the wound is healing, he advises us to introduce a leaden tube smeared with some suitable ointment to prevent adhesion. (vii, 28.)

Albucasis makes mention of a singular substitute for the leaden tube recommended by Celsus: "Coeat mulier omni die ut non consolidetur locus vice alia!!" The same advice is gravely given by Rhases (Cont. xxii), and by Alsaharavius, who, as we have formerly stated, was probably the same person as Albucasis. (Pract. xxv, 2, 19.) But when the obstruction arises from a fleshy tumour, Albucasis recommends us to make use of the leaden tube. (Chirurg. ii, 72.) Alsaharavius directs us to remove the obstruction by corrosive medicines or with the knife.

Rhases briefly describes the phimus, and directs us to perforate it with an instrument of iron, and then to introduce a tent moistened in some styptic wine.

Haly Abbas states that obstruction of the uterus may arise either from a natural, that is to say, a congenital impediment, or from the effects of ulceration. He recommends us to make the midwife clear away the obstruction with a scalpel or any other convenient instrument. The Arabians were very delicate in allowing male practitioners to perform surgical operations about the genital organs of women. (Pract. ix, 66.)

LXXIII—ON ABSCESS OF THE WOMB

When the abscess is situated at the mouth of the womb, so as that it can be operated upon, we must not be in haste in having recourse to incision, nor until the disease be ripened, and the inflammation has increased to its utmost, and the vascular bodies which surround it have become attenuated, owing to the importance of the uterus in the system. In operating, the woman should be placed on a seat in a supine posture, having her legs drawn up to the belly, and her thighs separated from one another. Let her arms likewise be brought down to her legs and secured by proper ligatures about the neck. The operator, sitting on her right side, is to make an examination with a speculum proportionate to her age. The person using the speculum should measure with a probe the depth of the woman's vagina, lest the stalk (fistula) of the speculum being too long it should happen that the uterus should be pressed upon. If it be ascertained that the stalk is larger than the vagina, folded compresses are to be laid upon the alæ pudendi, in order that the speculum may be placed upon them. The stalk (fistula) is to be introduced, having a screw at the upper part, and the speculum is to be held by the operator, but the screw is to be turned by the assistant, so that the laminæ of the stalk being separated the vagina may be distended. When the abscess is exposed, if it be soft and thin (which may be ascertained by touching it with the finger), it is to be divided at the top by a scalpel or needle, and after the discharge of the pus, a soft oblong tent well smeared with rose-oil is to be introduced into the incision, or rather external to the opening into the woman's vagina, so as not to produce compression. And externally to the alæ pudendi and the region of the pubes and loins unwashed wool, or clean wool dipped in oil, is to be applied. On the third day she is to be placed in a hip-bath of warm oil or water, or of a decoction of mallows; and having wiped the parts, we introduce the tent gently into the opening, spread with the ointment tetrapharmacon, either alone or with clarified honey; its strength, however, ought to be reduced with butter or oil of roses. The external parts are to be covered with cataplasms until the inflammation subside and the sore become clean. If it is got cleansed with difficulty, an injection of the decoction of iris, of birthwort, or of honey, may be thrown up with an ear-syringe. The healing process may be promoted by the calamine ointment diluted with wine and applied upon a pledget. But if the abscess be within the mouth of the uterus, we must decline operating.

Commentary. A similar description of the method of opening abscesses in the vagina is given by Aëtius. (xvi, 85.) The only difficulty in comprehending his description or our author's arises from our unacquaintance with the construction of the ancient dioptræ or specula. Drawings of several sorts of them are given in the surgery of Albucasis and by Scultet. (Arsenal de Chirurg. tab. 18.) One of the simplest of them consists of two laminæ or plates so united that by turning a vice or screw they separated to the proper distance. Albucasis evidently copies our author's description. (Chirurg. ii, 71.) The account given by Haly Abbas is quite similar. (Pract. ix, 57.)

LXXIV—ON EMBRYULCIA AND EMBRYOTOMY

We have described the treatment of difficult labours in the Third Book. If the process of parturition be not rectified by the means there laid down, we must proceed to the surgical operation, after having formed a probable conjecture whether the woman will survive or not; and if she may be saved, then we are to operate; but if not, we must decline attempting the operation. Those in a dying state are affected with coma, lethargy, and loss of muscular motion; they are difficult to rouse, or if roused by loud cries, they return a feeble answer, and again sink into a comatose state. Some have convulsive contractions, or subsultus tendinum, or insensibility to food. The pulse is found to be greatly inflated, but obscure and feeble. Those who are to recover have none of these symptoms. Having placed the woman in a supine posture, with her head rather depressed, her thighs are to be kept elevated by women on each side, or by certain assistants; or if they are not at hand, her chest is to be first fastened to the bed by ligatures, so that when the fœtus is pulled the woman's body may not follow, and diminish the force of the pulling. Then the alæ pudendi being separated by an assistant, we must introduce the left hand lubricated with some unctuous substance, the fingers being contracted, to the mouth of the uterus, and dilate it, and having got it relaxed by lubricating it with oil, we seek for the most convenient place for fastening the hook (embryulcus). The most convenient places in presentations of the head are—the eyes, the occiput, the roof of the mouth, the chin, the clavicles, and the parts about the sides and hypochondrium; and in feet presentations, the bones of the pubes, the middle of the ribs, or, again, the clavicles. The hook is to be held in the right hand, and its curvature grasped with the fingers, and it is to be gently introduced with the left hand, and fixed on some of the aforementioned places, being pushed to the cavity of the uterus. And another is to be applied opposite to it in order that the pulling may be straight down and not to one side. Then we are to pull gently, not only straight-forward but also from side to side, as in the extraction of teeth; and there ought to be no relaxation of the pulling in the intervals. Then introducing the index-finger or more fingers besmeared with fat between the mouth of the womb and the impacted body, we must lubricate it all around. When the hook comes down properly it must be changed to a part above, and so on until the fœtus is completely extracted. When a hand presents, and is so impacted that it cannot be returned, we must wrap a cloth round it so that it may not slip, and pull it so far, and when it is properly fallen down it should be cut off at the shoulder. The same thing is to be done when two hands fall down into the vagina; and in like manner, when the feet come down, and the rest of the body does not come along, we must amputate at the groins, and then endeavour to turn the rest of the body. If the impaction take place owing to the head being larger than natural, if it be a hydrocephalous fœtus, we must open its skull with a polypus-scalpel, or a needle, or a sharp-pointed knife concealed between the fingers, in order that it may collapse when evacuated; but if it be a naturally large head, we must open the skull in like manner, and break down its bones with a tooth-forceps or a bone-forceps, and if the bones project they ought to be extracted. If, after the head has been delivered, an impediment should take place at the chest, the parts about the clavicles should be divided down to the cavity of the thorax with the same instrument, so that the thorax may collapse when its fluid contents are discharged; but if it do not collapse we may divide the clavicles and extract them, when the thorax will collapse. If the belly be inflated, owing to the death of the child, or its being dropsical, we must evacuate its contents with the intestines in the same way. In presentations by the feet the wrong direction may be easily rectified at the mouth of the womb. But if the fœtus stick at the chest or belly, we must wrap a cloth about it and draw it down, and making a division in the same manner, evacuate its contents. If, after the other parts are cut off, the head retreat backwards and is retained, we must introduce the left hand, and if the mouth of the womb be open, push up the hand to the cavity of the womb, and having found the head, bring it down with the fingers fixed in the mouth, and extract by one or two hooks fixed in it; but when there is inflammation at the mouth of the womb we must use no violence, but lubricate the parts with unctuous and fatty applications, and have recourse to hip-baths, embrocations, and cataplasms, in order that when the mouth is dilated extraction may be accomplished in the manner described above. Cross presentations, if they can be rectified, may be treated according to the afore-mentioned methods; but if not, the whole fœtus must be cut asunder within, and extracted in pieces, taking care that none of the parts of it be left behind. After the operation we must have recourse to the treatment for inflammations of the uterus. If hemorrhage come on, you have already had the management of it described.

Commentary. There is a curious treatise commonly published along with the works of Hippocrates on the extraction of the fœtus; but, as it is not mentioned by Erotian and Galen, it is now generally admitted not to be genuine. The author of it directs us, when the arm presents, to pull it down and amputate at the shoulder-joint; after which the head is to be brought to the proper position and delivery accomplished accordingly. This is not now the general rule of practice, and yet we were once compelled by necessity to deliver in this way, after we and an intelligent assistant had been foiled in all our attempts to turn the child. We have known of similar cases happening in the practice of other surgeons; and, in fact, this method of procedure was advocated lately by a sensible writer in the 'Edinburgh Medical and Surgical Journal.' The author of the ancient treatise in question recommends us to bring down the head in its natural state, if possible, but if this be found impracticable, to break it down. He directs us to give for drink a white, sweet, undiluted wine.

Celsus gives an interesting account of this subject, and his practice is deserving of much consideration. He recommends us, when the position is unnatural, to turn the child either to the head or the feet; adding, afterwards, that delivery may generally be accomplished easily enough by the feet. In arm presentations, he approves of turning to the head, that is to say, in cases when it is ascertained that the fœtus is dead. If the head is at hand, a smooth hook with a small point is to be fastened at the eye, the ear, the mouth, or the forehead, and its body is to be thus dragged down. This, however, must not be attempted when the mouth of the womb is not properly dilated. The right hand is to be employed in dragging down the fœtus, and the left in directing the instrument and the fœtus. When the body of the fœtus is distended with a fluid, it is to be let out, and the body brought down with a hook. If the child lie across and the position cannot be got rectified, the hook is to be inserted at the armpit, and extraction gradually performed. In extreme cases he recommends us to cut the neck asunder, and extract the parts separately, beginning with the head, for fear of its being left in the uterus. Should such an accident occur, however, he directs us to get the belly compressed so as to force the head down to the os uteri; after which it may be extracted with a hook in the manner described above. (Smellie relates histories of such cases.) When one foot presents, and the breech sticks at the os uteri, he recommends us, when the other foot cannot be found, to separate the one which protrudes; after which the body of the child may be pushed up, and the other leg found and brought down. It is to be recollected that this practice is only recommended when the child is dead. He adds, that other difficulties may give rise to the necessity of performing embryotomy. (vii, 29.)

Aëtius has an interesting chapter on the Extraction of the Dead Fœtus, copied from the works of Philumenus. His description of embryotomy is similar to our author's. He directs us to apply two hooks to certain parts of the head, such as the eye, mouth, and chin, and thus to drag down the body. If the head is large or hydrocephalic, he advises us to open it and evacuate its contents; and if even then it is found to be too large for the passage, he recommends us to break down the bones of the skull and remove them with a forceps, after which the instrument is to be fixed and the fœtus dragged down. If obstruction to the delivery take place at the chest or the belly, he directs us to evacuate their contents in like manner. When an arm or both present, he recommends us to amputate at the shoulder-joint. If the child come down doubled, and the position cannot be got rectified, he advises us, if the head can be reached, to break down its bones, and then extract the other parts accordingly; but if the legs are got at most easily and cannot be brought down, they are to be amputated at the hip-joint, and then the head will be got delivered. When the body is so impacted in a doubled state that it cannot be moved, he directs us to separate the vertebra at the neck, and then to drag down the lower part of the body; after which the head is to be sought for by the hand introduced into the uterus, and brought along with two hooks. (xvi, 23.)

No ancient author has described the operation of embryotomy so accurately as Soranus; but as his account of the process is lengthy and does not differ essentially from that of Aëtius, (indeed the latter evidently copies from Soranus,) we need not seek to give any outline of it. (Op. 51, 52, 53.)

Avicenna takes his chapter on the extraction of the dead fœtus from our author. (iii, 21, 2, 24.) We have mentioned in the Third Book that he was acquainted with the forceps.

Albucasis, in like manner, takes his account of embryotomy from Paulus. He relates a singular case that came under his own knowledge of an extra-uterine conception; the most remarkable circumstance about which was, that the bones of the fœtus after a time were discharged at the umbilicus. The work of Albucasis contains drawings of the instruments used in his time for obstetrical operations. There are several forcipes among them, but as they all have teeth, it is to be presumed that they were used only for delivering the fœtus when dead. It is to be regretted that he has entirely omitted the forceps mentioned by Avicenna. (See Chirurg. ii, 76 and 77.)

Rhases directs us when the child's head is large and cannot be brought down with fillets, to open it and deliver with hooks. When it is ascertained that the child is dead, he recommends us to break down the bones of the head and evacuate the brain. In preternatural presentations he recommends us to deliver, if possible, by the head or feet, but if this cannot be got accomplished, he directs us to cut off the protruding part. Upon the whole his rules of practice are much the same as our author's. (Cont. xxii.)

Haly Abbas gives ample directions for the management of these cases. When the head presents (the child being dead and delivery found otherwise impracticable), he directs us to fix hooks in the hollows of the eyes, neck, or jaw-bone; or if the feet present, at the tops of the thighs. The body of the child is then to be dragged along. When a hand presents, he recommends us to pull down the arm and amputate at the shoulder; and in like manner he directs us to amputate at the hip-joint when in footling presentations the delivery cannot be otherwise accomplished. When the head is preternaturally large, he directs us to open it and evacuate its contents; and to do so in like manner with the chest when any obstruction takes place at it. He makes no mention of any instrument resembling the modern forceps. (Pract. ix, 57.)

LXXV—ON RETENTION OF THE SECUNDINES

Often, after the removal of the fœtus, the placenta (which is also called the secundines) is retained in the uterus. When the mouth of the uterus is dilated and the placenta separated, and rolled into a ball in some part of the uterus, the extraction is most easy. The left hand warmed and anointed is to be introduced into its cavity, and the secundines extracted as they present. But if they adhere to the fundus uteri we must introduce the hand in like manner, and grasp them and pull them along, not straight down for fear of prolapsus, nor with great violence, but they are to be moved gently, at first from this side to that, and afterwards somewhat more strongly, for thus they will yield and be freed from their adhesion. If the mouth of the uterus be found shut we must have recourse to the same treatment. If the strength is not sunk, sternutatories and fumigations with aromatics in a pot may be used; and if the mouth of the womb dilate, the hand is to be introduced and an attempt made to extract the placenta, as aforesaid. If even in this way it cannot be extracted, one need not be alarmed, for after a few days it will putrefy, dissolve into sanies and drop off. But since the fetid smell affects the head and disorders the stomach, we must use suitable fumigations, among which cardamom and dried figs are much approved.

Commentary. We have mentioned in another place that Hippocrates' practice in retention of the placenta consisted in suspending weights from the end of the umbilical cord.

Celsus directs us, when the placenta is not cast off soon after the delivery of the child, to draw down the umbilical cord gently with the left hand, taking care not to break it. The right hand is then to follow it up to the secundines, and their veins and membranes being separated from the womb, the whole are to be extracted along with whatever coagulated blood may be in the uterus. (vii, 29.)

Our author merely abridges a fuller account of the subject given by Aëtius from the works of Philumenus. (xvi, 24.)

Moschion reprobates the ancient practice of using sternutatories, pessaries, and fumigations, and of suspending scales or weights from the cord, because these means sometimes occasion hemorrhage. He recommends the midwife, if the mouth of the womb be still open, to introduce her left hand, and to take hold of whatever part of the placenta presents: then, if it does not adhere to the fundus uteri it is to be extracted; but if it is not separated it is to be moved gently hither and thither without violence. When the mouth of the uterus is contracted, he advises her to use those liquors and injections which are applicable for inflammations of the womb. (Section liv.) His method of securing the umbilical cord after delivery is nearly the same as that now adopted. After the child has been allowed to lie on the ground for a few minutes, two ligatures are to be applied round the cord, the nearest being four fingers from the belly; it is then to be cut with a scalpel or any sharp knife. He disapproves of using instruments of wood, glass, or reeds, and hard crusts of bread, as practised by the ancients. (lxv.) He directs lacerations of the perineum to be treated by applying ointments composed of wax, oil of roses, litharge, ceruse, and alum, with suitable bandages. (lvii.)

The practice of Soranus in these cases is most judicious, and such as can scarcely be improved upon at the present day. He disapproves of all violent attempts at extraction, but when the placenta cannot be got otherwise removed from the womb, he approves of introducing the hand well lubricated to extract the secundines gently. He directs us when the mouth of the womb is shut to open it if possible with the fingers in a gentle manner. This is the case now incorrectly called the hour-glass contraction.

Avicenna repeats the directions given by Paulus and Aëtius, but seems to have considered the introduction of the hand into the uterus as a painful, and, in general, an unnecessary operation. (iii, 21, 2, 16.)

Albucasis follows our author's practice. (Chirurg. ii, 78.)

Haly Abbas directs us to introduce the hand well lubricated with oil of violets, or the like, into the uterus, and extract the placenta if it be separated; but if it still adhere it is to be moved from side to side, and not pulled straight downwards. He adds, that when not extracted, it becomes putrid. (Pract. ix, 59.)

Rhases directs us when the secundines do not come away after delivery to make the woman sneeze, and if they are still retained, to pare the nails, and having introduced the hand into the uterus to pull cautiously so as not to give pain. When they cannot be removed in this way, he recommends us to throw injections into the womb so as to promote putrefaction of the placenta. In another place he mentions, that when long retained, the placenta putrefies and comes off in pieces. (Cont. xxii.)

LXXVI—ON BURNING THE HIPS

As in the case of the shoulder, so also the hip-joint getting dislocated from a collection of humours requires burning. Wherefore Hippocrates says: "When dislocation at the hip-joint takes place from long-continued ischiatic disease, the leg wastes, and the patients are lame unless burnt." Burning, therefore, is to be performed more particularly at the place where the joint is dislocated, for thus the redundant humour will be dried up, and the part being condensed by the cicatrix will no longer be able to receive the bone, wherefore the burning should be carried to a considerable depth. The moderns form three eschars by burning; one behind in the hollow of the buttocks, another a little above the knee on the outside, and a third on the outside of the ankle in the fleshy part.

Commentary. Hippocrates recommends us to burn the parts over the hip-joint with crude flax. (De Affectionibus.) The author of another of the Hippocratic treatises directs us to burn the bony parts with fungi and the flesh with a red-hot iron. (De Affect. Int.)

Aëtius, upon the authority of Archigenes, recommends burning in this case with irons, the roots of fuller's herb and birthwort, or with goat's dung. (xii, 3.)

Cælius Aurelianus, in cases of ischiatic disease, speaks of forming issues over the hip-joint by the actual and potential cauteries. His potential cauteries, with which he mentions that eschars were burnt, appear to have been the ashes of herbs, that is to say, impure preparations of the caustic alkali, to which quicklime was sometimes added. They must, therefore, have been nearly the same as the *calx cum kali* of modern use. He states, that some burned the part with the root of fuller's herb; others with pieces of iron shaped like the letter Γ; that some raised the skin in a fold and transfixed it with heated irons; that some burned it with fungi, and others with a piece of linen cloth folded and laid on the part. (Pass. Tard. v, 1.)

But the fullest account which we have of the ancient modes of burning the hips for diseases of the joint is that which is given in the book 'Euporistôn,' ascribed to Dioscorides. Mention is there made of the methods of burning with goat's dung, and with wool smeared with oil. Some, it is said, form a ball of clay, and, having laid it on the place, apply to it a burning staff as long as it can be borne. Others, having stretched the skin over the affected joint, transfix it with a heated style or writing pen. The Libyans performed the operation with shavings of the lote tree, sulphur, and elaterium. The Marmaridæ are said to have done it with green pieces of the wood of olive trees. The Parthians used a leaden tube, the extremity of which they smeared with dough, in order to prevent the oil in the inside from escaping; then hot cauteries, to the number of forty or fifty, were introduced, and the burning continued as long as it could be well endured. Care in the meantime was taken to cool the face with cold water; and it was attended to, that the tube was not over-filled with oil, lest it should run over. (Euporist. i, 242.)

Albucasis describes minutely the process of burning with red-hot irons. (Chirurg. i, 43.) Haly Abbas in like manner directs us to burn an eschar over the joint, and to keep it open for a considerable time. (Pract. ix, 81.)

Asclepiades (apud Nicetæ Collect.) mentions that he had seen two cases in which dislocation had taken place at the hip-joint without any accident. The editor of this work, Anthony Cocchi, states that he had met with only one such case in the whole course of his practice. We need scarcely remark that such cases, however, are by no means of rare occurrence.

LXXVII—ON FISTULÆ AND FAVI

The present occasion requiring us to treat of fistula in ano, it will not be improper to give an account in the first place of fistulæ in general. A fistula then is a callous sinus, attended with little or no pain, and forming in most parts of the body. It generally originates in abscesses not properly healed. The callus is compact and white, the flesh dry, and therefore insensible, neither vein nor nerve passing to it. Sometimes the sinus is dry and sometimes filled with a discharge. The discharge is sometimes constant, and sometimes at intervals, the mouth of it being at one time shut up, and at another time open. Sometimes the fistula terminates on a bone, sometimes on a nerve, or some other important part; and it is either straight or crooked; has either one orifice or many. Those therefore that terminate upon large arteries, or nerves, or tendons of considerable size, or the pleura, or any important part, are either not to be meddled with at all, or with great and skilful caution; but the others may be operated upon in this manner. We first examine them if they be straight with a sound (specillum), or if crooked with a double-headed specillum of a very flexible nature, such as those made of tin, and the smallest of those made of copper. When there are two or more orifices, we must not trust to the examination with a specillum, but injecting the sinus by one of its openings we ascertain from the manner in which the injection comes out whether it be one fistula with many orifices, or if there be several fistulæ. After the examination, if the sinus be superficial and narrow, it is to be distended by the introduction of a specillum, and the callus is to be cut off with a properly-shaped scalpel, or pared with the nails or the point of a scalpel. If it is also broad the redundant parts are to be dissected away. If it is not superficial, but deep and straight, we must cut off the callus all around as far as we can make incisions, and if any part remain, destroy it with a caustic medicine; or if the callus be large, and do not yield to medicine, we must form a slough by burning it with hot irons. If the fistula terminate with a bone, and if it is not diseased, we need only scrape it, but if it is carious, or otherwise corrupted, the whole diseased portion is to be cut out with counter perforators, and if necessary we may bore a hole with a wimble (trephine?) whether the bone be diseased only to the diploe or as far as the marrow. If a bone project, as after a transverse fracture, we must saw it off. Taking, therefore, two bandages, we apply the middle of the one to the projecting bone itself, and get it kept stretched by an assistant; the other being thicker, or formed of wool, we are to take in like manner, and apply the middle of it to the flesh under the bone, and taking its ends below, we give directions that the flesh below be retracted by this band lest it be torn by the teeth of the saw, and in this manner we accomplish the sawing. When any vital part is situated below, such as the pleura, spinal marrow, or the like, in cutting or sawing the bone, we must use the instrument called meningophylax for protecting them. If the bone is not diseased, but is denuded of flesh all around, it is to be sawn in the same manner, for bones which are disengaged from the other parts all around cannot possibly incarnate. In like manner, the extremity of a bone near a joint, if diseased, is to be sawn off; and often, if the whole of a bone, such as the ulna, radius, tibia, or the like, be diseased, it is to be taken out entire. But if the head of the thigh-bone, or pelvis, or a vertebra of the spine be diseased, we must not attempt to operate upon them for fear of the adjoining arteries. We must proceed in this manner in every particular case, attention being paid to the situation, proximity, and connexions of the affected parts, the extent of the disease, the strength and powers of the patient. The favus being a fistulous sinus with a milky discharge must be subjected to the same operation and treatment as fistula.

Commentary. For an account of the practice of Hippocrates we refer to our notes on the 49th section of the Fourth Book.

Celsus states that if fistulæ spread deep, are crooked, or are numerous, they are to be cured by an operation rather than by medicines. Wherefore, if it spread transversely, he recommends us to introduce a specillum, or sound, and cut down upon it. But if it is crooked, its bendings are to be followed out and cut open in the same manner. When the operator has reached the end of the fistula, all the callus is to be cut out, and the lips of the wound secured by clasps and agglutinative applications. When the fistula terminates with a rib he directs us to saw out a piece of it lest it affect the adjoining parts. Fistulous sores about the abdomen he pronounces to be highly dangerous. He recommends us, however, to attempt a cure by making an incision, and uniting the edges of the wound by sutures. (vii, 4.)

Aëtius lays down nearly the same rules for the treatment of fistulæ as our author. When the sinus runs transversely along the skin, he directs us to lay it open. When it penetrates downwards he advises us to cut off the callus; and when the ulcer terminates with a bone to remove the diseased lamina of it. (xiv, 55.)

Albucasis delivers the surgical treatment of fistulæ at great length. He is very particular in inculcating the necessity of making free incisions, and of removing any pieces of diseased bone which may happen to be found at the bottom of the sore. He relates a case of fistulous ulcer in the thigh, to cure which he removed large pieces of bone, sawing it down as far as the marrow. Some of his saws are very ingeniously constructed, and one of them is not unlike the saw introduced into the practice of surgery by the late Mr. Hey, of Leeds. He enumerates nine causes which prevent sores from healing; and as they appear to be of some practical utility we shall briefly mention what they are: 1, a deficiency of blood in the body; 2, cachexy, or bad condition thereof; 3, fungous flesh, which prevents the union of the edges of the sore; 4, much sordes in the ulcer; 5, putridity, or any other bad quality of the fluids; 6, improper applications; 7 and 8, the pestilential state of the atmosphere and the insalubrity of the place where the patient resides; 9, a diseased bone. When none of these causes are present, the restorative principle of nature will of itself effect the cure of any solution of continuity. (Chirurg. ii, 88.)

Rhases gives extracts from Antyllus, and many other authors, on this subject, but as their principles of treatment are much the same as those delivered by Paulus, we need not occupy much room with an abstract of them. Antyllus forbids us to use the knife when the fistula is situated in the groin or fundament. When it is not judged expedient to have recourse to an operation, one of his Arabian authorities, Aaron, recommends a powder composed of equal parts of quicklime, cantharides, arsenic, sandarach, sal ammoniac, and ginger. (Cont. xxviii.)

LXXVIII—ON FISTULÆ IN ANO

Fistulæ in ano are discovered, if they are *blind*, from their being attended with pain, although no orifice appears; from there being a purulent moisture about the anus, and in most cases from their being preceded by symptoms of abscess; or, if they are *open*, by the introduction of a sound or swine's bristle; for the instrument will pass down into a cavity and meet the index-finger introduced into the anus if the fistula has penetrated to the inside; but if it has not penetrated, the instrument does not come in contact with the finger but the intermediate substance between them remains imperforated. The fistula is known to be crooked and winding from the instrument's passing down but a short way, while a great quantity of pus is discharged in proportion. Those near the intestines are known by an abdominal worm or fæces sometimes passing through the mouth of them. In almost all cases some callus appears about the orifice of the fistula. A fistula is incurable that perforates the neck of the bladder, or extends to the joint of the thigh, or to the rectum. A fistula is difficult to cure when it has no orifice, is *blind*, ends with a bone, and has many windings. All the rest are, in general, easily cured. We proceed with them thus: having placed the patient in a supine posture, with the legs elevated, so that the thighs may be bent upon the belly, as when an injection of the bowels is administered, if the fistula terminate superficially, having introduced a sound or ear-specillum through the orifice of it, we cut the skin which covers it at one incision. But if the fistula terminate deeply in the anus, having introduced a specillum into the mouth of it, and if we find that it has perforated the gut, by introducing the finger into the anus opposite the affected buttock, we take hold of the head of the specillum, and bending it, bring it to the outside, and with one simple division cut asunder the parts which lie over the sound. If the fistula is found not to have as yet perforated the gut, and to have terminated only deeply in the fundament, and if upon examination we find that a scaly or membranous substance intervenes between the index-finger and the extremity of the sound, we must perforate it violently with the head of the sound, and forcing the sound through the rectum, we must again, as formerly described, cut asunder the intervening parts with a scalpel; or, having perforated the bottom of the fistula in ano with the sharp part of a falciform instrument for operating upon fistulæ, we bring the instrument out at the anus, and so divide all the intermediate space with the edge of the instrument; and after the incision, having taken hold of the surrounding parts, which mostly consist of callus, with a common forceps, or one called staphylagra, we cut them out all around, avoiding the sphincter muscle; for some cutting deep in an unskilful manner, have wounded it, from which the patient has had an involuntary discharge of fæces. Those who from timidity, avoid a surgical operation may be treated with the ligature, as recommended by Hippocrates. For Hippocrates directs us to pass a raw thread, consisting of five pieces, through the fistula by means of a probe having a perforation, or a double-headed specillum, and to tie the ends of the thread and tighten it every day until the whole intermediate substance between the orifice be divided and the ligature fall out. If it remain long, the thread may be sprinkled with the detergent powder called psarum, or some such powder, and drawn in. Some insert a thread into the opening of the falciform instrument for operations on fistulæ, and pass it through in the manner described, which I think ought not to be done. For by avoiding an operation, in addition they incur the inconvenience of a slow recovery. With regard to blind fistulæ, Leonides says: "When the fistula is deep, and penetrates the sphincter, whether beginning in the fundament, or arising from a distance and terminating in the sphincter, after the examination which has been described, we dilate the anus as we do the female vagina, with the instrument for that purpose, or the small specillum. When the orifice of the fistula is discovered, the end of an ear-specillum is to be passed through it, and pushed deep into it, and cutting down upon it where it presents, the whole fistula is to be divided with a semispathula or a spathula for operating upon fistulæ." We having met with this state of the disease, have found it impossible to practise this mode of operating, because we could not discover the cavity of the fistula. For it was situated between the anus and sphincter towards the right side, and the dilator rather obscured the operation. But having dilated the wrinkles about the anus a certain fissure appeared among them, being as it were the defluxion of the fistula, for the pus passed out by it we saw to pass the head of the specillum into the fistula by it, which served as a director; and having passed the index-finger of the right hand to the sphincter, and having found a certain thin substance intervening between the finger and the sound, by pressing the sound violently to the finger, we perforated the bottom of the fistula, which was turned upwards; and passing with the finger the head of the instrument outwards, the whole of the substance between the mouths of the fistula, (I mean the one so situated as to favour the defluxion, and that now made by us,) we divided with a scalpel and cut out the sound.

Commentary. Hippocrates describes minutely the apolinose, or the cure with the ligature, in his work 'De Fistulis.' We must mention, however, that Kühn and Sprengel do not admit this among the genuine treatises of Hippocrates, although they allow that it is ancient. Littré also, though with some hesitation, has rejected it from his list of the genuine works of Hippocrates. And yet, considering that it was received as such by Galen and Erotian, it seems bold in any modern critic to refuse its claims.

Celsus likewise describes distinctly the method of applying the ligature. The process, he says, is slow but free from pain. It may be expedited by smearing the thread with some escharotic ointment. The same thing, he adds, may be accomplished by means of a scalpel guided upon a specillum (sound). When many sinuses open by one mouth, he directs us to cut open a straight fistula with a scalpel, and then the others being thereby exposed are to be tied with a thread. The diet is to be of a diluent nature, with a liberal allowance of water for drink. (vii, 4.)

Aëtius gives, from Leonides, a full account of fistulæ in ano, as we have explained in another place. He recommends us to introduce a specillum, and having cut open the fistula upon it, to pare away the callous parts of it. (xiv, 11.)

Actuarius approves of the same practice as the others. He cautions against making large incisions lest the sphincter ani be wounded. (Meth. Med. iv, 6.)

Albucasis delivers nearly the same rules of treatment as our author. According to circumstances he approves of the knife, the cautery, or the apolinose. (Chir. ii, 80.)

Haly Abbas describes only the operation by the incision. He also states that if the sphincter ani be wounded, it will occasion irretention of the fæces. (Pr. ix, 60.) See also Rhases (Ad Mansor. ix, 80; Cont. xxviii); and Avicenna (iii, 18, 1, 18.) Avicenna prefers twisted hairs or bristles of a hog, as they will not putrefy.

Upon the whole no other of the ancient authorities has treated so efficiently of fistulæ in ano as Paulus.

See an excellent account of the operation in Sprengel's 'History of Medicine.' John de Vigo trusted to septics, such as arsenic and the ægyptiacum. Ambrose Paré approved of the apolinose and incision. Severinus was an advocate for the cautery. Foubert and Camper likewise practised the apolinose—the one with a leaden thread, the other with a silk one. Guido de Cauliaco and Rogerius approve of the ligature. Brunus and Theodoricus prefer the actual cautery, but describe the others. The surgeons of this country have now generally rejected the methods with the ligature and the cautery.

The following account of the ancient specillum by the learned Harduin will serve to illustrate our author's description of the operation. We overlooked it in the commentary on the fifteenth section. "Quid sit specillum Varro explicat (Lib. 5 de Lingua Lat.) *Quo oculos inunguimus quibus specimus* (hoc est, aspicimus), *specillum est*. Græcis μηλὴ dicitur. Aëtius Serm. 8, 14, *cum specillo instrumento, quod melam Græci appellant*. Instrumentum parvum ac teres, quo utuntur ad vulnerum aut fistularum viam aut profunditatem pernoscendam. Une sonde de chirurgien." (Ad Plin. H. N. vii, 54.) If the κοπάϱιον, however, was the same as the μηλὴ or the specillum, it was evidently used for cutting with as well as for cutting upon.

LXXIX—ON HEMORRHOIDS OR PILES

The existence of hemorrhoids is rendered manifest to us by the discharge from them. Before proceeding to the operation we must use frequent clysters with the view of evacuating at the same time the contents of the intestine, and, by irritating the anus, of rendering it more disposed to eversion and protrusion of the gut. Having, therefore, laid the patient on his back in a clear light, if we are to use the ligature we pass a very thick thread round the lips and secure each of the hemorrhoids with this ligature, leaving one as an outlet to the superfluous blood (for so Hippocrates directs.) After the application of the ligature, using a compress that has been dipped in oil and the bandage adapted for the anus, we order the patient to remain quiet, and treat the bowels with tepid oil and honied water, and afterwards we use a cataplasm made of crumbs of bread and saffron; and after the falling off of the hemorrhoids the cicatrization is to be promoted by wine. Leonides has not recourse to the ligature, but having seized the hemorrhoids and held them for some time with the forceps used for operations on the uvula he cuts them off with a scalpel. After the operation we must use manna and starch with chalcitis, or the plaster of burnt sponge with pitch, and the trochisk called faustinum, in order to burn it completely. Others by filling the cavity of the instrument called staphylocaustes, with caustic medicines, have burnt hemorrhoids like a scirrhous uvula.

Commentary. Hippocrates directs us to pass a needle armed with a very thick thread through the hemorrhoids, and tie them with it. Septic applications are afterwards to be made to them. (De Victu Acut. 67.) The author of another of the Hippocratic treatises recommends us to cure them by burning with red-hot irons. (De Hæmorr.)

Celsus directs us when the base of a hemorrhoid is narrow to tie it with a thread where it joins the anus, and to apply over it a sponge squeezed out of hot water until it become livid, when it is to be scraped off with the nail or a scalpel. Sometimes, however, he says, the ligature occasions great pain and retention of urine. If the hemorrhoid be large and its base broad, he directs us to seize it with a hook, and dissect it out a little above its base: the part is to be secured with a thread. When there are many hemorrhoids he advises us not to operate upon them all at one time. When there is a discharge of blood it is to be stopped by the application of a sponge. The day after the operation he recommends us to use the tepid bath and catalapsms. (vii, 30.)

Aëtius approves of cutting off hemorrhoids, and describes the operation minutely. He directs us to seize the pile with a hook, grasp it firmly, and bind it with a thread, after which it is to be raised and cut off. To stop the bleeding a piece of sponge bound round with a thread is to be introduced into the anus. Suitable dressings and bandages are then to be applied, (xiv, 6.)

In the 'Isagoge' ascribed to Galen, the method of treating hemorrhoids by the ligature is particularly commended.

Albucasis prefers excision and burning, but if the patient will not submit to these methods of cure he approves of having recourse to the ligature. Excision is performed by seizing the hemorrhoid with a hook and cutting it at its base, after which some styptic application is to be made. The ligature is applied by transfixing the base of the hemorrhoid with a needle armed with a thread. (Chirurg. ii, 81.) He gives particular directions about the process of burning. (p. i, 37.)

When the hemorrhoid is internal Rhases directs us to evert the anus, and having laid hold of the tumour to cut it out. He also describes the process of tying them in the same terms as the other authorities. (Contin. xxiv.) The directions given by Avicenna are quite similar.

Haly Abbas recommends excision or the ligature. (Pract. ix, 61.)

Fabricius makes mention of all these methods of treatment, but speaks of the application of the cautery as being dangerous. Upon the whole he appears to have entertained great apprehensions from stopping the discharge of piles. (Œuv. Ch. ii, 94.)

Theodoricus and Brunus recommend excision, the cautery, and the ligature, according to circumstances. Theodoricus also makes mention of applications for consuming and drying them up.

LXXX—ON CONDYLOMATA OR EXCRESCENCES, AND FISSURES

Condyloma on the fundament differs in situation alone from that on the female parts of generation, being a wrinkled excrescence of the anus, either from a preceding inflammation or fissure. At first, then, it is called an excrescence, but when it becomes callous, condyloma. These also, like the former, are to be taken hold of with a forceps and cut out, and the cure completed with escharotics. Fissures are occasioned principally by hard fæces, and being slow of granulating owing to their callosity, must be converted into recent ulcers by paring them with the nails or a scalpel, when they may be made to granulate by proper applications.

Commentary. Celsus briefly directs us to seize the condyloma with a forceps and cut it out by the roots. Should any fungous flesh arise it is to be kept down with the squama æris. (vii, 30.)

Aëtius gives a fuller account of these affections than our author. The condyloma, he says, is a tubercle which forms in the soft wrinkled skin about the anus. When it becomes hard and callous he recommends us to take hold of it with a forceps and cut it out by the roots. Old fissures he directs us to treat by paring their edges and applying suitable dressings. (xiv, 3.)

The same treatment is recommended by the Arabians. See Haly Abbas (Chirurg. ix, 62); Albucasis (Chirurg. ii, 81, 82); Rhases (Contin. xxiv.)

LXXXI—ON IMPERFORATE ANUS

In new-born children the anus is sometimes found imperforate, being blocked up by a membrane. If possible, then, the membrane is to be ruptured with the fingers, but if not, we must cut it with the point of a scalpel, and accomplish the cure with wine. And since often in adults, owing to an ulcer not properly cured, a stricture takes place at the anus, we must break it with a convenient instrument, and treat it properly with a pipe of lead, or some wedge-shaped tent introduced into the anus until the cure be completed, lest contraction should again take place. The wedge-shaped tent is to be anointed with some healing ointment.

Commentary. Soranus describes this operation in very distinct terms. (p. 164.)

Albucasis evidently copies our author's account, recommending us to break or divide the membrane, and introduce a canula of lead into the opening to prevent adhesion. (Chirurg. ii, 79.)

Haly Abbas, in like manner, directs us to make an opening and introduce a leaden tube or a piece of sponge. (Pract. ix, 63.)

LXXXII—ON THE EXCISION OF VARICES

The varix is a dilatation of a vein occurring sometimes in the temples, sometimes in the hypogastric region below the navel, sometimes in the testicles, but more especially in the legs. For the most part it derives its origin from a melancholic humour. The operation for those of the testicle we have already described when treating of cirsocele, and those in the leg may be operated upon in a similar manner, making the attempt upon those in the inner parts of the thighs, where they generally arise; for below this, as they are divided into many ramifications, they are more difficult to succeed with. Wherefore, having washed the man, and applied a ligature round the upper part of the thigh, we are to direct him to walk about, and when the vein becomes distended we are to mark its situation with writing ink or collyrium, to the extent of three fingers' breadth or a little more, and having placed the man in a reclining posture with his leg extended, we apply another ligature above the knee; and where the vein is distended we make an incision upon the mark with a scalpel, but not to a greater depth than the thickness of the skin, lest we divide the vein; and having separated the lips of the wound with hooks, and dissected away the membranes with crooked specilla, like those used in the operation for hydrocele, and laid bare the vein, and freed it all around, we loose the ligatures from the thigh, and having raised the vessel with a blind hook, and introduced under it a needle having a double thread we cut the double of it, and opening the vein in the middle with a lancet, evacuate as much blood as may be required. Then having tied the upper part of the vessel with one of the ligatures, and stretched the leg, we evacuate the blood in the limb by compression with the hands. Then having tied the lower part of the vein, we may either cut out the portion intermediate between the ligatures, or suffer it to remain until it drop out of its own accord with the ligatures; then we have to put a dry pledget into the wound, and apply over it an oblong compress soaked in wine and oil, and secure them with a bandage, and accomplish the cure by the treatment applicable in cases of suppuration. I am aware that some of the ancients do not use ligatures, but cut out the vessel immediately after it is laid bare, whilst others stretch it from below and tear it out by force. But the mode of operating now described is of all others the safest. Varices on the hypogastrium may be treated in like manner, and those on the temples as described in the operation of angiology.

Commentary. Hippocrates directs us to make small punctures in varices of the leg, but forbids to open them freely. (De Ulceribus, 16.) In the Hippocratic treatise entitled 'Hippiatrica,' it is recommended to burn varices in the legs of horses.

Celsus treats ingeniously of varices on the head (aneurism by anastamosis) on the belly (cirsocele?), and on the leg. With regard to the treatment, he says, in a word, that they are all either to be burnt or cut out. If the varix be straight, or if, although transverse, it consist of a single vein of moderate size, it will be better, he says, to burn it. If crooked and convoluted, and if it consist of a multitude of veins, it will be more useful to cut them out. He directs us, in burning them, to make an incision in the skin, and having laid bare the vein to touch it with a slender blunt piece of iron red-hot, taking care not to burn the edges of the wound which are to be drawn aside with hooks. This is to be done at intervals of about four fingers along the whole extent of the varix, and then the dressings for burns are to be applied. The varix is cut out in this way. The vein is to be exposed as above directed, and dissected with a scalpel from the surrounding parts (care being taken not to hurt it); a blunt hook is then to be introduced below it; and the same thing is to be done at the same interval as mentioned above. When this has been performed wherever there are varices, the vein is to be cut asunder at one of the hooks, and drawn towards the next hook, and then torn out. The leg being in this way cleared of the varices, the lips of the wound are to be united, and an agglutinative plaster applied above. (vii, 31.) It will be remarked that our author makes mention of this method of treatment but disapproves of it.

Aëtius describes the excision of varices in exactly the same terms as our author. He also makes mention of the treatment by the actual cautery. (xiv, 84.)

The operation of extracting varicose veins is briefly described in the 'Isagoge' of Galen. Albucasis describes accurately the different modes of operating upon varices. He says there are two methods of performing the operation with the knife, that is to say, by incision or by extraction. The former method is done by applying a piece of fillet round the upper part of the thigh, and at the inferior part near the knee, and then opening the vein in one, two, or three places, and evacuating the blood in it: the limb is then to be bound up. In performing extraction, the veins are first to be made to swell by putting the limb into hot water, applying fomentations, and taking strong exercise; and then a longitudinal incision is to be made in it, either at the knee or the ankle. The vein is afterwards to be dissected from the neighbouring parts and suspended with a blunt hook. The vein is to be laid bare in like manner at the distance of three fingers' breadth, and in more places if required. At last, it is to be cut asunder at the ankle and drawn out. Afterwards wool dipped in wine and rose-oil is to be applied. When the varix consists of a congeries of tortuous vessels he recommends us to dissect it out entire. (Chirurg. ii, 92.)

Haly Abbas briefly inculcates the same treatment as Albucasis. (Pract. ix, 64.) Avenzoar considers the complaint nearly incurable.

Rhases directs us, in the first place, to bleed and purge, and then to expose the vessel or cut it out. He also approves of compression. (Cont. xxviii.)

It is related that the operation here described was performed upon the celebrated Caius Marius. See Cicero (Tusc. Disput. ii.) Pliny (H. N. xi, 104); and Plutarchus (in Mario.) It seems to have been a very painful operation, since it is mentioned as a proof of his fortitude that he submitted to it without being bound. It would appear that the learned and ingenious Aurelius Severinus used to perform it. (V. Mangeti Bib. Chir. xvi.)

LXXXIII—ON THE DRACUNCULI OR GUINEA-WORMS

The treatment of dracunculi being principally accomplished by medicines, we have given an account of it in the Fourth Book.

Commentary. We have treated fully of this subject at the end of the Fourth Book.

LXXXIV—ON AMPUTATION OF THE EXTREMITIES

Sometimes the extremities, such as a hand or a foot, having mortified, so that the bones themselves are corrupted, either from having been fractured by some external means, or from having become putrid owing to some internal cause, it is necessary to saw them off; before doing which the parts surrounding the bones must be divided. But since, when this is done first, as a considerable time is required for the sawing, there is danger of a hemorrhage taking place, Leonides properly directs us not to divide all the parts at once unless they are completely mortified, but first to cut the part where not many nor very large veins or arteries are known to be situated, down to the bone quickly; then to saw the bone as expeditiously as possible, applying a linen rag to the parts which have been cut lest they be torn by the sawing and occasion pain, and then having cut through what remains, to apply red-hot irons to the vessels and stop the hemorrhage thereby with compresses of lint, and to apply proper bandages with the dressings suitable to suppurations.

Commentary. Hippocrates and Galen recommend amputation to be performed in general at a joint. (De Articulis, Galeni Comment. t. v, p. 650, ed. Basil.) Hippocrates says complete excision may be performed at the joints of the hand and foot, and at those of the wrist and ankle, and generally with safety, unless the patient be cut off by fainting, or continual fever supervene on the fourth day. When gangrene attacks a fractured limb, his rule of practice is to let the parts drop off, and he remarks, many persons thus recover, even when the fracture is seated in the femur. When gangrene comes on without being preceded by fracture, he directs the soft parts, as soon as they have lost all sensibility, to be removed at the nearest joint below, and the surgeon is to wait until the bone also separates. He says he had seen the bone of the thigh thus separate on the eightieth day; in that case the limb below had been removed at the knee on the twentieth day. In a similar case of gangrene of the leg, the bones separated on the sixtieth day. He pronounces gangrene of the extremities to be more formidable in appearance than in reality. He recommends a mild and anti-inflammatory treatment, and that the limb should be laid in an elevated position as long as there is any fear of hemorrhage. Violent attacks of dysentery are apt to come on, but do not generally prove obstinate. (De Artic. 69.) It would appear from Thucydides and Lucretius that it was not uncommon to amputate in cases of gangrene in the days of Hippocrates. (See their Descriptions of the Plague of Athens.)

In cases of gangrene Celsus directs us to make an incision of the flesh, between the sound and corrupted part, down to the bone, which is to be sawed across, and after the asperities have been removed from the end of the bone, the skin is to be brought over the stump. (vii, 33.) He gives us no particular description, however, of amputation of the extremities. We turn, therefore, to the celebrated fragments of the works of Archigenes and Heliodorus, preserved in the collection of Nicetas, published by Cocchius. (Chirurgici Græci, Florent. 1756.)

Archigenes begins by stating the circumstances which require recourse to be had to amputation. They are, the presence of some intractable disease, such as gangrene, necrosis, putrefaction, cancer, certain callous tumours, and sometimes wounds inflicted by weapons, and the like. Before attempting the operation he recommends us to consider well if the patient's strength will enable him to endure it. The operator must then tie or sew the vessels which pass to the parts; in certain cases a ligature is to be applied round the whole limb, cold water is to be poured upon it, and some are to be bled. Amputation near the joints is not to be attempted. In such as are of a full habit of body, a circular band is to be put round the limb, to draw up the skin with, and to direct the incision. After cutting down to the bone, the tendons are to be retracted, and the bone scraped and sawn. When much blood is discharged, red-hot irons are to be applied, and a double compress laid on the part from which the blood proceeds. Having loosened the band, a cataplasm of leeks, bread, and salt is to be applied to the stump; and the parts about the jaw-bone are to be anointed with cerate of iris and old oil, doubtless in order to obviate the danger from tetanus.

Heliodorus states that a limb may require to be amputated owing to gangrene or any other cause that occasions the death of it. In the extremities, then, he remarks, amputation may be performed with less danger; but above the knee or elbow the danger of hemorrhage from the great vessels being wounded is very considerable. Some, he says, from too great anxiety for despatch, cut through all the bodies (the soft parts?) at one incision, and then saw the bones. But this method of removing the limb is not unattended with danger, as many vessels pour forth blood at the same time. "Wherefore," he adds, "it appears to me better first to divide those parts of the limb where there is least flesh, as on the anterior part of the leg, and then to saw the bone; and I myself am in the practice of first applying a ligature above the part of the limb which is to be sawn across, and then of operating in the manner described. In sawing the bone the plate of the saw ought to be applied even, in order that the sawing of the bones may be even. When the bones are sawed the other parts which remain undivided are straightway to be cut through with a scalpel, and large pledgets applied along with suitable compresses. External to these, sponges with suitable bandages are to be put on. After the third or fourth day, when all fear of hemorrhage is over, suppuration is to be promoted by suitable dressings."

In no other of the Greek medical works which have come down to us is there any description of amputation of the extremities.

Avicenna mentions the operation of sawing off the bones of the extremities, but in such general terms as gives us no information in what manner it was performed. (iv, 4, 4, 10, 11, 12.)

The description given by Haly Abbas is more complete. A limb, he says, is amputated thus. The operation is to commence with first cutting the skin, and then when the bone of a limb is to be sawn, you must not cut through the whole flesh at once, lest an immoderate discharge of blood take place from the veins and arteries so as to occasion the death of the patient and interrupt the process of sawing the bone; except the flesh of the limb be wasted or putrid. But you ought first to divide that part of the flesh where no great arteries and veins are situated, cutting them down to the bone, which is to be sawn across as quickly as possible, the fleshy parts in the mean time being retracted with a piece of linen, lest the saw should tear them and occasion bleeding and pain; when the bone is sawn across, whatever portion of the flesh remains undivided is to be cut, and then the veins and arteries are to be burned. When the bleeding is stopped a pledget with suitable bandages is to be applied. (Pract. ix, 65.)

Albucasis represents amputation as necessary in cases of mortification, as indicated by the smell and discoloration. When the disease is seated in the hand, he recommends us to amputate at the fore-arm; when in the forearm, at the elbow; and if the arm itself be affected, he pronounces the case to be hopeless. In like manner, with regard to the lower extremities, he pronounces all cases incurable in which the disease is seated above the knee. In performing the operation he directs us to apply two bandages around the limb, the one above and the other below the place at which it is to be cut off. These bandages are to be pulled, the former upwards and the latter downwards, by two assistants, so as to put the skin upon the stretch; the fleshy parts are then to be divided with a large scalpel down to the bone, which is afterwards to be cut out, or sawed across, and during this part of the process a piece of linen is to be applied around all the fleshy parts, to prevent them from being injured by the sawing. Should any hemorrhage occur during the operation, he directs us to apply the cautery, or a styptic powder; and after the operation he recommends us to bandage the limb in a suitable manner, until the stump is healed. He relates a case, from which the timidity of his own practice is rendered very apparent. A person who had a spreading mortification in the foot, cut it off at the ankle-joint himself, and was cured for the time. The disease next attacked the hand, upon which he applied to Albucasis, requesting that he would cut it off in the same manner, but this he refused to do, for fear that the man's strength might not be able to endure the operation. He afterwards learned that the man had cut off his whole hand, and had recovered. (Chirurg. ii, 89.) The history of this case proves decidedly that the operative surgery of the Arabians, in the days of Albucasis, must have been very defective; this he himself frankly confesses, for he declares that all knowledge of this art had been lost, except what vestiges of it had been preserved in the works of the ancient authors, whose descriptions, he complains, had been mutilated and corrupted. (Prefatio.) We mention this, in order that the ignorance which prevailed in his time may not be imputed to all preceding ages, nor may be used as an argument against the genuineness of the extracts from the works of Heliodorus and Archigenes, given above.

Rhases makes some interesting remarks on the sawing of bones. He directs us to stretch the flesh upwards and downwards, with a piece of cloth, so that it may not come in the way of the teeth of the saw. When it is necessary to saw a rib or a bone, near any important membrane or organ, he recommends us to use a plate (tabella), to protect the soft parts from the saw. When the bone connected with a joint is diseased, he directs us to extract it at the joint. When the os brachii, or tibia, is diseased, he recommends us to extract it entire, but forbids to meddle with the head of the femur or the vertebræ. In another place he declares it as his opinion that when a joint is swelled, and the bone diseased, (in cases of white swelling?) it will be impossible to effect a cure unless the whole diseased portion of the bone be cut out. (Cont. xxix.) From these passages it is quite obvious that the ancients practised excision of the bones of joints. See also what our author says on this subject in the seventy-seventh section of this book. A Cooper or a Liston could not recommend a bolder plan of treatment in such cases.

Theodoricus, Guy of Cauliac, and the other surgical writers of that age, follow closely in the footsteps of the ancients, especially of the Arabians. When the mortified part is near to a joint, they recommend amputation at it. In other cases they direct us to make an incision between the sound and the dead parts, to saw the bone with a fine saw, and to stop the bleeding with a heated iron. Theodoricus recommends stupifying medicines, such as opium, hyoscyamus, mandragora, or cicuta, before the operation. Ambrose Paré has undoubtedly the merit of introducing the use of the ligature into modern practice in amputations, and, in fact, Archigenes seems to be the only ancient authority who mentions it in such cases. We have shown, however, in another place, that the ligature was freely used by the ancients for stopping bleeding from wounds.

LXXXV—ON PTERYGIA ABOUT THE NAILS

The pterygium is a fleshy excrescence about the nails, covering part of the nail, and being commonly formed in the large fingers and toes. But those in the feet arise most commonly from an accident, whereas, those in the hands arise from whitlow, the inflammation being neglected and turning to pus. For, the pus being allowed to remain, corrodes and corrupts the root of the nail, and often destroys the whole of it, but generally the one half, while a portion of it uncorroded is left at the root of the nail, and sometimes the whole root is left uncorroded. Sometimes, too, it corrupts the bone, when a disagreeable smell arises from it, and the extremity of the finger becomes swelled and appears livid. They are to be treated, then, by cutting and removing all the remaining part of the nail with the point of a scalpel, and then burning both the ulcerated and cut part with cauteries. For, the pterygium is a spreading disease, and does not stop unless burnt, so that, if neglected, it affects the whole finger. If, while the nail and bone remain sound, the inner angle of the nail sink down and pierce the adjacent flesh, it occasions inflammation; and in this case the irritating portion is to be raised upon a thin probe, or some such thing put under it, and removed with the point of a scalpel, and the excrescence eaten down with an escharotic medicine. And most cases are cured by being treated in this way. But if larger, it is first to be cut out with a scalpel, and then the medicine is to be used.

Commentary. We have given an account of the ancient treatment of pterygia by medicines towards the end of the Third Book.

Celsus recommends excision with the knife and the application of cauteries or strong caustics afterwards. (vi, 19.)

Aëtius and Oribasius trust to septic and caustic applications without an operation. Antyllus (apud Rhasis Cont. xxxvi,) recommended excision and burning when the discharge from the ulcer is fetid.

Albucasis, like our author, recommends us to cut off the piece of nail that is attached, and then to apply a burning iron to the part. The burning, he adds, is of great consequence. When the bone is diseased he directs us to take it out, which generally may be done at the joint. (Chirurg. ii, 9.)

Haly Abbas likewise directs us to cut off the piece of nail and apply the cautery. He says, if this be neglected the bone is apt to become diseased. When pus is seated below the nail, he recommends us to introduce the head of a probe under it, and cut upon it with a knife; after which a caustic medicine is to be applied to the flesh. (Pract. ix, 66.)

LXXXVI—ON A BRUISED NAIL

Since, owing to nails having been bruised by accidents, pains supervene, which compel us to operate upon them, it will be sufficient to give you Galen's account of the matter. He says, then: "When the nails are contused we have found the evacuation of the blood a palpable remedy for soothing the pain, when it and the throbbings are very violent. But we must make an oblique incision, not straight from above downwards, with a sharp scalpel, so that when the blood is evacuated the divided part of the nail may serve as a cover to the parts under it. But if you make a straight incision from above down to the fleshy excrescence, as it is called, another body is formed from the flesh below the nail shooting out through the division of the nail, whence pains again invade, as in the complaint we call paronychia, owing to the flesh under the nail being compressed by it. Wherefore, one may see the patients immediately relieved from pain by this section. On the following days we may gently raise the divided part of the nail, and press the sanies from under the nail, and then again, as I said, apply the nail as a cover to the flesh below. The rest of the treatment of the finger should be soothing and discutient."

Commentary. Avicenna and Rhases approve of the plan of treatment here recommended, upon the authority of Galen. Rhases, in fact, gives the very words of Galen. (Cont. xxxvi.)

Albucasis directs us, in the case of a bruised nail, first to have recourse to venesection, and then to make a transverse (oblique?) incision through it. (Chirurg. ii, 91.)

See our remarks in the sixtieth section of this Book on the confusion of the terms *transverse* and *oblique* by the translators of the Arabians.

The same treatment is recommended by Haly Abbas. (Pract. ix, 67.)

LXXXVII—ON CLAVI, MYRMECIA, AND ACROCHORDONES

The clavus is a round callus, white, resembling the head of a nail, and occurring in all parts of the body, but more especially on the soles of the feet and the toes, occasioning pain and lameness in walking. Wherefore, having scarified around the clavus or corn, and taken hold of it with a forceps, we cut it out by the roots with a sharp-pointed scalpel or lancet for bleeding. Some, in order that they may not grow again, use heated cauteries. The myrmecia is a prominence of the skin, small, callous, round, thick, spreading deep at the base, and, if rubbed, occasioning a sensation like the bites of ants, and being formed in all parts of the body, but more especially in the hands. Wherefore, some, among whom is Galen, advise us to scarify around the myrmecia with the stalk of a hard feather, such as those of old fowls, of geese, and of eagles, and to push it down so as to remove the myrmecia from the root. Others do the same thing with a copper or iron tube. The moderns are satisfied to scarify around it, and, having seized it with a forceps, to cut it out like corns with a scalpel. The acrochordon is a small rising of the surface, free of pain, callous, for the most part round, and having a narrow base so as to appear to hang. It is so called from its resemblance to the end of a cord. Having stretched out the protuberance then we may cut it out; or, otherwise, we may tie a thread or a hair round it. I have known many who consumed this and all the afore-mentioned protuberances with what is called the cold cautery.

Commentary. We have already treated fully of these diseases towards the end of the Third Book and in the Fourth, to which we refer the reader for further information on this head.

Celsus recommends us merely to shave the clavus or corn. The others he directs us to remove by caustics, such as the lees of wine (potass?), or a mixture of alum and sandarach. The acrochordon, he says, when cut out leaves no roots behind. (v, 28.)

Albucasis particularly recommends burning for the cure of clavus and myrmecia. This may be accomplished either with fire or hot water. If the former method is preferred, an iron proportionate to the size of the corn is to be heated red-hot and applied to it, and the burning carried to such an extent as to occasion suppuration. In the other method a funnel of copper or iron, or else the quill of a vulture is to be applied to the corn, and then filled with boiling water. By these means, he says, the corn may be eradicated. (Chirurg. i, 55.)

See also Haly Abbas (Pract. ix, 12) and Rhases (Cont. xxxvi.) Rhases does not state very distinctly the difference between the myrmecia and acrochordon. He speaks of scraping them out with a hard pen, and of tying them at the base; but upon the whole he approves most of taking hold of them with a forceps and dissecting them out.

Avicenna recommends us to cut out the clavus and then apply a caustic medicine to the part. (iv, 7, 4, 14.)

LXXXVIII—ON THE EXTRACTION OF WEAPONS

That the extraction of weapons is a most important department of surgery is declared by the Poet Homer, when he says:

> "The man of medicine can in worth with many warriors vie,
>
> Who knows the weapons to excise, and soothing salves apply."

We must first describe the different kinds of weapons. Warlike instruments, then, differ from one another in material, figure, size, number, mode, and power. In material, then, as the shafts are made of wood or of reeds; and the heads themselves are either made of iron, copper, tin, lead, horn, glass, bones, and of reeds, too, or of wood: and such differences are found especially among the Egyptians. In figure, inasmuch as some are round, some angled (as triangular), some pointed and lance-shaped, as some have three points; some are barbed and some are without barbs; and of the barbed, some have the barbs turned backwards, so that in attempting to extract them they may fasten in the parts; and some forwards, so that when pushed they may do the same thing: some have them diverging in opposite directions like the forked lightning, in order that whether pulled or pushed they may fasten in the parts. Some missiles have their barbs united by a hinge, which being expanded in the extraction, prevent the weapon from being drawn out. They differ in size, inasmuch as some are three fingers' breadth in size, and some are as small as one finger, which are called *micca* in Egypt, and some are intermediate between them. In number, inasmuch as some are simple and some compounded. For certain small pieces of iron are inserted in them, which, in the extraction of the weapon, remain concealed in deep-seated parts. In mode, as some have the sharp extremity fixed to a tail and some to a shaft; and some have it carefully inserted in the shaft, and some carelessly, so that in the extraction they may separate and leave the head behind. In power, as some are not poisoned and some are poisoned. Such are the differences of weapons. We now proceed to treat of the extraction, both in cases of those who have been wounded in war and those not in war, whether voluntarily and involuntarily, under whatever circumstances, and of whatever materials they may be composed. There are two modes of extracting weapons from fleshy parts; either by pulling them backwards, or pushing them forwards. When the weapon is fixed superficially the extraction is made by pulling it back, and in like manner when it is lodged deep, but the opposite parts, if wounded, would occasion danger from hemorrhage or sympathy. It is to be pushed forwards when lodged deep, and the intervening substances between it and the opposite side are of small size, and neither nerve, bone, nor any such thing is an obstacle to the division. When a bone is wounded, the mode of extraction is by pulling; if, therefore, the head of the weapon be in sight, we make the extraction immediately; but, if it is hid, we must, says Hippocrates, get the wounded person to put himself in the same posture as when he received the wound, and thus make the examination; or, if this cannot be done, he is to be placed in the nearest possible to it, and thus it is to be examined with a sound. If the head of the weapon has fixed in the flesh, it is to be drawn out with the hands, or by laying hold of the appendage, which is called the shaft, if it has not fallen off. This part is mostly made of wood. When it has fallen off, we make the extraction by means of a tooth-extractor, or a root-extractor, or an instrument for extracting weapons, or any other convenient instrument. And sometimes we make an incision in the flesh around it in the first place, if the wound do not admit the instrument. And if the head of the weapon has passed to the opposite side, and it is found impossible to extract it by the way in which it entered, having divided the parts opposite we extract it through them, either drawing it out in the manner mentioned, or we make a hole with the weapon itself, pushing it either by the shaft, or, if it has come away, by an impellent instrument, taking care not to divide a nerve, vein, artery, or any important part, for it would be disgraceful if, in extracting the weapon, we should do more mischief than the weapon itself had done. If the weapon has a tail, which is ascertained by examination with the probe, having introduced the female part of the impellent instrument and fixing it, we push the weapon forwards, but if it has a shaft, the male part. And if the head when extracted appear to have notches, so that other small pieces of iron might be inserted in them, we make an examination again with the probe, if we find them we extract them in the same manner. And if the weapon has barbs in opposite directions, which do not yield to our pulling, we must make an incision in the adjacent parts, if no important vessel or the like lie there, and when the weapon is laid bare, we extract it without trouble. Some apply a tube about the barbs, so that when they draw out the weapon the flesh may not be torn by the barbs. If the wound does not become inflamed, we may use sutures, and heal it up like a bloody wound; but if it inflame we may remove the inflammation by embrocations, cataplasms, and the like. If the weapon be poisoned we must, if possible, cut off all the flesh which has imbibed the poison, which is known by its being altered from the sound flesh, for it appears pale, livid, and as it were dead. They say that the Dacians and Dalmatians touch the points of their weapons with elecampane, called also *ninum*, and that when it thus becomes mixed with the blood of the wounded animal it proves fatal, although it is eaten by them with impunity. If, again, the weapon fix in a bone, we make trial with the instrument, and, if flesh prevent the extraction, we cut it off, or separate it; but if it be lodged deep in the bone (which we know by its being so firm that it cannot be shaken with a considerable force) we first remove the remaining part of the bone with a cutting instrument, or bore it with trephines if it has considerable thickness, and thus disengage the weapon. If a weapon be lodged in any important part, such as the brain, heart, throat, lungs, liver, stomach, intestines, kidneys, womb, or bladder, and fatal symptoms have already shown themselves, as the extraction would occasion much laceration we must decline the attempt, lest while we do no good we expose ourselves to the reprobation of ignorant people. But if the result be dubious, we must make the attempt, having first given warning of the danger. For in many cases, when an abscess has formed in some vital part, recovery has unexpectedly taken place; and the lobe of the liver, part of the omentum and peritoneum, and the whole uterus are said to have been taken away, and yet death was not the consequence. And we often open the windpipe intentionally, in cases of angina, as we mentioned under the head of Laryngotomy. To leave the weapon then as it is, occasions certain death, and exhibits the art in an inhumane light, whereas by extracting it we might possibly save a life. It is not difficult to ascertain when an important part is wounded, this being discovered by the peculiarity of the symptoms, the discharges, and situation of the parts. When, therefore, the membranes of the brain are wounded, there is intense pain of the head, the eyes are fiery, the tongue red, and there is aberration of intellect; but if it is attended with a wound of the brain, there is prostration of strength, with loss of speech, distortion of the countenance, vomiting of bile, a discharge of blood from the nostrils, an evacuation of a white and pultaceous fluid by the auditory foramen, and of ichor, if it can find a passage by the wound. If the weapon has penetrated to the cavity of the chest, and sufficient room is left for it, the breath passes out. When the heart is wounded, the weapon appears at the left breast, and feels not as if in a cavity, but as fixed in another body, and sometimes there is a throbbing motion; there is a discharge of black blood if it can find vent, with coldness, sweats, and deliquium animi, and death follows in a short time. When the lungs are wounded, if the opening be sufficiently large, a frothy blood passes out at it; but if not, it is rather vomited up, the vessels of the neck are swelled, the tongue changes colour, and there is an urgent desire of cold things. When the diaphragm is wounded the weapon appears lodged about the false ribs, there are large inspirations with pain, sighs, and heavings of the parts about the shoulder-joints. If the viscera of the abdomen are wounded, the nature of the injury will be apparent from the discharge, if the wound be sufficiently large, or if the weapon be extracted, or if the shaft be broken internally; for chyle is evacuated from the stomach, and fæces from the intestines; sometimes the omentum or an intestine protrudes. When the bladder is wounded urine is discharged. When the membranes of the brain or the cerebrum itself is wounded, we extract the weapon by trepanning the skull, as will be described presently in fractures of the bones of the head. If the weapon is lodged in the chest, and does not come out readily, it is to be extracted by means of a moderate incision in the intercostal space, or by cutting out a rib with the assistance of the instrument called meningophylax. In like manner, when the stomach, bladder, and other deep-seated parts are wounded, if the weapon come out readily it is to be extracted without more ado; but if not, we must enlarge the wound, and afterwards use the dressings for fresh wounds. In wounds of the abdomen, gastroraphé as formerly described may be had recourse to, if necessary. But if the weapon has lodged in any of the larger vessels, such as the internal jugulars or carotids, and the large arteries in the armpits or groins, and if the extraction threaten a great hemorrhage, they are first to be secured with ligatures on both sides, and then the extraction is to be made. If parts have been fastened to one another, such as the arm to the chest, or the fore-arm to the other parts of the body, or the feet to one another, if the weapon (as a spear) do not penetrate through both parts, we are to take hold of the weapon externally and extract as if only one part were affected, but if it has passed through both, having sawed the wood through the middle, we extract each part singly, in the most convenient direction. But since often stones or the sharp points of rocks, or pieces of lead, or the like, are lodged in the body, either being impelled with force from a sling, or happening to be acuminated, they are to be known by the swelling being hard and irregular, and by the solution not being everywhere straight, but larger than common, and having the skin bruised and livid, and the pain being attended with a sense of weight. They are, therefore, to be dislodged by means of suitable instruments, or scraped out with the concave part of a specillum or of an ear-specillum adapted for wounds; or, if they can be applied, a tooth-extractor or a root-extractor may be used for pulling them out. In many instances weapons lodged in the body lie concealed, and a long time after, when the wounds are healed up, the part having suppurated bursts, and the weapon drops out.

Commentary. Hippocrates considered the extraction of weapons to be one of the most important departments of surgery. It is to be fully learned, he says, only by attaching oneself to a foreign army. (De Medico.) He makes some interesting remarks on the subject in his treatise 'De Capitis Vulneribus.'

We must now attempt to give an abstract of Celsus's very interesting chapter on the Extraction of Weapons. Every weapon is to be extracted either by the part at which it enters or by that to which it tends. If it is not deep-seated, or if it has not passed any great vessels or nerves, there is no better plan than to draw it out as it entered. But if there is a greater space through which it must return than there would be to push it out, and if it has already passed the vessels and nerves, it will be better to open what remains undivided, and extract it in this direction. If the weapon is to be drawn backwards, the opening is to be enlarged by a scalpel, which will occasion less inflammation and obstruction of the parts than if they are torn by the weapon itself. In whichever way it be extracted great care ought to be taken that no nerve, large vein, or artery be divided. If any of these parts be detected in the wound they are to be drawn aside with a blunt hook. These are his general directions. He then subjoins instructions for extracting particular kinds of weapons. An arrow being a slender body, and generally impelled with great force, is often lodged deep, and is to be extracted for the most part rather by the opposite side to which it entered, especially as it has barbs, which tear most if drawn backwards. The flesh about the weapon is to be separated by means of a suitable instrument, and then if the head (mucro) appear with the shaft (arundo) fixed to it, the weapon is to be propelled until it can be laid hold of at the opposite side and extracted; or if the shaft has fallen out and only the iron remain lodged within, the head is to be seized with the fingers or a forceps, and removed, and it is to be extracted by the opening at which it entered, upon the same principles; for the wound being enlarged, the weapon is to be drawn back by the shaft if it remain, or otherwise by the iron itself. If there appear to be barbs upon the arrow, and if short and small, they are to be broken off with a pair of pincers; or, if larger and stronger, they are to be covered with split writing-pens (fissis scriptoriis calamis) to prevent them from tearing the flesh during extraction. And here we may mention, that the common *calamus scriptorius* of the ancients was made from an Egyptian reed. See Montfauçon (Palæographia Græca, p. 3.) When the weapon which is lodged in the body is large it must not be extracted by the opposite side, as it would make the wound too large. He directs us to draw it back by means of an instrument invented by Diocles, of which he gives a description. Another class of weapons which must sometimes be extracted are leaden balls, stones, or any such thing which breaks the skin, and is buried within. In all such cases the wound, he says, must be enlarged and the body extracted with a forceps. A complication which increases the difficulty of extraction arises from the weapon being lodged in a bone, or between two bones at a joint. When lodged in a bone it is to be moved about until loosened, when it is to be grasped with a forceps and extracted in the same way that a tooth is pulled out. It rarely happens that the weapon cannot be removed in this way; but if it remain fixed in the bone, it is to be struck with some iron instrument until it be shaken from the place where it is lodged. When other means do not succeed, the bone is to be perforated with a trephine. When the body is lodged in a joint between two bones, the two members about the wound are to be wrapped round with strips of cloth, or leathern thongs, and thereby separated by pulling in opposite directions, by which means the space between them will be slackened, and then the weapon may be removed without difficulty. When the weapon had been poisoned, these things must be done with all possible despatch, and the remedies applied which are used when a poison has been swallowed, or a person has been stung by a serpent. The wound from which a weapon has been extracted requires no other treatment than what is applicable for ordinary injuries. (vii, 5.)

Albucasis borrows mostly from our author the account which he gives of the construction of weapons and the symptoms occasioned by the wounds which they inflict. He also relates some interesting cases of recovery from very severe wounds. An arrow entered at the root of a man's nose and was extracted by Albucasis behind his ear; and the man recovered without having sustained any injury to the eye. He extracted another large arrow which had lodged deep below the eye of a Jew; and in this case also the sight was not impaired. He extracted a barbed arrow which had lodged in the throat of a Christian, by enlarging the wound, and the man recovered. An arrow had lodged in a man's belly, so that, at first sight, Albucasis considered the case as hopeless; but, after thirty days, as no mortal symptoms had supervened, he enlarged the wound and extracted the weapon. He saw a man who had got an arrow lodged in his back; the wound healed, but after an interval of seven years the weapon came out below his buttocks. He knew a woman who had an arrow lodged in her belly, and the wound healed, and the weapon never afterwards occasioned her any inconvenience. He knew a man who had an arrow lodged in his face, and the wound healed up, and never gave him much trouble. He relates that he extracted an arrow which had been buried in the nose of a prince, after making various fruitless attempts for the space of four months. He then delivers general directions for the extraction of weapons, borrowing, as usual, very freely from our author. When a weapon cannot readily be got extracted at the time, he recommends us to let it alone until it become loosened by the putrefaction of the surrounding parts. When impacted in a bone, he directs us either to move it about until it is loosened, or to perforate the bone with a trephine. When lodged in the cranium, it is to be removed in like manner with a trephine, provided the dura mater is not injured, for if it is wounded the case must not be interfered with. When a weapon is lodged deep in any part of the body where there are no large nerves, veins, or bones, he directs us to enlarge the wound and extract the weapon; but if it has barbs, the fleshy parts about it must first be carefully separated to prevent them from being torn. When a weapon passes through a limb, or attaches one part of the body to another, he directs us to cut off the part which projects, and then extraction may easily be accomplished. If fastened in a bone, he advises us to turn it round so as to loosen it; and if that does not suffice, he recommends us to leave it for a few days, when it may be extracted without difficulty. If the shaft or wooden part of a weapon be broken off, he directs us to apply to the head an impellent instrument with a concave extremity, so as to adapt itself to the form of the body which is to be extracted. When the weapon is poisoned, he recommends us, if possible, to cut out the flesh around it. When a weapon lodges in the breast, belly, bladder, or side, and can be felt with a probe, he directs us to cut cautiously upon it, taking care not to wound a vein or nerve. He concludes with giving drawings of forcipes and impellents. (Chirurg. ii, 96.)

Rhases gives sensible directions for the management of these cases, but they are so similar to those of our author that we need not dwell upon them. If the size of the wound permit, he directs us to introduce a forceps to the iron head and draw it out. If the opening be too small, he recommends us to enlarge it. When the weapon has nearly passed through the limb, he advises us to push it out at the opposite side. Thorns and such like sharp things are to be removed by the application of extractive plasters. (Ad Mans. vii, 25.)

Avicenna gives a literal translation of the present chapter of Paulus, and supplies nothing additional of much interest. (iv, 4, 2, 10.)

The account given by Haly Abbas is full, but like that of Albucasis. He mentions that he had seen cases in which an arrow had been lodged in the intestines, and although fæces were discharged by the wound, the patient recovered. He adds that others relate cases in which recovery took place although the liver or omentum had been wounded. (Pract. ix, 15.)

The rules for the extraction of weapons laid down by Theodoricus and all the earlier authorities are mostly copied from the ancient authors. (i, 22.)

It would be naturally expected that we should give some account in this place of the surgery in the heroic ages, as far as it can be learned from the poems of Homer and the Commentary of Eustathius. The Commentator remarks that three methods of extracting weapons are mentioned by Homer: 1. By evulsion or pulling the weapon backwards, as in the case of Menelaus. (Iliad, iv, 214.) 2. By protrusion or pushing it forwards, as in the case of Diomedes. (Iliad, v, 112.) 3. By enlarging the wound and cutting out the weapon, as practised by Patroclus in the case of Eurypylus. (Iliad, xi, 218.) He further remarks that it appears to have been a common practice to suck a wound with the mouth; and, he adds, that this method was still in use among a barbarous people in his days. (Iliad, iv, 219.) The weapons used in the Trojan war were swords, spears or javelins, stones flung by the hand or by a sling, hatchets or axes, as used by the Trojans on certain occasions (Iliad, xii, 590), and arrows. Eustathius remarks, however, that there would appear to have been very few bowmen. In his Commentary on the Odyssey he states that poisoned arrows were never employed in war, but only for killing wild beasts. (Odyss. i, 260.) We believe that no weapons of iron were used in the war of Troy, and that they were all made of copper. (See Jameson's Mineralogy, iii.) Little transpires from Homer with regard to the internal treatment. In one place (Iliad, xi, 638) mention is made of a mixture of wine and cheese having been given to a wounded warrior, which practice, Eustathius says, had given rise to a variety of conjectures. Some supposed that the wound in the case referred to was so slight as not to render the administration of stimulants improper; others rather believed that the loss of blood had been so great as to call for the use of wine to support the strength. But many, he adds, were of opinion that men in the heroic ages lived so temperately that their constitutions readily bore things on extraordinary occasions, which in after ages were reckoned to be of too inflammatory a nature. This explanation is advocated by Athenæus. (Deipnos, i.) In the Odyssey, mention is made of a hemorrhage being stopped by incantation, which shows, as Eustathius remarks, that amulets and incantations were as ancient as the heroic ages.

LXXXIX—ON FRACTURES AND THEIR DIFFERENCES

Having described the surgical operations on the fleshy parts, we have next to give an account of those which relate to the bones, I mean the treatment of fractures and dislocations; for these also fall under the department of surgery. And first, of fractures, beginning with fractures of the bones of the head, because they hold an intermediate place between the operations on the fleshy parts and the bones, and because the cranium overtops all the other parts. In general terms, then, a fracture is a division of a bone, or rupture, or excision of it, produced by external violence. The differences of fractures are many. A bone, then, is said to be fractured *raphanatim, scandulatim, in unguem, polentatim,* and *per defractionem.* A fracture *raphanatim* is a transverse one through the thickness of the bone, and is called also *cucumeratim* and *caulatim,* because cucumbers and cabbages break in this way. *Scandulatim* is a longitudinal fracture of a bone. *In unguem* is a fracture at one part straight, and at its extremity lunated, and it is also called *arundatim. Polentatim* is a fracture of a bone into small pieces; and it is also called *nucatim* by some: *Defractio* or *præcisio* is when part of a bone is taken away with tearing of the skin, so that part is removed and is wanting. These are the differences of fractures.

Commentary. The following is a list of the ancient authors who have treated of fractures and dislocations: Hippocrates (de Fracturis; de Articulis; de Vulner. Capit.; Officina Medici); Galen (Comment. in eosdem, Meth. Med. vi.); Celsus (viii); Oribasius (de Machinamentis, &c.); Nicetæ Collectio ex Chirurg. Græc.; Apollonius Citiensis (Scholia in Hippocrat. ed. Dietz); Avicenna (iv, 5, 23); Rhases (ad Mansor. vii, 26; Divis i, 140; Cont. xxix); Averrhoes (Collig. vii, 36); Avenzoar (ii, 6, 1); Haly Abbas (Pract. ix, ad finem.)

Hippocrates does not make use of the technical terms explained by our author in this section, and Galen hints that he thinks his Master did better in confining himself to words generally understood. Galen defines only a few of these terms. He calls that kind of fracture in which the end of a bone at an articulation is entirely taken away, *âbruptio* (ἄπαγμα.) A transverse fracture with a complete separation of the broken portions is called a fracture *caulatim* (καυληδὸν.) A longitudinal division not attended with an entire separation of the parts is called *scandulatim* (σχιδακηδὸν.) He thinks the later writers on the subject who had introduced the use of such terms as *raphanatim* (ῥαφανηδὸν) and *polentatim* (ἀλφιτηδὸν) had refined too much.

All the terms mentioned by our author occur in a fragment of Soranus, preserved in the collection of Nicetas. They are also treated of very elaborately in the fragments of Heliodorus, contained in the same collection.

Celsus, who was studious of perspicuity and elegance, avoids all technical terms as much as possible. He thus defines the varieties of fractures. A bone, he says, may be split longitudinally like a piece of wood, or it may be broken transversely or obliquely, and its ends may be blunt or sharp, which last variety is the worst of all, as they cannot be easily made to unite with the other parts, and are apt to wound the muscles and nerves. Sometimes the bone is broken into fragments, and in certain bones a fragment is occasionally separated entirely from the broken bone.

The Arabians, especially Avicenna, Haly Abbas, and Albucasis, adopt the terms used by our author. Albucasis remarks, that the fracture of a bone is recognised by the derangement of the broken pieces, by their projection, and the crepitus produced upon pressure. He says, however, that there may be a fissure without derangement or crepitus.

XC—ON FRACTURES OF THE BONES OF THE HEAD

In particular, then, a fracture in the head is a division of the cranium, sometimes simple and sometimes complex, occasioned by some external violence. The differences of fractures of the head are these: a fissure, an incision, an expression, a depression, an arched fracture, and, in infants, a dent. A fissure, then, is a division of the skull, either superficial or deep, when the inward bone is not removed out of its place. An incision, or slash, (ἐγκοπὴ) is a division of the skull with refraction of the fractured bone (if the injured bone be broken off some call the affection *deasciatio,* i. e. as if done by a hatchet). An expression is a division of a bone into many parts, with a sinking down of the fractured pieces upon the membrane of the brain. A depression (ἐγγίσωμα) is a division of a bone with a sinking downwards of the fractured bone from its natural position towards the meninx. An arched fracture (καμάρωσις), as Galen says, is a division of the skull attended with elevation of the fractured pieces in the middle, and depression around the edges of the sound parts, like as in expression. Such is his opinion. Some enumerate also the capillary fracture, but it is a very narrow fissure which eludes the senses, and therefore, being often overlooked owing to the symptoms of it not being obvious, it occasions death. An indentation is not a division of a bone, and, therefore, such an injury is not properly called a fracture, but is, as it were, a protrusion and bending of the skull inwardly, forming a hollow without a solution of continuity, as when vessels made of copper, or the raw hide of an ox, are struck on the outside. There are two different kinds of indentation, for either the bone is depressed through its whole thickness, so that often a separation of the membrane of the brain takes place, or it is pressed upon by the skull throughout; or sometimes the indentation does not affect the skull through its whole thickness but only its outer plate down to the diploe. To these differences some also add that by repercussion, which happens, say they, when a fracture of the cranium takes place opposite to the part which received the blow. But they are in a mistake, for what happens to glass vessels does not, as they say, happen here; for, this happens to them from their being empty, but the skull is full and otherwise strong. But when many other parts of the head have been struck, as in a fall, and a fissure of the skull takes place without a solution of continuity of the skin, an abscess afterwards forms in it, and being opened, this fissure is discovered, which appears to them to have been occasioned by the blow on the opposite side; and this is to be cured like the fissure first mentioned. If a fracture, then, occur in the head, it is discovered by the sharpness, weight, hardness, or violent force of the body which struck it, and by the symptoms which supervene upon the person who has been struck, such as vertigo, loss of speech, and sudden prostration, more particularly if it be a fracture with depression, or contusion, or expression, or the internally-arched fracture, owing to the compression of the brain. It is also discovered by its appearances to the senses; for if there be a considerable division of the skin we ascertain the occurrence readily thereby; but if there be no division, or a very narrow one, and we suspect a fracture, we make an incision in the skin and ascertain it by the sight, or by probing it with an instrument. If then it be any of the other kinds of fracture it will readily be apparent, but if it is only a narrow capillary fissure which eludes the sense, having poured on the part some black liquid medicine, or the common writing ink, we scrape the bone, for the fissure appears black, and we must go on scraping until the symptoms of the fissure disappear; but if it extend to the membrane we must desist from the scraping, and endeavour to ascertain whether the membrane has separated from the bone or remains fixed. For if it remain, the inflammation of the wound continues moderate, the patient gets gradually freed from the fever, and the pus appears concocted. But if the membrane has separated, the pains increase and the fever in like manner, the bone changes colour, and then unconcocted pus is discharged; and if the person who has the charge of it neglect the case, and has not recourse to perforation, still more grievous symptoms will come on, vomiting of bile, convulsions, disorder of intellect, and acute fever, under which circumstances one must decline operating. But if these are not present, and the membrane has not separated, and if the fracture be a mere fissure, it may be cured by scraping alone, although it be of considerable depth. If it extend to the diploe only it is to be scraped down to it, or the broken bone removed, as will be described. If broken into small pieces, these also are to be extracted with a convenient instrument. And if the membrane separate, and you have treated the patient from the commencement, and if it be winter, endeavour by all means to effect the removal of the bone before the fourteenth day; but, if in summer, before the seventh, while the afore-mentioned symptoms have not come on you may operate in this way:

The Operation.—Having first shaved the head about the wound, we make two incisions intersecting one another at right angles like the Greek letter X, one of them being the wound already existing; then dissecting the four angles at the top, so that the bone about to be perforated may be wholly laid bare, if there be bleeding we apply pledgets moistened in oxycrate, but if not dry ones; and then applying a compress out of wine and oil, we use a proper bandage; and next day, if no new symptom supervene, we proceed to perforate the affected bone. Wherefore, having placed the patient on a seat, or in a reclining posture suitable to the wound, and stuffed his ears with wool in order to avoid the noise of the perforation, we loosen the bandage from the wound, and having removed all the dressings and sponged it, we direct two assistants with small twisted bands to retract the four angles of the parts lying over the fracture, and if the bone be weak, either naturally or from the fracture, we cut it out with counter-perforators, beginning first with the broader ones and changing to the narrower, and then using those which are of the form of a specillum, striking gently with the mallet to avoid shaking the head. But if the bone be strong it is to be first perforated with that kind of perforators called abaptistæ, which have certain eminences projecting a little above the point that prevent them from sinking down to the membrane, and then, by using the chisels, we remove the fractured bone not at once, but by pieces, if possible with the fingers, or otherwise with a tooth forceps, or bone forceps, or hair-nippers, or some such instrument. The space between the perforations should be as great as the breadth of the largest head of a specillum, and its depth should be until it is near the inner surface of the bone, taking care that the perforator (trepan?) do not touch the membrane. Therefore, in order to suit the thickness of the bone with the size of the perforator, several ought to be previously prepared for the purpose. But if the fracture extend only to the diploe the perforation should be carried no farther. After the removal of the bone, having cleared away any asperity that remained after the cutting of the bone with a carving instrument, or the extremity of a perforator, using the meningo-phylax as a protector, and bringing away carefully the small bones and spiculæ which remain, we proceed to the application of the dressings. This is the more common, and at the same time the easiest and least dangerous mode of operating; but the method of performing it with a sort of incisor called lenticular is greatly praised by Galen, being performed without perforation after the part has been scraped all round with hollow chisels (κυκλίσκοι). Wherefore he says thus: "If you have once laid bare the place, then applying the incisor, which has a projection at the extremity like a lenticular, blunt and smooth, but sharp longitudinally, when you apply the broad part of the lenticular to the meninx, divide the cranium by striking with the small hammer. For we have all that we require in such operations; for the membrane, even if the operator were half asleep, could not be wounded being in contact only with the broad part of the lenticular, and if anything adhere to the cranium, the round part of the lenticular removes its adhesion without trouble. And behind it follows the incisor, or knife itself, dividing the skull; so that is impossible to discover another mode of operating more free from danger or more expeditious." But the mode of operating with saws and the instruments called chœnicides or modioli (trepans?) is condemned by the moderns as a bad one, and the operation may be done as we described for fissure. The same mode of removing bones will be applicable in the other fractures of the cranium. But regarding the amount of bones requiring extraction Galen informs us, writing thus plainly: "What parts of a fractured bone are to be removed I will now explain to you in order. When it is greatly bruised it is to be taken out entire, but if certain fissures extend from it farther, as sometimes they appear to do, we must not pursue them to their termination, well knowing that no harm will result from them if everything else be properly done." After the operation, having dipped a simple linen rag of the size of the wound in oil of roses, we lay it over the membrane as a cover, and in like manner, having dipped a small ball of wool in oil of roses, we put it over the aforesaid rag, and then having moistened a doubled compress in wine and oil, or in the same oil of roses, we apply it to the whole wound, taking care that they be not too heavy for the meninx. We then have recourse to a broad bandage, which also must not be made tight, but so as merely to preserve the pledgets. And the regimen is to be what is called anti-inflammatory and such as is applicable for fevers, frequently bathing the membrane with oil of roses. After the third day loosing them and sponging the part we pursue the treatment applicable for recent wounds and the anti-inflammatory; sprinkling upon the meninx some of the powders called cephalics until it incarnate, and sometimes scraping the bone, if it require it, on account of certain projecting spiculæ, or for the sake of incarnation itself. And we may apply medicines of the ingredients recommended for wounds.

On inflammation of the membrane of the brain. Often after the operation the membrane is inflamed, so as not only to rise above the skull but likewise above the skin, and is attended with hardness, and obstructs the natural pulsatory motion of the brain, in which case convulsions and other severe symptoms, or death, for the most part supervene. It becomes inflamed either from the irritation of some sharp projecting piece of bone, or from the weight of the dressings, or from cold, or from eating too much, or from drinking wine, or some other cause not apparent. If then the cause be obvious it is to be speedily removed, or, if it is not, it will be proper to contend strenuously against it, either by having recourse to venesection, if nothing prohibit it, or to a diet suitable for inflammation. We must also use topical remedies, such as warm embrocations with hot rose-oil, and bathing the part with the decoction of marshmallows, or of fenugreek, of linseed, of camomile, and such like, and cataplasms of raw barley flour, or of linseed with the aforementioned decoction and the grease of a fowl; and irrigations with wool to be poured upon the head and occiput, and some anti-inflammatory oil is also to be poured into the meatus auditorius. The viscera also are not to be neglected, but suitable cataplasms are to be applied to them. And care is to be taken of the whole body, putting the patients into warm baths and anointing them. If the inflammation continues and nothing else prohibit, Hippocrates directs us to purge them with cholagogue medicines.

On blackness of the meninx. When the meninx turns black, if the blackness be superficial, and has been brought on by medicines which have that property, we may remove it by applying three parts of honey with rose-oil upon pledgets, along with the other suitable treatment. But if the blackness has come on spontaneously, more particularly if deep-seated, and be attended with other dangerous symptoms, then we must refrain from using them, for these appearances indicate a dissolution of the natural heat. I knew a person who had his skull trephined a year after the accident, and recovered. The fracture was from a weapon, and was situated on the bregma, and the discharge having an outlet, the meninx was thereby preserved free from injury.

Commentary. Hippocrates very properly lays it down as a rule that no injuries of the head are to be considered as trifling, since wounds affecting only the integuments will sometimes prove dangerous if neglected. He treats distinctly of fissures, contusions, and fractures of the cranium, which is an excellent arrangement of these accidents. Our limits, however, will not allow of our entering minutely into an explanation of his modes of treatment. In fractures of the head he forbids liquid applications, especially wine. He calls the trephine by the name of τρύπανον; and makes mention of a raspatory (ξυστὴρ). It would appear that his object in applying the trepan was altogether preventive; that is to say, that he had recourse to the operation in order to prevent inflammation and swelling of the brain, and not to remove the effects of them. He holds that severe contusions without fracture and fissures are more dangerous than injuries attended with depression and considerable separation of the fractured portions, and it is in the former class of cases that he recommends trepanning. When the bone is broken into several pieces, he says it stands in no need of the trephine. One of the varieties of fracture, which he describes with surprising accuracy, is the separation of the bones at a suture. It, he adds, seldom requires the use of the trephine. He remarks, that convulsions often occur in consequence of injuries of the head, and that the convulsions are in the opposite side to that in which the injury of the brain is seated. He gives an excellent account of erysipelas of the face supervening upon injury of the head, and recommends it to be treated with cholagogues. Altogether, his work 'On Injuries of the Head' bespeaks extensive acquaintance with the subject, and we need have little hesitation in pronouncing it to be one of the most valuable relics of antiquity. In one of his aphorisms, he states that concussion of the brain occasions loss of speech; that is to say, as Galen explains his meaning, superinduces apoplectic symptoms.

Galen mentions three sorts of instruments for operating upon the cranium, namely the cyclisci, the lenticulars, and the narrow raspatories. Fractures are classed by him into those which extend only to the diploe, and those which penetrate to the inner surface of the bone. He likewise divides them into simple fissures, contusions, and depressions inflicted by the body, which occasioned the injury. When the fissure extends down only to the diploe, he directs us to scrape down the bone with raspatories, and then to apply the medicines called cephalics, consisting of Illyrian iris, the farina of tares, manna, birthwort, and panacea. Of the fractures which extend to the meninx, if a simple fissure, it may be treated in the same manner by raspatories; but if attended with contusion, by perforating it all round with an auger (trepan?), and then using the scalpel, or by means of the cyclisci at once. Some, he says, instead of these instruments, use the abaptista, which had a circular border projecting a little above the sharp extremity of the perforator. Some, he says, from timidity, use only the instrument called chœnix (modiolus). Of all modes, however, he prefers that by the lenticular, as stated by our author. He then defines the engeisoma and camerosis, which we have translated the depressed and the arched fractures, the former being attended with depression, and the latter with elevation in the middle of the fracture. These are to be taken out entire by means of a lenticular or bone forceps. This, by the way, was the practice of the celebrated Heliodorus, of whose opinions on this subject we will give a short abstract below. (Nicetæ Collectio.) Such is Galen's general treatment of fractures of the skull. In a word, he lays it down as a rule, that parts which are greatly comminuted, must be entirely removed; but that fragments, which extend far, must not be followed to their extremities. He forbids the use of bandages. He mentions having trepanned the head occasionally, but states that he generally left this task to the Roman surgeons. Sprengel remarks, that Galen was averse to the use of the trepan, and preferred the two instruments called by him φακωτὸς and κυκλίσκος. The latter, he remarks, was, properly speaking, a hollow chisel (un ciseau creux), which he drove in with a hammer. The former was a true lenticular-knife, resembling that described by Petit and Bell (Hist. de la Méd., 18.)

We will now attempt an abstract of Celsus's lengthy account of these accidents. When the skull has been struck, he recommends us in the first place to inquire whether the person has vomited bile, has experienced dimness of vision, with loss of speech, or a discharge of blood from the nose and ears; whether he fell down at the time, and if he lay in a comatose and senseless state. These symptoms, he says, indicate a fracture of the bone, and the accident is to be looked upon as serious. But if torpor has come on, with mental aberration, paralysis, or contraction of the tendons, it is probable that the membrane of the brain has been injured, and little hopes of recovery need be entertained. In order to ascertain whether or not the bone be fractured, nothing answers better, he says, than making an examination with a specillum (sound), that is neither too sharp nor too blunt. If the bone is felt to be everywhere smooth, we are certain that it is sound; but if roughness is detected, we know that it is occasioned by a fracture. He warns us, however, not to mistake a suture for a fissure, as was once done by Hippocrates, upon whom he bestows a merited eulogium for this frank confession of his own blunder. When this method of inspection does not succeed, he advises us to pour writing ink on the part and to scrape the bone, which will appear black when there is a fissure. Sometimes, however, he adds, the blow has been sustained on one part of the skull, and the fissure occurs in another. This is the case of fracture by repercussion, of which we will make further mention afterwards. Celsus says, we ought to suspect the existence of it when symptoms of fracture have occurred without our being able to detect one in the part which received the blow. He also recommends us, if softness and swelling be detected in any part, to examine it, as it is likely that a fissure of the bone may be found there. (By the softness and swelling, of which he speaks, he probably meant the *puffy tumour*, described by Mr. Pott, in his work on 'Injuries of the Head.') Sometimes, he adds, but rarely, although the skull be safe, a vessel in the membrane of the brain bursts and pours forth much blood, which, becoming coagulated, occasions great pain and dimness of sight. In such a case, he says, the pain will point out the seat of the extravasation, and if an incision be made in the skin, the bone will be found to be pale—"eo loco cute incisâ, pallidum os reperitur." (Heliodorus, in like manner, states that when extravasation has taken place within the cranium, the bone will be found to be pale—Nicetæ Collectio.) The fact that in cases of extravasation below the skull the bone is pale, that is to say, does not bleed, is pointed out by Mr. Abernethy as an unerring guide to practice in such cases. He says, "unless one of the large vessels of the dura mater be wounded, the quantity of blood poured out will probably be inconsiderable; I believe that a bone so circumstanced will not be found to bleed." Celsus then proceeds to the description of the operation. If the injured portion of the bone is not sufficiently exposed, he directs us in the first place to enlarge the wound of the integuments. The periosteum is then to be scraped away with a raspatory. The form of the incision, if made solely by the operator, is to consist of two cross lines intersecting one another like the letter X, from the extremities of which the skin is to be dissected away. If there be a discharge of blood it is to be stopped by a sponge dipped in vinegar, or by compresses, while the head is elevated. In cases of fracture and fissure of the cranium, the ancient surgeons, he says, had immediate recourse to instruments for cutting out the part; but he recommends the surgeon, in the first place, to try the effect of applications for allaying the irritation, such as suitable plasters, with wool soaked in vinegar, proper bandages, and the like. This treatment is to be continued for five days, and on the sixth the part is to be fomented with a sponge soaked in warm water. If the skin begin to heal, and the fever to abate, and if the appetite return, with sound sleep, he recommends perseverance in the use of these applications. In this manner, he adds, fissures will often be filled with callus; thus, also, bones more extensively fractured may become united with callus, which forms a much better cover to the brain than the common integuments after a piece of bone has been cut out. But if, on the other hand, fever set in at the first with disturbed sleep, a copious discharge from the wound which shows no appearance of healing; if the glands of the neck swell, or if violent pain comes on, with loathing of food, the surgeon must proceed forthwith to the operation. Dangerous consequences, he adds, may arise either from a fissure or a depression. A fissure may allow fluids to descend to the membrane of the brain, and thereby give rise to pain and inflammation. A depression in like manner may occasion irritation, and spiculæ of bones by wounding the brain may prove particularly troublesome. As a general rule, he recommends as little of the bone as possible to be removed. If the one edge overtop the other, it will be sufficient to remove with a raspatory the prominent part; for when it is taken away there will be a sufficient opening for the cure. If the edges are firmly compressed together, a hole is to be bored with a wimble (terebra) on its side, at the distance of a finger's breath, and from it two lines are to be cut to the fissure with a raspatory (scalpel), in the form of the letter V, so that its vertex may be at the hole, and its base at the fissure. If the fracture be long, more of these holes must be cut out. In cases of depression the whole depressed portion must be removed. In whatever way the pieces of bone are cut they are all to be removed by means of a suitable forceps. But we will not occupy more space in explaining his method of operating, as we have been already more than usually prolix. Enough has been said to show that the practice of Celsus was sensible, and in many respects not very different from that which is now followed in such cases. It will be seen that he was not forward to perforate the skull, and that many of the rules of treatment lately laid down as new discoveries are distinctly mentioned by him. For a description of the instruments used by him, namely, the modiolus, terebræ, and scalper excisorius, we must refer the reader to the original work. (viii, 3.)

The different kinds of fracture to which the skull is subject, and the treatment of them, are given very minutely in the Fragments of Heliodorus, published by Cocchi (Ch. Vet. 100, &c.); but as the views of the subject there laid down are nearly the same as our author's, we shall only give a few specimens of the doctrines he inculcates. He describes very distinctly the species of fracture called *diastasis*, namely, the separation of two bones of the head at a suture. He directs that the head should be moulded into its former shape, and secured with compresses and tight bandaging. When matter forms he recommends it to be cut down upon. When depression of the bone without fracture occurs in children, it is not to be much interfered with, if no untoward symptoms come on. But if any collection take place, it is to be evacuated, even if trepanning should be required for this purpose. He says, in the treatment of simple injuries of the scalp, that the cure *by the first intention* is the quickest, but the suppurative the safest. In the same Collection there are a few fragments of Archigenes, containing some curious and important matter. He describes *diastasis* of the bones with more minuteness than any other ancient author, but does not touch upon the treatment. He appears to treat of *hernia cerebri* under the name of *hypersarcosis*, and recommends the excrescence to be removed, with septic medicines or the scalpel, down to the membrane (*dura mater*); after which a light dressing dipped in rose-oil is to be applied, and the part surrounded with a circular bandage. (Chirurg. Vet. p. 119.) Effusion of blood within the cranium is indicated by fevers coming on with chills, inordinate heat, disturbed sleep, eyes glossy, muddy, and red, loss of flesh, &c. In such cases, he remarks, if operated upon speedily, they exhibit promises of recovery, but generally soon die. (Ibid. 117.)

Albucasis enumerates the same varieties of fracture as our author, and his description of the operation is little different. The drawings which he gives of the surgical instruments used by the ancients in operations on the head are interesting, as they tend to illustrate the descriptions of Paulus and the other authorities. We may remark, by the way, that his *abaptista*, which he calls *terebra non profundantia*, are a sort of spear-shaped instruments, having a globular ball a short way above their extremity. They, therefore, had no resemblance to a modern trephine with a conical crown.

Avicenna gives a very full account of injuries of the head, but it is taken almost word for word from Galen and our author. Nearly the same may be said of Haly Abbas.

Avenzoar states that trepanning the skull will be proper when there is fracture with depression; but laments that in his time it would be difficult to find a surgeon capable of performing the operation. Averrhoes likewise intimates that he did not know a surgeon who could trepan the skull. This is an additional proof to what we have mentioned in the section on amputation that the Arabians in general were very timid operators.

Rhases strongly inculcates the propriety of having recourse promptly to the operation, when the bone is fractured and depressed, before dangerous symptoms have come on. Unless there be pressure on the brain, however, he does not approve of having immediate recourse to the operation.

It will be remarked that Celsus affirms, and our author denies, the occurrence of fracture by repercussion. It is the same as *la fracture par contre-coup* of the French medical authors, or the *counter-fissure*, namely, the *fractura per resonitum* of the earlier authorities. Soranus, who, like Celsus, believes in its occurrence, defines it to be a fissure which takes place in the part of the cranium opposite to that which received the blow. (Nicetæ Collectio.) Hippocrates himself makes mention of the counter-fissure, and pronounces it to be incurable, as the surgeon has no certain data to discover its existence. (Vul. Cap. viii.) Tulpius, Paré, and Van Sweiten have related cases of the counter-fissure. (See Comment. in Boerhaav. Aph. 254.) Heister also believed in its occurrence. (Chirurg. i, 1, 14.) For cases of it he refers to D. Wagnerus, (Dissert. de contra-fissura,) and Le Maire (De resonitu.) He is mistaken, however, when he quotes Ægineta as an authority for it. Sabatier relates a case of fracture *par contre-coup* in the sternum occasioned by a fall on the back. (Mémoires de l'Institut Natural, ii, 120.) See also Sprengel (Hist. de la Méd. 17.) Garengoit further relates various cases of the *contre fissure*. Bertaphalia defines it in much the same terms as Soranus. (v, 5.) Mr. Guthrie treats learnedly of this subject; but although he quotes many instances from the earlier authorities of fracture on one side of the head from a blow on the other, he states that in later years there is little proof of such an occurrence taking place. He admits, however, as indisputable the occurrence of fracture at the base of the skull from a blow on the vertex or back of the head. (Injuries of the Head, 65.) He also states that the term ἀπήχημα of our author, and that of 'resonitus,' as used by Latin authors, was applied to that species of fracture when the inner plate of the skull is knocked in or fractured, without the outer one being injured. (Ibid.) It does not appear, however, that the ancients applied the term in this sense. Thus Soranus, as stated above, defined it to be a fissure produced in the parts of the skull opposite to those which have received the blow. See the learned note of Cocchi. (Ap. Chirurg. Vet. 47.) Galen's definition is to the same effect. (Ibid. 107.)

The treatment here recommended for inflammation of the membranes of the brain is so judicious, that even at the present day scarcely any improvement could be made on it. Our late authorities have shown the utility of cholagogue purgatives in such cases, and it will be remarked that they are recommended by our author and Hippocrates. (De Cap. Vuln. 27.)

Celsus directs us, when the dura mater gets inflamed and swelled, to pour tepid rose-oil upon it; and if it rise above the bone to apply lentil or vine leaves pounded with fresh butter or the grease of geese. He enjoins us to avoid all kinds of food requiring mastication, also smoke and sternutatories. When the brain projects beyond the bone (a case called hernia cerebri by modern surgeons), he advises us to sprinkle it with squama æris, and to use cicatrizing applications. A person who has sustained a fracture of the skull is advised to avoid the sun, wind, frequent baths, and the free use of wine until the wound is healed.

Aëtius recommends bleeding and laxative clysters. (vi, 47.)

Heliodorus recommends abstinence at first, and afterwards spare diet, water for drink, bleeding, when the inflammation is violent and the patient full, light dressings, cataplasms of melilot, linseed, and oil, and fomentations with decoctions of fenugreek or mallows. Archigenes directs us when there is a fungous tumour projecting above the bone, to remove it with septics or the scalpel, and then to apply pledgets. (Nicetæ Collect.)

Avicenna and Albucasis repeat our author's directions. Haly Abbas follows in the same strain, recommending us to remove any cause of irritation, to pour refrigerant oils on the place, and to have recourse to venesection. (Pract. ix, 85.)

Our author having alluded to the pulsatory motion of the brain, we will state briefly the opinions of the principal ancient and modern authorities on this matter. Besides our author, Hippocrates, Galen, Oribasius, and Aëtius, among the ancients, mention a certain movement of the brain, namely, a swelling up during expiration, and a falling down during inspiration. Fallopius, Vesalius, Voltherus, Coiter, and Boerhaave maintained that this opinion is unfounded. But Columbo, Piccolomini, Dulaurens, Riolan, Littré, and more recently, Schliting, Lamure, Haller, Lorri, Vic d'Azyr, and Dumas, have reproduced this ancient truth. We once had an opportunity of observing the pulsatory motion of the brain in the case of a poor boy who had lost a considerable piece of the skull by exfoliation.

This would appear to be the most suitable occasion which we shall have to introduce an account of the osseous tumour, nearly all the information regarding which is derived from a fragment of Heliodorus. He describes it as a hard resistent tumour, immoveable, without pain, or change of colour. He says it occurs on all parts of the body, but more especially on the head, about the temples, when if one is formed on each side they are called horns. He directs that the tumour should be cut out from the very base, and the bone scraped with a raspatory. The wound is to be healed by glueing (the first intention?), if possible, but otherwise by suppurative applications. (Ch. Vet. 124.)

XCI—ON FRACTURE AND CONTUSION OF THE NOSE

The under part of the nose being cartilaginous does not admit of fracture, but it is liable to be crushed, flattened, and distorted; but the upper part being of a bony substance is sometimes fractured. In such cases Hippocrates prohibits bandaging, which only increases the flatness and distortion, unless when from a blow the parts about the middle of the nose protrude. For in these cases he applies a suitable bandage with medicines, in order to give the nose its proper shape. When, therefore, the nose is fractured in its under parts, having introduced the index or little finger into the nostril, push the parts outwards to their proper position. When the fracture is of the inner parts this is to be done with the head of a probe immediately, during the course of the first day, or not long afterwards, because the bones of the nose get consolidated about the tenth day. But they are to be put into the proper position with the index-finger and thumb externally. In order to prevent the bones from changing their position, two wedge-like tents, formed of a twisted linen rag, are to be applied, one to each nostril, even if but one part of the nose be deranged, and these are to be allowed to remain until the bone or cartilage gets consolidated. And some sew the quills of the feathers of a goose into the rags, and thus introduce them into the nose, in order that they may preserve the parts in position without obstructing the respiration; but this is unnecessary, as respiration is carried on by the mouth. If the nose become inflamed we may use some anti-inflammatory application to it, such as that from juices (diachylon), the one from vinegar and oil, and such like; or a cataplasm of fine wheaten flour boiled with manna or gum may be applied, both for the sake of the inflammation and in order to keep the nose in position. When the nose is distorted to either side, Hippocrates directs us, after it has been restored to its proper position, to take a piece of leather of a finger's breadth, and having spread one of its ends with taurocolla or gum, to fasten one extremity of it on that side of the nose to which it inclines, and after it dries to bring the thong by the opposite ear to the occiput and forehead, and to fix the other end of the thong firmly there, so that the nose being drawn sideways may take the proper position in the middle. This practice, however, is not much approved of by the moderns. If the bones of the nose are broken into small pieces we must make an incision or enlarge the wound, and having removed the small bones with a hair forceps, unite the divided parts with sutures, and use the applications for recent wounds and those of an agglutinative nature. If there be a sore within the nose it is to be cured with the pledgets called lemnisci, spread with suitable ointments. Some also use leaden tubes until it cicatrize, lest a fleshy excrescence should arise from the ulcer.

Commentary. Some account of Hippocrates's practice is given by our author. As here mentioned, he strongly disapproves of bandages which, he says, never fail to disappoint the expectations of both surgeon and patient. He directs us to replace the broken parts, either with the fore-finger or a specillum. He also describes the application of the piece of thong; a distinct account of which is given by our author. (De Articulis, 30.)

Galen, in his 'Commentary,' explains the obscurities in the text, but supplies no additional facts or views of practice. He greatly disapproved of agglutinative applications and bandages. (Fragmentum ap. Nicetæ Collect.)

Celsus gives a full account of fractures of the nose, but as he follows the plan of treatment recommended by Hippocrates, it will be unnecessary to dwell long upon it. When the cartilages are fractured, the pieces are to be replaced with a specillum, or with two fingers pressing on both sides; then oblong tents sewed round with a thin soft skin are to be introduced into the nostrils; or a large quill smeared with gum, or artificers' glue may be applied in like manner. He speaks of the leathern thong, but uses it under somewhat different circumstances than those for which our author recommends it. He directs us to fasten the middle of it to the nose, and the extremities to the temples on either side. When any fragment of a bone does not coalesce properly with the rest, he recommends us to extract it with a forceps. The case, he properly states, is more dangerous when there is an external wound; but in this case he recommends us to apply one of the plasters adapted for recent wounds; like the others he disapproves of bandages.

Rhases, Avicenna, Haly Abbas, and Albucasis lay down exactly the same rules of practice as Hippocrates and our author.

The recent authorities consider the introduction of the tents into the nostrils unnecessary, and even prejudicial. (See Bell's Operative Surgery; Cooper's Surgical Dictionary.) But the earlier modern writers adopt exactly the practice of the ancients. Theodoricus recommends us to turn the nose to its proper shape when distorted, by means of a strip of linen fastened to its extremity with ichthyocolla, or the gluten of hides, as directed by the ancients. (ii, 29.)

XCII—ON FRACTURE OF THE LOWER JAW, AND CONTUSION OF THE EAR

We have treated of contusion of the ear in the Third Book, as this affection is not of the nature of a fracture. But the lower jaw is fractured from many causes. If, then, it be only fractured externally, and is not divided into two, as it occasions a curvature inwardly, the symptoms of it are obvious. Wherefore, having introduced the index and middle fingers of one hand—of the right, if the right jaw be fractured, and of the left, if it is the left—we push outwards the internal curvature of the fracture, which is to be secured with the other hand externally. The bones of the jaw are ascertained to be set straight by the equality of the teeth. When the jaw is fractured completely across, (*that is to say, caulatim,*) it is to be set by making extension and counter-extension, with the aid of an assistant; and the teeth, separated at the broken part, are to be fastened together, as Hippocrates says, and bound with gold, namely, with a ligature or thread of gold. But since this is not readily procured by everybody, a strong flaxen thread, a piece of fine linen, horse-hairs, or the like, may be substituted. If the fracture be attended with an external wound, we must examine with a probe and ascertain whether a piece of bone be broken off, and if this be found to be the case, and the wound is small, it is to be enlarged and the broken piece or pieces removed with some suitable instrument, and the lips of the wound united with sutures; then dressings suitable to recent wounds with bandages are to be applied. If there be no wound, a simple cerate is to be applied to the jaw along with suitable bandages. In applying the bandage, the middle of it is to be placed on the occiput, and the fold of it brought along by the ears on both sides to the chin, and then from the chin to the occiput again, and then again to the chin, and thence by the cheeks to the bregma, and then again to below the occiput, where the bandage must terminate. Upon these again a cover, that is to say, another bandage, is to be applied to the forehead and fastened behind the head, in order to secure the aforementioned bandages. Some, also, apply a light splint, or a piece of leather of proper size, to the jaw, and bandage it as we have described. Others use the bandage called a muzzle. If both sides of the jaws are separated at the symphysis, having removed them a little asunder with both the hands, adapt them again to one another, and having fastened the teeth together as aforesaid with a ligature, and applied the proper bandages, order the patient to be nourished with thin soups, because mastication is hurtful in this case. And, if you suspect that it has been deranged from its position, loose the bandages on the third day, and apply them again, and do in like manner until the callus be formed. The callus of the jaw-bone is generally formed within three weeks at most, because it is spongy and full of marrow. If any inflammation come on, we must not neglect the embrocations and cataplasms suitable to it; which practice is to be observed in all cases.

Commentary. Our author's account of fractures of the lower jaw is taken almost word for word from Hippocrates. (De Articulis.) He divides them into external fractures, and fractures *caulatim* (or *cauledon*), which, agreeably to the explanation of this term, given in the 89th section, Galen interprets to be a complete separation of the fractured portions. He directs us to fasten the teeth with a gold thread; and in other respects also his practice is exactly the same as our author's. His account of fracture at the symphysis is very correct.

Soranus gives a very sensible account of this subject. A transverse fracture, he says, often takes place, but a longitudinal one seldom, and in certain cases it is not attended with any distortion. It is to be recognized by examination with the fingers, when any displacement of the parts and crepitus will be recognized. Fracture in the ramus may be distinguished from dislocation, by there being mobility in the former case, whereas there is none in the latter. (Chirurg. Vet. p. 49.)

Celsus says, that in fractures of the jaw-bone the separated portions are never completely disjoined. When the bone is fairly broken transverse, the tooth at the fractured part protrudes, and is therefore to be secured to the adjoining one with a hair. He then recommends us to apply a double compress, moistened in wine and oil, with agglutinants; and afterwards a bandage or soft piece of leather is to be put on with its middle at the chin, and its extremities fastened above the head. In this, as in every other species of fracture, he recommends at first abstinence, and afterwards, liquid food; not allowing a full diet until the inflammation has subsided. He says, a fractured jaw-bone gets consolidated between the 14th and the 21st day.

Albucasis evidently copies from our author; and Avicenna and Rhases do so avowedly.

Haly Abbas gives a similar account, recommending us to secure the teeth with a thread; and then to apply bandages, and occasionally a compress, as directed by our author.

By the first variety, described by all the ancient authorities, was meant, we suppose, a fracture of the condyle.

XCIII—ON FRACTURE OF THE CLAVICLE

The clavicle in its natural position is united to the sternum at its inner extremity, and at its outer it is articulated with the acromion; and, therefore, as it supports the shoulder and the arm itself, if it undergo a fracture in any part whatever, the portion of it united to the shoulder sinks down, being dragged along with the arm. It is better, then, that the fracture be transverse, and not longitudinal, or partly straight with a lunated extremity, according to the opinion of most surgeons. For that which is fractured transversely, can, by extension and compression with the fingers, be readily restored to its proper position; but the other kinds of fracture have prominences not easily arranged. If, therefore, it be broken in any way through its whole thickness, let one assistant take hold of the arm connected with the fractured clavicle, pulling it at the same time outwards and upwards; and let another pull the opposite shoulder, or at least the neck, and let them make counter-extension. The surgeon then, with his fingers, is to set the fracture, pushing down what is prominent, and drawing outwards what is situated too deep. If more counter-extension be required, a ball of rags, wool, or something such, may be applied below the armpit, and the elbow brought to the rib adjoining to it; and the other things may be done as described already. But if it is found impossible to raise up the end of the clavicle connected with the shoulder that is lodged down below, having laid the man on his back, and placed a moderate cushion under his back, let an assistant push the shoulders downwards, so that the bone of the clavicle which is lodged below may be bent upwards, and then set the fracture with the fingers. But if part of the clavicle be broken off and unconnected, and if we find it irritating the parts, we must make a straight incision with a scalpel and remove the broken portion, and smooth the remainder with chisels, taking care that the instrument called meningophylax, or another chisel be put under the clavicle to make it steady; and if no inflammation is present, we may use sutures, but otherwise, pledgets. And having prepared various splenia (compresses), we must apply the larger and thicker to the projecting part of the bone; and these, when inflammation is present, are to be dipped in oil, but otherwise they are to be applied dry. And having put a moderate ball of wool under the nearer armpit, we apply a suitable bandage round by the armpits, the fractured clavicle and the scapula, bringing the folds in a proper direction; and if the part of the clavicle connected with the shoulder fall downwards, the middle of a broad thong is to be put under the elbow of the same side, and the whole arm suspended by the neck, and the hand is to be slung in another bandage as in cases of bleeding at the elbow. But if, which rarely happens, the outer part be uppermost, we must not have recourse to this arrangement of the arm. The patient must lie in a supine position, and live upon a spare diet, and if necessary, embrocations and other suitable applications are to be made until the callus is formed. The callus of the clavicle is formed in about twenty days at most.

Commentary. Hippocrates gives such an account of this accident as clearly bespeaks his intimate acquaintance with the subject. Transverse fractures, he says, are easily healed, whereas such as are oblique prove more difficult to manage. He justly remarks, that the deformity occasioned by this injury appears at first very great, and annoys both the patient and his physician, but that it gradually becomes less, and the patient, feeling little inconvenience from it, grows careless, and the physician, seeing no evil consequences result from this neglect, acquiesces in it, and presently it is found that proper callus is formed. Hippocrates further exposes the mistake of those who endeavour to push down the projecting bone, which, he justly remarks, cannot be effected. The part which projects, as he states, is almost universally the extremity attached to the sternum, the other portion being dragged down by the weight of the arm; and hence the mistake is obvious of those who attempt to push down the upper extremity. He recommends the patient to lie in bed until adhesion takes place, which generally occurs between the fourteenth and twentieth day. (De Articulis, 16.)

Galen directs us to apply four splenia or oblong compresses intersecting one another like the letter X. (Comment, et Fragment, apud Nicetæ Collect.) When the fracture is near the shoulder, Galen recommends the spica bandage (De Fasciis), for a drawing and description of which, see Heister's 'Surgery,' (p. iii, c. 4, §1, c. 3.)

Celsus agrees entirely with the account of the matter given by Hippocrates. When the bone is broken transversely, he says, it will sometimes unite readily without the application of a bandage. In general, as he explains, the upper end of the fractured portions is the part attached to the sternum, the other being attached to the shoulder and dragged down along with the arm. He mentions that this is so generally the state of the parts, that some great masters of the art had declared that they had never seen a case in which the end attached to the shoulder projected, but that Hippocrates, who is rich in information upon these subjects, had affirmed upon his own authority that such an occurrence is to be met with. In setting the fracture he properly directs us to raise the shoulder; and his mode of bandaging would seem to have been little different from that now generally followed. He directs us to fill the armpit with wool, and to apply over the fractured portions of the bone a compress three times folded, and moistened in wine and oil; or, if the bone is broken into many fragments, a splint formed of cane (ferula). If the bones incline to the common position, the arm is to be fixed to the side, but if the outer end has a tendency upwards, the arm is to be tied to the neck. The man is to be laid on his back. All spiculæ of bones are to be cut out, if it is found that they are wounding the flesh.

Albucasis follows our author closely. He particularly enjoins the surgeon when there are any projecting spiculæ, to make an incision and cut them out; after which, a suture may be used to heal the integuments, provided the wound is large. A compress, soaked in rose-oil, vinegar, and wine, is to be applied to allay inflammation. He directs the patient to sleep on his back with a pillow under his armpit.

Rhases, Avicenna, and Haly Abbas give exactly the same account of the accident as Albucasis and our author.

XCXIV—ON THE SCAPULA

The scapula is not fractured in its broad and tabular part, but a fracture may sometimes take place at its spine. The fracture being sometimes what is called by expression, sometimes a simple fracture, and sometimes a piece is broken off. The expression, then, is ascertained by the touch, exhibiting a hollow, and occasioning torpidity of the adjacent arm and a throbbing pain. Simple fracture is known by its roughness and local pain. Both are to be managed according to the anti-inflammatory plan of treatment. When a piece is broken off, which also may be ascertained by the touch, if it gives no disturbance it may be fixed by a convenient bandage, but when it moves about and produces irritation, it is to be removed by an incision, and sutures used, as described above. Bandages like those for the clavicle are to be applied, and the patient is to be laid on the opposite side.

Commentary. Hippocrates has not treated particularly of this fracture.

Celsus treats in general terms of the cheek-bone, breast-bone, the broad bone of the scapula, the spine, os sacrum, &c. If there be an external wound, it is to be healed with suitable dressings; after which the fissure or hole in the bone will fill up with callus. If the skin be entire, he merely enjoins rest, a suitable cerate, and gentle bandages.

Albucasis and Avicenna, as usual, copy from our author. The former states that fractures of the scapula are healed in twenty or twenty-five days. Haly Abbas, like the others, directs us to remove any spiculæ which occasion irritation, to apply soothing cataplasms, and suitable bandages. Rhases remarks that the body of the bone is little subject to fractures, but that its extremities may be broken off. A fracture of the hollow portion of it is ascertained by a rising in the part; fissures are recognized only by the local pain.

XCV—ON THE BREAST-BONE

The middle of the sternum is fractured by simple division and by expression, and the extremity of it is broken off. When, therefore, the fracture is deranged, pain and inequality of the place follow, and there is crepitus upon pressure with the fingers. When by expression, there is violent pain, dyspnœa, and cough, owing to the pleura being irritated; and rarely there is vomiting of blood, a hollow in the fractured place, and yielding thereof. The same treatment is to be applied as that recommended for the scapula. When the fracture is by expression, we may practise Hippocrates's mode of setting which he recommended for the clavicle when it inclines inwards, having recourse to the supine posture, the application of a cushion upon the back, pressing down the shoulders, and drawing the sides together with the hands. The sides being covered with wool, we apply a circular bandage, having first put on two thongs straight from the shoulders, so that afterwards the two ends may be united in a proper manner, and prevent the circular bandage from falling off.

Commentary. Hippocrates holds injuries of the sternum to be more dangerous than those of the ribs. He recommends in this case a light diet, rest, silence, bleeding at the arm, and so forth. (De Artic. 50.)

Celsus directs this fracture to be treated upon general principles, as explained in the preceding section.

The Arabians evidently follow our author. Albucasis speaks of applying thin splints.

The reader will find, upon reference to the ninetieth section, that a fracture by expression is a comminuted fracture with depression.

XCVI—ON THE RIBS

Of the ribs, called also spathæ, those which are long admit of a fracture in any part, but the false only at the spine, because there only they are of a bony nature; for at their anterior part they are cartilaginous, and are liable to be crushed, but not fractured. The diagnosis is not difficult, for an inequality presents itself to the fingers of the examiner, and there is crepitus with derangement at the fractured part. When the fractured parts incline inwards there is a violent pungent pain, more severe than that in pleurisy, from the pleura being wounded as with a sharp instrument; there is difficulty of breathing, cough, and often vomiting of blood. The other modes of displacement, then, may be rectified by the fingers, but in that inwards this cannot be done, owing to the difficulty of applying distension. Wherefore, some direct us to give much flatulent food, in order that by the inflation and distension occasioned by it the fracture may be propelled outwards. But this is not necessary, for there is no communication between the chest and the organs of nutrition, and besides, the inflammation will be augmented by repletion. Others apply a cupping instrument, which is not amiss, unless a collection of humours should be occasioned by the suction, and the fracture be thereby pushed more inwardly. Wherefore, Soranus says, "Let the parts be covered with wool dipped in hot oil, and let the intercostal space be filled with compresses, in order that the circular bandage applied, as in the case of the sternum, may lie smooth. And let everything be done, as in pleurisy, according to the degree of accident. But if any great necessity compel us, owing to the pleura being irritated, we must divide the skin and lay bare the broken part of the rib; and then putting the instrument for protecting membranes under, to prevent the pleura from being wounded, cut off properly, and remove the irritating pieces of bone. After this the parts which are not inflamed are to be united and cured as recent wounds; but such as are inflamed are to be covered with pledgets dipped in oil. The diet and treatment must be anti-inflammatory, and the patient is to be laid in the easiest posture."

Commentary. Hippocrates gives a full and accurate account of this accident. He remarks that when the broken ends of the bone are not pushed inwards, it seldom happens that fever or any unpleasant symptoms supervene. When fever is not present he thinks that abstinence by occasioning an emptiness of the belly, proves rather prejudicial by removing what otherwise tends to support the part affected, which is thereby made to hang unsupported. In this case a slight bandage will be sufficient. The ribs, he says, become united in about twenty days. When the skin about the ribs is bruised by a blow or any other such cause, much blood, he says, is often vomited up. Galen, in his commentary on this passage, states that when the vessels of the pleura are wounded and blood effused into its cavity, a spitting of blood may take place although the lungs themselves have not been injured. The treatment recommended by Hippocrates consists of bleeding at the elbow, enjoining silence, applying folded compresses with broad bandages, neither too tight nor too loose. He directs us to use a double-headed bandage, and to commence at the seat of the fracture. He approves of gentle aperients and restricted diet for ten days, after which period nourishing food is to be given. He adds, that when the proper treatment is neglected, even if no other inconvenience should result from it, a viscid collection is sure to form in the part. When, in addition to this swelling, a chronic pain gets seated in the part, he advises the actual cautery to be applied. (De Articulis.)

Celsus, with his characteristic elegance and terseness, expounds the rules of practice delivered by Hippocrates. He directs us to apply a bandage, to bleed from the arm, to open the belly; to avoid noise, speaking, tumultuous passions, smoke, dust, and whatever is calculated to excite coughing and sneezing. Gruels only are to be taken before the seventh day, after which bread may be used. When the pain is violent he directs us to apply a cataplasm made from darnel, or barley with fat figs. Should a collection of matter take place it is to be opened with a red-hot iron. When mucus forms about the fracture, he recommends the application of the cautery. The above is but an imperfect outline of his admirable chapter on fractures of the ribs.

Avicenna professedly copies from our author. Haly Abbas, Rhases, and Albucasis give nearly the same account, without the slightest addition of any importance. They all approve of making an incision and extracting the pieces of bones which may happen to be irritating the pleura. Albucasis gives a drawing of the meningophylax, or instrument for protecting membranes during the sawing of bones.

XCVII—ON THE BONES OF THE HIPS AND PUBES

The bones of the ischium or hips are rarely fractured indeed, but admit of the same varieties as those of the scapula. Their extremities, then, are sometimes broken off; there may be fracture along their length, and the middle may be fractured by expression. They are attended with a local pain, a pungent and throbbing sensation, and torpor of the leg on that side if from expression. It is to be set in the same way as that of the scapula, only it does not admit of the extraction of broken pieces by an operation on account of the external parts. If necessary, it is to be set by the fingers, and afterwards we must apply the other convenient treatment, using embrocations, and filling up the hollows of the loins with compresses, in order that the circular bandages which are put on may lie even. The same things may be said with respect to the bones of the pubes, for we have nothing more particular to say of them.

Commentary. The other authorities do not treat of these cases so minutely as our author, whose account of them is sufficiently accurate.

Celsus merely directs us to treat them upon general principles.

Albucasis recommends the same plan of treatment as our author, with the addition of splints made of wood or leather. These, however, cannot be very much required. He directs the patient to lie on his back or on the sound side.

Avicenna does not treat of these cases of fracture. Haly Abbas and Rhases abridge our author's account.

XCVIII—ON THE VERTEBRÆ, SPINE OF THE BACK, AND OS SACRUM

The round bodies of the vertebræ may sometimes be crushed, but rarely undergo fracture, in which cases the membranes of the spinal marrow or the marrow itself being compressed, sympathetic nervous affections take place, and death speedily follows, more particularly if the vertebra of the neck be affected. Wherefore, having first given warning of the danger, we must, if possible, attempt to extract by an incision the compressing bone, or if not we must soothe the part by the anti-inflammatory treatment. But if any of the processes of the vertebræ, of which the spine, as it is called, consists, be broken off, it will readily be felt upon examination with the finger, the broken piece yielding and returning again to its position, and, therefore, we must make an incision of the skin externally and extract it, and having united the wound with sutures, pursue the treatment for recent wounds. When the os sacrum is fractured the index-finger of the left hand is to be introduced into the anus, while with the other we manage as we best can the fractured bone; or if we feel any piece broken off, we make an incision and lay hold of it, and apply bandages and suitable treatment.

Commentary. Celsus remarks that when a piece of one of the vertebræ is broken off a hollow is felt in the place, it is attended with pain, and the person is compelled to bend inwards. The treatment is to be conducted upon general principles, as explained under fractures of the scapula.

Albucasis lays it down as a rule that when a fracture of the cervical vertebræ produces paralysis and insensibility of the arms, the case may be abandoned as hopeless. When, after a fracture of the dorsal vertebræ, it is remarked that there is paralysis and insensibility of the lower extremities, and that the alvine and urinary discharges are passed unconsciously, he, in like manner, pronounces the case to be desperate. When a piece of bone is broken off and occasions great irritation, he recommends us, like our author, to make an incision and take it out.

Haly Abbas and Avicenna borrow everything from Paulus.

Rhases gives many curious remarks upon injuries of the spine, but several of them are borrowed from Galen. (De Locis Affectis.) Galen relates many cases to show that retention of the urine and fæces is a common effect of an injury of the spine. He also mentions that loss of speech is sometimes the consequence of the upper part of the spine being injured. Rhases relates the case of a man who lost the sensibility of his arms from an injury of the last vertebra of the neck, produced by a fall from a horse. He states, that when the injury is below the neck the respiration is never affected. He inculcates that whenever there is paralysis of the limbs, or of any part after a fall, it arises from some injury of the spine. (Cont. i.)

When the sacrum or os coccygis is fractured, he directs us to replace the parts by introducing the finger *per anum*. (Cont. xxix.)

XCIX—ON THE ARM

When the arm is broken Hippocrates makes the extension thus: he says, "We must take an oblong piece of wood, such as that which is put into the holes at the end of spades, and fastening ropes to its extremities, suspend it transversely from some beam, and placing the man upon some elevated object more erect than what is called the erect sleeping posture, we pass his hand over the above-mentioned piece of wood, so that the middle of the wood may be fitted to the armpit, and his arm being bent at a right angle, an assistant stooping down takes hold of the hand, and then some heavy object, such as a stone, a leaden ball, or the like, is to be fastened to the elbow, and being allowed to hang suspended, in this way you must set the fracture, or instead of a weight an assistant may pull down the arm, and instead of the above-mentioned piece of wood some use the step of a ladder." Soranus, however, proceeds thus: Having placed the man in a chair, or, which is better, as it occasions less disturbance, in a supine posture, then having put a ligature round the wrist and suspended it from the neck so as to preserve its angular figure, we direct two assistants, the one to apply his fingers below the fracture and the other above, and thus to make the extension. Or if we require stronger pulling we apply two equal pieces of thong to the arm, the one above the fracture and the other below, and giving one of the pieces of thong to the assistant who stands above the patient's head, and the other to the one at his feet, we order them to make counter-extension. If the fracture be near the top of the shoulder we apply the middle of the thong to the armpit and direct the assistant at the head to hold it, and, while the other pulls in the opposite direction, we make the counter-extension as above. And when the fracture is at the elbow, the ligature is to be applied there or at the wrist. The bones of the fracture being properly set, the extension is to be relaxed, and it is to be bound up according to the method of Hippocrates. When the fracture is free from inflammation and recent, we must use linen bandages of a proper length, and three or four fingers in breadth, which have been soaked in water or oxycrate, but when there is inflammation, thin soft pieces of wool steeped in oil are to be used. And if the fracture be at the middle of the arm the bandaging must commence at the fracture, and after two or three turns the bandaging is to be carried upwards, in order, as he says, that the overflow of blood to the part may be intercepted; and it is to terminate there. A second bandage is then to be applied with its head at the fracture, and, having done as in the former case, carry it from above downwards, and again reverting from thence upwards let it terminate there. There should be a moderate degree of tightness according to our own feeling and that of the patient. If the fracture be near the top of the shoulder, the first bandage should take in the acromion, scapula, and sternum, so as to form what is called the crane bandage. The second one is to extend to the elbow, and reverting from thence to the upper parts it is to take in, with the acromion, the scapula and sternum, like the first bandage. If the fracture be at the elbow, the fore-arm is to be taken in with the bandage, the figure of the elbow-joint being preserved. And so in like manner with the other members, such as the fore-arm, the thigh, and the leg; and when the fracture is in any part near a joint, and not in the middle of the limb, the joint is to be bound along with it. After the bandaging the moderns immediately apply splints, in order to preserve the bones which have been set in their proper shape, tightening them agreeably to the patient's feeling and the swelling occasioned by the inflammation. But the ancients did not apply the splints until after the seventh day, within which period, as the inflammation had declined, the limb had become less swelled. Hippocrates orders the bandages to be loosed every three days, lest, owing to the part being constantly covered up, distension and pruritus should come on, and that the insensible perspiration might not be obstructed after the bone has become firm; for that by these means not only does a painful pruritus take place in certain cases, but ulceration of the skin is occasioned by the acrimony of the sanious humours. He directs us, therefore, to bathe with tepid water, so as to dispel the humours, but after the seventh day to loose the bandages at greater intervals, because the parts no longer require the expulsion of the humours; the formation of callus thus goes on properly. The splints are to be applied in this manner. Compresses, thrice folded and dipped in oil, are to be put upon the bandages, and if the limb be of equal thickness this is to be done even; but if it is of unequal thickness, the hollow parts are to be filled up with the compresses so as to make the arm of equal thickness for the application of the splints; then the splints being wrapped with a moderate quantity of wool or flax, we apply them around the fracture, being not more than a finger's breadth distant from one another, binding them moderately tight, and taking care, as much as possible, that the splints do not come in contact with a joint, and being more particularly careful of the inner part of the joint, for there they sometimes occasion ulcers and inflammations of tendons. But there the bandaging must be made slacker; and stronger, on the other hand, where the fracture swells up. It is better that the chest should be moderately bound with the arm, lest by its motions it should derange the position. If inflammation should come on (which we know by the swelling and redness around, and from the limb being more tightly bound than formerly), or if the fracture become deranged, or if, without these occurring, the bandages become slacker, or, on the other hand, tighter than proper, the bandages are to be loosed and everything rectified. The patient is to be laid in a supine position, with his hand upon his stomach, and a soft pillow is to be placed under the arm having a skin upon it to receive the embrocations which run from it. The part is to be bathed with warm oil every day, more especially if inflammation be present, and during the time of inflammation he is to be fed sparingly, and afterwards moderately, to promote the growth of callus. He must lie quiet until the callus is formed, which, in the arm and leg, takes place about the fortieth day. After this the bandages are to be loosed, and after using the bath he is to be treated with plasters suitable to fractures. This mode of procedure is applicable in almost all cases of fracture of limbs.

Commentary. Hippocrates's account of fracture of the os humeri, as quoted by Paulus, is from the eighth chapter of his work 'De Fracturis,' but our author has used considerable liberties in making the extract. The mode of using the piece of wood for suspending the arm is easily understood, from his own description without the commentary of Galen. (See p. 541, t. v, ed. Basil.) In the edition by Littré it is, moreover, well illustrated by a drawing. (T. iii, p. 445.) He directs the splints not to be applied until the seventh day, in order to give time for the inflammation and swelling to subside. He says, the bone gets consolidated in about forty days. He justly remarks, that when distortion of the arm takes place it is to the outside, that is to say, backwards. His method of bandaging for fractures of the arm and fore-arm was the same. He directs us in the first place to put a cerate to the part, and then to apply the first bandage, beginning at the fracture, and carrying it two or three turns upwards, so as to prevent the blood from falling down into the part. The second bandage is to commence above the fracture, and is to be carried downwards. Afterwards splenia or oblong compresses, spread with cerate, are to be laid over them, and these are to be secured by strips of linen cloth. These bandages are to be removed when they become slack, generally about the third day. On the seventh the ferulæ or splints are to be applied, the limb by that time having lost its swelling, and they are to be allowed to remain until the 24th day after the accident. When swellings arise on any part of a limb from pressure, they are to be anointed with cerate or wine and oil, and wrapped in soft wool; and if the splints be hurting the limb they are to be removed for a time. (De Fract. 21.) When the bandages are taken off, he directs that hot water should be poured upon the limb. He recommends a spare diet unless there be a wound of the integuments. (De Fract. and Galen. Comment.) It may be proper to give some more account of the splenia and ferulæ (νάρθηκες), used by Hippocrates in fractures of the extremities. In his work entitled 'The Surgeon's Shop' (ἰήτρειον), he directs the length of the splenia to be made proportionate to the part which they are applied to, their breadth three fingers, their thickness three or four folds, and their number such as to encircle the limb without doing either more or less. It appears quite clear that they consisted of folded linen. The intention of them was to give some support to the part. He directs the splints to be smooth, even, concave, and somewhat shorter than the length of the bandages, in order not to hurt the sound skin. It appears, then, that the whole apparatus used by Hippocrates in the treatment of fractures, consisted, 1st, of two under-bandages, 2d, of splenia or folded compresses, 3d, of the ferulæ or splints, 4th, of an outer bandage to secure the splints. With regard to the cerate used in the Hippocratic system of bandaging, it is important to state that, from a passage in his treatise, 'Officina Medici,' it would appear that the cerate was not only applied to the skin, but that, for the sake of greater security, every fold of the bandages was rubbed with it. See Galen's Commentary on the work, (T. v. p. 692, ed. Basil,) and Littré's Hippocrates, (T. iii, p. 316.) It remains to be mentioned, that the bandages were secured by means of a thread or with a needle. (Off. Med. 8.) Nothing can surpass the judgment and precision with which Hippocrates lays down his rules for the application of the bandages. (Ibid.)

Galen describes the splenia as being pieces of linen folded three or four times, which are to be laid along the arm longitudinally. He directs us to spread them with cerate. He says that they support the limb. He says distinctly that all the folds of the bandages should be rubbed with cerate in order to give greater support. All his directions for the treatment of a broken limb are most judicious. When at first there is much pain and inflammation, he recommends bleeding and purging; but when the callus begins to form, he directs the patient to use a nourishing diet. Spiculæ and scales of bone are in general to be allowed to exfoliate of themselves, and not removed forcibly by the surgeon. (Comment. and Fragment. ap. Nicetæ Collect.)

Celsus lays down the principles of treatment in fractures of the arm, fore-arm, thigh, and leg so circumstantially, that we can afford room only for an outline of them. He recommends no time to be lost in getting the displaced parts properly reduced. For this purpose, if the limb be strong, two assistants may be required to pull in contrary directions; and if other means do not succeed, thongs of leather, or linen bandages, may be attached to each end of the broken limb to make extension and counter-extension with them. When the ends of the bone have been adjusted, (which is known by the pain and deformity being removed,) the limb is to be wrapped in linen cloths folded two or three times, and dipped in wine and oil. Six bandages or rollers (fasciæ) are then to be applied. The first is the shortest, which is to be three times rolled round the limb upwards in a spiral direction, and three times generally will be sufficient. The second must be one half longer, and is to commence wherever the bone projects; or if there be no projection, at any part of the fracture; and is to be carried first downwards and then upwards, so as to terminate a little above the former. These are to be secured by a broader linen cloth spread with cerate. The third and fourth bandages are then to be applied upon the principle, that the latter is to be put on in the contrary direction to the former; and further, it is to be observed that the third bandage terminates below, whereas all the others terminate above the fracture. Upon the whole, he adds, it is better to secure the limb with many than with tight bandages, these being apt to occasion mortification. When properly applied they ought not to be loose on the first day, yet such as not to give pain; slacker on the second, and loose on the third day. They are then to be removed and again applied, and a fifth bandage is now to be superadded to them; and again, these are to be taken off on the fifth day, and six bandages put on, in such a manner that the third and fifth may terminate below, and all the others above. Whenever the bandages are taken off, the limb is to be bathed with hot water, and proper fomentations applied to allay the inflammation, which will generally be found to have subsided about the seventh or ninth day. Then the bandages are again to be put on as directed above, and ferulæ or splints are also to be added, taking care to put on a stronger and broader splint at the side to which the fractured bone has a tendency to be protruded. These must all be rounded where they come in contact with a joint, to avoid injuring it; they are only to be secured with such tightness as to keep the bones in their place, and when they get loose their thongs are to be tightened. The bandages are to be removed gradually. These are his general directions for all fractures of the extremities, and it is to be remarked that his mode of treatment is essentially the same as that of Hippocrates. He afterwards describes at considerable length the method of setting the broken ends of the os humeri. After this is accomplished he directs us to bind the arm gently to the side. With regard to the splints, he properly recommends the longest to be applied externally; shorter ones on the brawn of the arm (over the biceps muscle?), and the shortest under the armpit. He advises us to remove them frequently when the fracture is situated near the fore-arm; and at these times the arm is to be bathed with hot water, and rubbed with a soft cerate.

It will be seen that the methods of Hippocrates and Celsus, although the same in principle, differ in the following respects. Hippocrates uses three bandages, Celsus six: Hippocrates uses small compresses, Celsus large pieces of linen: Hippocrates uses cerate, Celsus wine and oil.

The Arabians conducted the treatment in much the same way as the Greeks. In cases of fracture of the arm, Albucasis directs us to make the bandages of soft, thin linen cloth; but of broader and firmer linen if the thigh or leg is to be treated. Below them is to be applied a smooth cloth spread with a suitable liniment. After the under bandages have been put on in the manner already described, the splints are to be applied, provided no swelling nor inflammation be present, for in that case they are to be deferred for a few days. These splints are to be constructed from the middle part of the alcanna, or of pine, or of the palm-tree, or of a tree which he calls *calingi*.

Avicenna directs us to form the splints of the wood of alcanna, or of oleander, or of pomegranate tree, or the like. The length of the splints is to be made equal to that of the limb, and their greatest breadth about three fingers. They are to be secured with another bandage and pieces of tape made of linen cloth. There is to be an interval of a finger's breadth between each splint. He says, it is best to apply four splints of such a length as to reach from joint to joint. They are to be smooth and even so as not to injure any part. In cases of fracture of the os humeri he directs us to surround the nearest joint with the bandages, and, if the fracture be in the middle, to make them take in both extremities. He recommends us to foment the limb with vinegar and water, or water alone. The arm is to be fastened to the side and the hand laid on the stomach.

Haly Abbas, in giving directions for the treatment of fractures in general, recommends the splints to be made of pieces of alcanna, or any hard wood. Afterwards he directs the limb to be laid upon a table having a pad (pannus) placed on it, which last is to be secured with fillets. He gives particular directions not to apply the splints over the processes of bones, and when inflammation comes on he forbids splints to be used at all; in that case the patient is to be kept upon restricted diet. The bandages are to be removed in the course of three days.

The directions given by the experienced Rhases about the bandages and splints are very similar to our author's, and therefore need not be repeated.

See an account of the ancient splenia, or compresses, and of the ferulæ, or splints, in Scultet's 'Arsenal de Chirurgie.' (29, 30.) See also Van Swieten's 'Commentary,' (354.) Van Swieten remarks, that although the eighteen-tailed bandage be supposed a modern invention, a similar one is described by Hippocrates, (De Fract.) and by Galen in his commentaries on the same.

Le Clerc gives a pretty full description of the Celsian method of treating fractures. (Hist. de la Méd.) See also Fabricius ab Aquapendente (Œuv. Chir. ii, 3, and i, 4). We are certain it will be generally admitted that the waxed apparatus of the ancients in the case of fractures was probably quite as efficacious as the starched bandages which have been introduced of late years with so much advantage.

C—ON THE ULNA AND RADIUS

The ulna and radius are sometimes both fractured together, and sometimes one of them only, either in the middle or at one end, as at the elbow or wrist. The worst of all is when both are fractured together, after that the ulna alone, but a fractured radius is, of all cases, the easiest cured. For, although it be larger than the ulna, yet it has this bone as a base and support to it. If only one be fractured, the extension must be applied principally to it, but if both, they are to be stretched evenly, the arm being put into an angular position, so that the thumb may be higher than the fingers, and the little finger lower than any of the others, for thus the ulna will be placed under the radius. If stronger extension be required, especially when both are broken, we must apply it not only with the hands but also with ligatures, as described when treating of the arm; and everything relative to the bandaging and the subsequent treatment, with the application of the splints, is to be done as in that case until callus is formed. The bones of the fore-arm have their callus formed in about thirty days at most. And the fore-arm is to be otherwise arranged in the same manner as the arm, with the exception of those things which are put under it.

Commentary. Whoever would wish to see a full exposition of the principles upon which these cases of fracture ought to be conducted may consult the first part of Hippocrates's work. (De Fracturis.) He shows, with a singular precision, the disadvantages of the prone and supine positions of the hand, both of which, it appears, had their advocates in ancient times. The bandages, compresses, and splints are to be applied in the manner described in the preceding section. He insists strongly on the necessity of having the arm and wrist carefully suspended in a broad soft sling, and that the hand be placed neither too high nor too low. Hippocrates takes notice of fracture of the olecranon, as will be explained afterwards.

Oribasius gives a description and drawing of a laqueus calculated to retain the splints, and secure the fore-arm in cases of fracture. (De Laqueis, 2.)

Celsus directs us to sling the arm, with the thumb a little inclined, towards the breast, in a convenient napkin (mitella), the broad part being applied to the arm, and the narrow ends tied behind the neck.

Albucasis treats of this case of fracture very accurately. He calls the ulna the larger of the bones. He directs the arm to be suspended with the thumb uppermost. When the fractured pieces of bone occasion irritation, he advises us to make an incision and extract them. When a troublesome pruritus seizes the arm, he recommends us to remove the bandages and bathe with hot water.

Rhases gives proper directions about not applying the bandages too tight or too slack. When the hand swells he recommends them to be slackened.

The accounts given by Avicenna and Haly Abbas are quite similar to our author's. Avicenna cautions us not to make the splints too long lest they hurt the hand. None of the Arabians, we believe, have noticed the fracture of the olecranon. Like most imitators, they often fall short of their originals.

CI—ON THE HAND AND ITS FINGERS

The bones of the carpus, metacarpus, and of the phalanges of the fingers, being of a spongy and porous nature, are often crushed but rarely fractured. The patient then being placed on a high seat, we are to direct him to lay his hand prone upon an even table, and the fractured pieces being stretched by an assistant, we arrange them with two fingers, that is to say, the thumb and the index-finger. A tight bandage is to be used at the time that inflammation prevails, for, owing to the porous nature of the bones, a redundance of callus is formed. If the phalanx or finger be simply broken, and it be the large one, called also the thumb, after suitable bandaging, it is to be bound to the palm that it may be kept at rest; but if any of the others, as for example, the index or little finger, it is to be bound along with the one next to it, or if one of the middle, it may be bound along with that on either side, or all may be bound altogether. For they are thus kept best at rest, as if the fractured bones had been supported with splints.

Commentary. Hippocrates recommends the general treatment applicable in all cases of fracture, with the exception of the splint, which, as Galen explains, is not admissible in these cases.

Celsus says, it will be sufficient when a finger is broken to bind it to one piece of splint (surculum) after the inflammation has subsided.

Albucasis recommends one small splint to be applied upon the thumb when it is fractured. If one of the fingers be broken, it is to be bound up with the others, or one small piece of splint may be used. Avicenna, Rhases, and Haly Abbas treat distinctly of these accidents, but supply no additional information.

CII—ON THE THIGH

The case of a broken thigh is analogous to that of the arm, but in particular, a fractured thigh is mostly deranged forwards and outwards, for the bone is naturally flattened on those sides. It is to be set by the hands, with ligatures, and even cords applied, the one above and the other below the fracture. When the fracture takes place at one end, if at the head of the thigh, the middle part of a thong wrapped round with wool, so that it may not cut the parts there, is to be applied to the perinæum, and the ends of it brought up to the head and given to an assistant to hold, and applying a ligature below the fracture, we give the ends of it to another assistant to make extension. If it is fractured near the knee, we apply the ligature immediately above the fracture, and give the ends to an assistant, with which to make extension upwards; and while we put a ligature round the knee to secure it, and while the patient lies thus, with his leg extended, we arrange the fracture. Pieces of bone which irritate the parts, as has been often said, are to be taken out from above; and the rest of the treatment we have already described in the section on the arm. The thigh gets consolidated within fifty days. The manner of arranging it afterwards will be described after delivering the treatment of the whole leg.

Commentary. Hippocrates has correctly stated the difficulty attending the management of a fractured thigh-bone, and the disgrace which an ill-managed case entails upon the surgeon. He directs him to make extension and counter-extension, and to apply the bandages and splints in the manner formerly described. He recommends a few turns of the bandage to be brought about the loins, in order to prevent the skin at the top of the thigh from being injured by the splints. He points out the extreme importance of attending to the position of the heel, as if improperly laid, it is capable of deranging the fracture entirely. It gets consolidated, he says, in about fifty days. (De Fracturis.)

Celsus pronounces it impossible to heal a fractured thigh-bone without deformity. The patient, he says, must ever afterwards tread upon his toes; and yet, he adds, the case will be worse if neglected.

Albucasis holds forth greater encouragement. He describes the process of treatment very minutely, directing the surgeon to stuff up all the hollow places in the limb with soft pads before applying the splints. He also recommends him to surround the whole limb with a bandage from the heel to the nates. We are inclined to think, although the language of his *barbarous* translator is not sufficiently precise, that his splints extended the whole length of the limb.

Rhases, and we believe, he alone of all the ancient authorities, directs the thigh to be laid in a somewhat bent position, and for this purpose he recommends something suitable to be put below it.

Haly Abbas and Avicenna, as usual, borrow everything from our author.

CIII—ON THE PATELLA

The patella is a porous bone kept firmly in its place by the parts above and below, and is often crushed but seldom fractured. It undergoes fracture also through its thickness, and is broken into small pieces, with or without a wound. The symptoms are obvious,—a solution of continuity, a hollow, and crepitation. The fracture is put in order by extending the leg, for thus the divided portions may be brought together with the fingers, until the lips of the fracture mutually touch, and are united to one another, and fractured pieces, when separated, are thus arranged together. For even if callus does not take place, owing to the parts being drawn in different directions by the muscles and tendons from the thigh and leg, which are inserted into it, yet the separation is much diminished. But it occasions much lameness to the patients; for, when they attempt to labour, the knee cannot sustain them long, and in walking their ascent upwards is impeded; but in moving along a plain their lameness is not perceptible. In ascending, however, as the knee cannot bend in raising and setting down the leg, the lameness becomes apparent. And in this case any bone that irritates is to be taken out where it protrudes, and proper treatment applied.

Commentary. None of the ancient authorities have given so full an account of this accident as our author. Hippocrates and Celsus have omitted it altogether. Soranus merely gives the symptoms, namely, a hollowness in the part and crepitus.

Albucasis recommends us, after arranging the broken pieces of bone, to apply a round splint over it if necessary. Rhases likewise speaks of applying a well-stuffed splint. Haly's account is distinct but similar to our author's, from which it is abridged. Neither he nor Avicenna makes any mention of a splint.

CIV—ON THE LEG

The treatment of fractures of the leg corresponds with that of the fore-arm, for it consists of two bones, the thicker of which bears the same name (tibia), and the small one, from its resemblance, has been called fibula. Its fractures also admit the same varieties, being deranged on all sides when both the bones are broken together, and to three when only one, namely, within, without, and the tibia backwards and the fibula forwards. Wherefore it is to be set in the same manner by the hands, or ligatures, sometimes applied to the leg itself, and sometimes to the thigh, (for the knee being a strong joint can bear the extension uninjured,) and ligatures are to be applied likewise below the fracture, as we mentioned under the head of the fore-arm. The case is to be managed otherwise, as described by us in the section on the arm.

Commentary. Hippocrates has treated of this case at considerable length. The bandages are to be applied as formerly described, and the leg laid on a level board with a soft cushion under it. It is clear that he did not approve of the bent position of the limb. The splints are to be applied on the seventh or eleventh day. Of the fractures of a single bone, that of the tibia, he remarks, is the worse, a fractured fibula being easily managed. He gives particular directions to attend to the state of the heel.

Celsus treats of these fractures in general terms, like those of the fore-arm. Albucasis directs us to apply two splints made of the wood of pines or palms, of moderate thickness, and of such length as to extend from the knee to the feet. One of these is to be placed below the leg and the other above; and they are to be tied in three places, namely, at the extremities and in the middle.

The other Arabians treat of these fractures in more general terms.

CV—ON THE FOOT

The astragalus cannot be fractured by any means, being guarded by bodies on all hands; by the tibia, the fibula, and the os cuboides. But the scaphoides, the bones of the tarsus, and those of the toes, and the cuboides itself, are fractured like those of the carpus, metacarpus, and the fingers of the hand, so that what was said of them is applicable here and need not be repeated.

Commentary. Hippocrates remarks that these bones can only be fractured by some sharp and heavy body. They are to be treated like fractures in general, only that they do not require splints. He recommends the recumbent position with the foot somewhat elevated, and states, in strong terms, the mischief brought on by unseasonable attempts at walking. (De Fracturis, 10.) Galen, in his Commentary, gives an accurate anatomical description of the bones of the foot.

Celsus is very brief on this case. He conducts the treatment on general principles. Albucasis directs us to make the patient put his foot on the ground, the surgeon is then to place one of his feet on it and stand on it. By this means the derangement of the bones will be rectified. He approves of a splint to the sole.

We find nothing worthy of notice in the works of the other authorities.

CVI—ON THE ARRANGEMENT OF THE LIMB

When the thigh or leg is fractured, the manner of arranging the limb will be as important a consideration to you as the other treatment. For the evenness of the fractured parts is especially preserved by this means when properly performed. Some, therefore, lay the fractured part upon a canal, either of wood or of earthenware, or else they lay the whole limb upon it; others apply it only in cases of fracture with a wound, because, say they, these cannot be bound with splints. But the moderns altogether reject the use of these canals for many reasons, but more especially on account of the pressure occasioned by their hardness. Nor is it improper to apply splints to fractured limbs with a wound, as we shall show afterwards. Let the patient, then, lie upon his back, and let a thick garment, equal to the limb in length, be laid under it, more especially where the fracture is, and let both its ends be convoluted and wrapped round so as to resemble the canal in its middle longitudinal cavity, and let it be covered with a soft skin for receiving the embrocations; and then let the limb be fitted to this canal-like cavity, and let other garments or wool be applied on both sides to prevent the limb from being moved to the sides. And let a small board, covered with rags for sake of softness, be fastened to the sole of the foot; and, for the sake of greater security, let the middle of two or three ligatures be applied under this canal-like garment, and let the broken limb be lightly bound along with it. But if the patient be unable to restrain himself from drawing in his leg, his foot should be fastened to the board by means of ligatures around the ankle, so that he may be prevented even from drawing in his leg involuntarily in his sleep. Some likewise cut out a hole in the middle of the bed, that the patient may void his urine and fæces by it without requiring to be moved until the callus has become formed.

Commentary. We have already mentioned that Hippocrates approved of the straight position of the limb. With respect to the *canals* (σωλῆνες) mentioned also by our author he expresses himself in equivocal terms. He says that they prove useful, but not to the extent generally believed. He properly remarks that they do not prevent the body from being moved, and that consequently they cannot be supposed capable of securing the limb entirely from derangement. He is decidedly of opinion that unless they extend from above the ham to the heel they do no good in fractures of the leg. (De Fracturis, 16, ed. Littré.)

Celsus gives the following description of the *canals*: "Is canalis et inferiore parte foramina habere, per quæ, si quis humor excesserit, descendat: et a planta moram, quæ simid et sustineat eam, et delabi non patiatur: et a lateribus cava, per quæ loris datis, moræ quædam crus femurque, ut collocatum est, detineant." Galen, in his Commentary on Hippocrates (l. c.)

describes these machines as being round externally and hollow within, so as to inclose the limb all around:—περιλαμβάνει τὸ σκέλος ὅλον ἐν κύκλῳ. From these words one might think that the canal of which he speaks was a complete cylinder or cone. But from our author's direction to lay the limb upon the canal, it would appear that the machine he speaks of was open above, and as such it is represented and described by Scultet (Arsenal de Chirurg. xxii, 6.) His words are: "Il faut que le canal embrasse plus de la moitié du membre;" this, therefore, is a sort of *trough*. Sprengel calls it a box (*boîte,* Fr. edit.) Littré translates it by *gouttière, l. c.* For an account of these and other machines anciently used in fractures of the lower extremities, see Van Swieten (Comment. 354), and Heister (Surgery, ix, 9.) Brunus and Theodoricus make mention of these *canals,* but do not much approve of them.

Galen informs us that the canals were made of different kinds of wood. He speaks of a surgeon in his time who made them from the wood of the phillyrea. He makes mention of a method of supplying their place by means of a bolster laid below the limb and tied round it with fillets. (Nicetæ Collect. and Comment. l. c.)

Avicenna and Albucasis take notice of these machines, but neither of them with approbation. They also speak of securing the limb in the way described by our author.

The canals would appear to be the machines which Rhases mentions by the name of *barangi*. (Cont. xxix.)

CVII—ON FRACTURES COMPLICATED WITH A WOUND

When a fracture is attended with a wound, if there be a hemorrhage it is to be first stopped; and if there be inflammation, we must use the applications suitable to it; and if there be contusion of the flesh, we must scarify the flesh to remove all apprehension of gangrene; or if gangrene or any other spreading mortification has come on, we must meet it with suitable remedies. The treatment of each of these cases you have had delivered in the Fourth Book. When none of these symptoms is present, nor much of the bone exposed, we may use hooks and sutures, and effect the cure by the treatment for recent wounds, having first cut out any broken pieces of bone which move about and produce irritation. But if a large bone project, which, for its size, cannot be brought into contact by the extension, it will require consideration. Hippocrates, then, in fractures of the thigh and arm, dissuades from replacing at once the protruding bones, predicting danger from it, owing to the inflammation or perhaps spasm of the muscles and nerves which are apt to be brought on by the extension. But time has shown that this attempt will sometimes succeed. Of whatever bones, therefore, we endeavour to replace the protruded ends, we must not meddle with them when in a state of inflammation, but on the first day, before inflammation has come on, or about the ninth day, when the inflammation has gone off. We may set them by an instrument called the lever. It is an iron instrument about seven or eight fingers' breadth in length, and of moderate thickness that it may not bend during the operation; with its extremity sharp, broad, and moderately bent. Its sharp extremity, then, is to be put under the protruding prominence of the bone, and by pushing at the other end while moderate extension of the limb is made, we bring the extremities of the fracture together; or, if we cannot do so, we must cut off the projections by counter-perforators (chisels), or saw them off in the manner described when treating of fistulæ. Having removed the spiculæ of bones and set the limb aright, we cure the wound by dressing with pledgets. But in those members which are double or in pairs, we must take care when the bones of either of them are sawn off, that no contraction of the limb take place, but that it be kept of its proper length by extension. The bandaging is to be thus applied: the circular folds are to be arranged on both sides of the wound, and oblique ones according to the length of the sore, so that they may intersect one another in the form of the Greek letter X, and prevent the lips of it from gaping. And when the ulcer is foul, we must apply dressing with cleansing ointments; but if clean, with incarnating, and the other articles of known efficacy. Hippocrates used the pitch-plaster, which is said to have been the same as the ointment, tetrapharmacon, called also basilicon. After the sore has incarnated we apply splints. Some apply them from the first, taking care not to hurt the parts about the ulcer, and tightening them according to necessity, or again slackening them. When a scale of bone is going to exfoliate, which we ascertain from the discharge being more copious and thin, we must remove the loose fungous flesh about it, and the bandages must be applied loose; but having removed the scale with a hook or some such instrument, we must have recourse to tighter bandages. During the whole time of the healing of the sore, the dressing called motophylax with some of the anti-inflammatory medicines is to be laid over the wound, to be kept on with a simple bandage, which is to be removed at each dressing; everything else remaining the same as described in the treatment of the arm.

Commentary. Hippocrates treats of these cases at great length. His method of rectifying the protruded ends of bones by means of a lever, is described by our author. He says, it may be done on the first or second day, but not on the third or fourth, after the inflammation is begun, for fear of occasioning convulsions. Compresses dipped in wine and oil, or soft bandages are to be used, but splints are not to be applied until the sore puts on a healthy appearance. He mentions that some were in the practice of bandaging the limb above and below the wound, and leaving it bare, in order to allow the discharges to escape; but this practice he greatly disapproves of, as tending to produce swelling in the place; and he recommends the whole limb to be well secured with bandages, but then not too tight. He states that all bones which are completely denuded, must exfoliate and come out. When a bone projects and cannot be replaced, he directs the surgeon to cut it off if it irritate the soft parts. No splints are to be applied when there is a bone which it is seen will exfoliate. If it be the summer season, the compresses applied to the wound are to be frequently soaked with wine; but if it be winter, greasy wool is to be dipped in wine and oil and applied. Compound fractures of the thigh or arm, attended with protrusion of the broken bone, are said to be peculiarly dangerous; for if replaced, they are apt to occasion convulsions; and if let alone, they give rise to acute bilious fevers. Some, however, he adds, recover when the bone is replaced. (De Fract. cum Comment. Galeni.) Galen explains, that the danger in cases of fractured femur and humerus arises from their vicinity to important blood-vessels and muscles.

Celsus lays down the rules for conducting the treatment in these cases with great precision. He states, that fractures complicated with a wound of the skin are generally dangerous, especially when it is the humerus or femur. In the latter case he directs us to saw off the ends of the bone. The case of a fractured humerus is more easily managed. The danger is greatly increased when the fracture is near a joint. He recommends us to divide any muscle which may run across the wound, to let blood, and put the patient upon a restricted diet. In other fractures the bones are to be gently replaced. The wound is to be dressed with a pledget dipped in wine, to which roses have been added. This application is borrowed from Hippocrates. The bandages are to be put on somewhat slacker than when there is no external wound. Neither splints nor canals must be used, but broad bandages. The parts are to be fomented with hot oil and wine, and the dressings renewed every day. When a small fragment of a bone projects, if it be blunt, he recommends us to replace it; but if sharp, he directs us to saw it off, and then replace the bones with the hands or a suitable instrument. Sometimes fragments of bones die, and after a time drop out; and sometimes sharp spiculæ irritate the soft parts, in which case he recommends us to enlarge the wound and cut off the projecting points.

The treatment recommended by Albucasis is very judicious. If inflammation be present, he directs us to subdue it by bleeding; and, in that case, reduction is not to be attempted until the ninth day; but in all other cases it is to be done at first. When it cannot be reduced by the hands, an iron instrument seven or eight fingers' breadth in length, and two fingers broad, is to be used as a lever for this purpose. When the ends of the fracture are sharp and cannot be replaced, they are to be cut off or sawed. His saw bears a considerable resemblance to that of the late Mr. Hey, of Leeds. He recommends an astringent wine as a suitable application, but condemns all cerates which contain oil. The bandages are to be put on very slack. Splints are not to be applied while the wound is irritable and ill-conditioned. When it does not heal, he says we ought to suspect that it is prevented by spiculæ of bones, which are to be sought out and extracted.

Avicenna and Rhases give very proper directions about removing spiculæ of bones, and applying slack bandages, but they evidently copy from Hippocrates and our author.

CVIII—ON THE REDUNDANT CALLUS OF FRACTURES

The superabundant callus of fractures occasions always a deformity, and sometimes also lameness if it be formed near a joint. If, therefore, the callus be newly formed, we use very astringent medicines, and bring it to its form by bandages; and sometimes we effect our purpose by applying a plate of lead to it. But if it is of a stony hardness we make an incision, and pare it off, removing the prominent part by chisels, if need be, and boring it with trephines.

Commentary. Celsus directs us to rub the limb with oil, salt, and nitre; to pour a great quantity of hot salt water upon it; to apply an emollient ointment; to bandage it tightly, and to give an emetic. He also recommends us to produce revulsion by the application of mustard to another part.

Albucasis recommends nearly the same plan of treatment as our author. When the case is recent, he directs us to make astringent applications, such as aloes, olibanum, and myrrh, with an astringent wine or vinegar. He also speaks of applying a plate of lead; and when the callus becomes hard, he approves of scraping and sawing it off, as directed by our author.

No additional information is to be got from the other Arabians.

Theodoricus, and the other surgical authorities of that age, describe the treatment exactly as the ancients. When the callus is hard, they direct us to scrape or saw it off.

CIX—ON DISTORTION FROM THE UNION BY CALLUS

When bones heal distortedly by callus, no little lameness takes place, more particularly if in the feet. The method then of breaking them over again is not at all to be admitted, as it may occasion the utmost danger;

but if the callus be newly formed, we must have recourse to the allusions of a relaxing nature, and to cataplasms, such as those from fat olives and pigeon's dung, and the other medicines for dissolving callus; and we also dispel it by friction with the hand, and bending it every way. But if it be of a stony hardness, we make an incision of the skin with a scalpel, and separate the union of the bones with chisels, and then cure the fracture as formerly said.

Commentary. Celsus approves of breaking the bones over again. With this intention he directs us, in the first place, to bathe the limb with much hot water, and rub it with liquid cerate; the callus is then to be moved with the hands, and the ends of the bone properly set; or if that cannot be thus accomplished, a rule is to be wrapped round with wool and bound upon the part, so as to restore it to its proper shape.

Avicenna agrees with Celsus in speaking favorably of breaking the bone over again. He also speaks favorably of the other treatment recommended by our author.

Rhases recommends emollient applications, and gentle attempts to restore the figure of the limb. Albucasis mentions the proposal of breaking the bone again with disapprobation.

CX—ON BONES WHICH HAVE NOT UNITED BY CALLUS

Sometimes fractured bones remain without forming adhesions, beyond the natural period, either owing to their being often loosed, or from too frequent bathing of the part, or from having been moved unseasonably, or from the number of the bandages, or from atrophy of the whole body, by which means the limb becomes emaciated. Wherefore we must endeavour to remove all the other causes, but more especially the atrophy, partly by calefacient applications which attract nourishment to the place, and partly by supplying a sufficiency of food and baths, and whatever also is of a refreshing nature. Among the other symptoms which follow the formation of callus, the bandages then become stained with blood, although no wound be present, which probably takes place from the substance about the callus, when it unites, squeezing out the drops of blood which were distributed to the hollows of the bones.

Commentary. When the fractured portions do not adhere after a certain time, Celsus directs us to extend the limb, and rub the ends of the bone together, in order to convert them again into the state of a recent fracture, taking care, however, not to hurt the muscles and nerves. The part is then to be fomented, and the splints applied on the fifth day.

Rhases recommends calefacient liniments, friction, and nutritive food.

CXI—ON LUXATIONS

We proceed to the treatment of luxations, which naturally follows that of fractures. A luxation then (to give a definition of it) is a displacement of a member from its proper cavity to an unusual place, by which means the voluntary motion is impeded. We have no other differences of it to mention, except that some are to a greater and some to a less degree. When the bone of a member, therefore, is completely removed from its place, the accident is called by the common name of luxation, but when only moved a little, or brought only to the brim of the cavity, it is called a subluxation.

Commentary. Celsus gives several important remarks upon dislocations in general, but as most of them may more properly be brought under particular heads, we shall notice them here but briefly. He distinguishes dislocations into two classes; the first consisting of a separation of two bones naturally united, such as the scapula from the humerus, the radius from the ulna, the tibia from the fibula, the os calcis from the bones of the ankle, which last is of rare occurrence, and the second being a removal of the bone of a joint from its proper place. When a dislocation occurs, as he remarks, the finger discovers a cavity in the part, and inflammation and fever come on, followed sometimes by gangrene and convulsions. If not reduced, the limb wastes. In a person who is lean, humid, and has weak nerves (muscles?) the dislocation is most easily reduced, but is more difficult to retain. The inflammation is to be reduced by the application of wool dipped in vinegar; by abstinence, a spare diet, and drinking tepid water. Afterwards friction, exercise, and a more generous diet are to be allowed. (viii, 11.)

See many curious remarks on this subject in Galen's Commentary on Hippocrates (de Articulis), and in Apollonii Citiensis Scholia in Hip. et Galen.; also Avicenna (iv, 5, 1); Haly Abbas (Pract. ix, 101); Rhases (Cont. xxix, 2.)

CXII—ON THE LOWER JAW

Beginning then again from the upper parts we shall treat of the lower jaw. For the upper being immoveable does not admit of dislocation; but the lower does not indeed readily admit of complete luxation, owing to its heads being firmly fixed to the upper jaw, but it often undergoes subluxation, for the muscles which are fixed to it being relaxed by the constant exercise of mastication and speaking, the jaw is readily slackened from the most common causes. For the term used by Hippocrates signifies *slackened*. In these cases the part returns to its natural place without trouble. With regard to the complete dislocation of the lower jaw, it will be sufficient to deliver Hippocrates's account, being, at the same time, brief, complete and clear. He says thus: "The jaw seldom falls out of the joint, but it is often slackened in yawning, as many other irregular actions of muscles and tendons do this. When it falls out of the joint it is marked principally by these symptoms; the lower jaw projects forwards, and is inclined in an opposite direction to the luxation; and the coronoid process of the bone swells out near the upper jaw-bone, and it is with difficulty that they shut their jaws. In these cases the suitable mode of reduction is apparent. For somebody must hold the patient's head, another grasps the lower jaw internally and externally with his fingers at the chin, while the patient yawns as much as he can conveniently; and we must first move the jaw with the hand hither and thither for a certain time, and order the man to relax the jaw and separate it; and then we must attend to perform three evolutions at the same time, we must move the jaw from its distorted shape to its natural; push the jaw backwards; and then shut the jaws close, and prevent yawning. This is the mode of reduction, and it cannot be performed by any other processes. Very little treatment will suffice afterwards. Having applied a waxed compress, it is to be secured with a loose bandage. But the surest process is to lay the man upon his back, and supporting his head upon well-stuffed pillows, that they may not yield, to get some person to hold the head of the patient. And if both ends of the jaw be dislocated, the treatment is the same, only the mouth cannot be so well shut, for then the jaw is more prominent, but less distorted from the teeth of the upper and lower jaws corresponding exactly together. Reduction is to be immediately performed, and the mode of it has been already described. If it cannot be restored, there may be danger of the life from continued fevers, torpor, and carus. For these muscles being altered and stretched in a preternatural manner produce carus. They frequently have evacuations by the belly, which are purely bilious, and small in quantity; and if they vomit, it is pure bile. These, for the most part, die on the tenth day." This mode of reduction we have often practised, having first used fomentations of warm water and oil, by a sponge along the dislocated jaw, more especially when there is any difficulty in restoring it to its position. Wherefore, having placed the man upon the ground, we stand behind and operate in the manner described by Hippocrates.

Commentary. The account here given of Hippocrates's method of reduction is taken from his work, 'De Articulis,' (31.) When a few of his technical terms are explained in the commentary of Galen, the description is sufficiently distinct, and is upon the whole a very correct account of the symptoms and treatment of this accident. The prominence of the coronoid bone is well described by Hippocrates. Galen remarks that the end of the jaw-bone slips under the zygomatic arch. It has been a matter of dispute what Hippocrates means by slackening, or incomplete luxations of the jaw. It is worthy of remark that such an accident is described by Sir Astley Cooper. (See further Littré's Hippocrates, t. iv, 29.)

Galen's description of the method of reduction is given in the Collection of Nicetas. (Chirurg. Vet. ed. Cocchius.) It is substantially the same as that of Hippocrates.

A mode of reducing the dislocation by means of a machine is described by Oribasius, in his work De Machinamentis, 30.

The account which Celsus gives of this accident is upon the whole very accurate, and corresponds very well with modern descriptions. If dislocated only at one end, the chin inclines to the opposite side, and the teeth of the upper and lower jaws do not correspond. If at both ends, the whole chin projects outwards, the lower teeth are more prominent, and the muscles appear stretched. The patient being properly seated, and his head held by an assistant, the surgeon having wrapped his thumbs with linen cloths, is to put them into the patient's mouth, while the fingers are applied externally. The jaw being firmly grasped, the chin is to be shaken, and then, at one and the same instant, the head is to be seized, the chin moved, the jaw forced into its place, and the mouth shut. After reduction, if pain in the eyes and neck has been brought on by the accident, he recommends us to let blood from the arm. The patient is to live upon liquids, and avoid talking.

Albucasis follows Hippocrates in distinguishing dislocations of the lower jaw into partial and complete. In addition to the symptoms already detailed, he mentions a flow of saliva from the mouth, and an inability to speak. When the dislocation is partial or incomplete, he says, it soon returns of itself to its proper place. When the luxation is complete, he directs us to reduce it by introducing the thumbs into the mouth, and grasping the jaw in the manner described by Hippocrates. He states that when not reduced the accident often proves fatal by superinducing fevers and coma. Avicenna, in like manner, affirms, that if not reduced, it may bring on fatal consequences. His account is borrowed entirely from Hippocrates. Rhases and Haly Abbas give exactly the same description of the symptoms and mode of reducing as Albucasis.

Monteggia, Fabricius ab Aquapendente, Sir Astley Cooper, and Mr. Samuel Cooper (the author of the well-known Surgical Dictionary) affirm that there is no foundation for the prognostic of Hippocrates, that the accident will prove fatal if the dislocation be not speedily reduced. We can say, however, from our own personal knowledge, that such fatal consequences do occasionally occur. We once knew a poor woman who was very liable to dislocations of the lower jaw, which we reduced three or four different times. At last, owing to circumstances which it is unnecessary to explain, an interval of more than a day elapsed between the accident and the reduction. By this time she was become seriously indisposed, and died a few days afterwards with all the symptoms described by Hippocrates. We may mention also that Heister states that fatal consequences may result from the accident. (Chirurg. p. i, iii, 4.) The same thing is affirmed also by Brunus (Chirurg. Mag. i); by Theodoricus (ii, 43); and by Guido de Cauliaco (v, 2.)

That species of sub-luxation described by Hippocrates, is mentioned by Guy of Cauliac in the following terms: "Mandibula quandoque mollificatur." (v, 2.)

CXIII—ON THE CLAVICLE AND ACROMION

The clavicle, at its inner extremity, is not liable to dislocation, for there it is articulated with the sternum, where it admits of no motion. But if from any sudden and violent force from without, it should be torn from its place, it is to be subjected to the same treatment as a fracture. And its extremity which is articulated with the shoulder does not readily fall out of the joint, being prevented by the biceps muscle and the acromion. But neither does the clavicle admit any strong peculiar motion of its own, being made solely for the expansion of the thorax, and hence man is the only animal which has a clavicle. If it should sometimes happen to be dislocated in wrestling, it is to be replaced with the hand, assisted by the application of many-folded compresses, together with convenient bandages. When the acromion is sub-luxated it may be restored to its proper place by the same treatment. It is a small cartilaginous bone connecting the clavicle to the scapula, which is not to be seen in the skeletons. This, if moved a little from its place, exhibits the appearance to inexperienced persons of the head of the arm being dislocated; for the top of the shoulder appears sharper, and there is a hollow from which it was removed; but the cases are to be distinguished from one another by the symptoms about to be enumerated.

Commentary. The dislocation of the outer end of the clavicle from the acromion is treated of by Hippocrates, who gives a very distinct account of the symptoms and mode of treatment. He warns the surgeon not to confound this accident with dislocation of the humerus, as he had frequently seen done. He directs the surgeon to push down the projecting end of the bone; and then to secure it with compresses, and bind the arm to the side. He holds that the accident always leaves some deformity. (De Articulis, 15.)

Galen mentions that this accident happens most commonly to young persons, and that when not reduced it occasions a wasting of the arm. The account which Galen in this place and, copying from him, our author have given of the accident to which they represent the acromion as being subject, has been the subject of much controversy among modern authorities. See Cocchi (Chirurg. Vet. 133); and Littré (Hippoc. iv, 12.) Hippocrates, whom they both evidently had in view, (de Artic. 13), clearly refers to dislocation of the scapular end of the clavicle; and probably Galen alludes to the same, complicated with separation of the acromion from the scapula in young subjects. We would beg leave to quote what Monro says of the acromion: "This is an epiphyse in children; and in some old subjects I have seen it joined by a cartilage to the spine." (Anat. of the Bones, p. 231.) Galen states decidedly that in young persons this process is sometimes bent along with the clavicle, and in them that replacement of the parts to their natural state is easily effected. He adds, "as dry wood is not adapted for bending, but such as is sappy and green bear this, in the same manner the bones of growing animals can be bent by force, and more especially such as are porous and fistulous, as the clavicle is." Galen relates that in his own person he met with the accident while wrestling in the Palestra, and that by using oily fomentations and light bandages, a cure was at last effected. He says he was then thirty-five years old, but adds, that he had never known another person cured who was so far advanced in life. (Ibid. 134.) Avicenna gives the same account of the acromion as the Greeks. (iv, 5,1, 10.)

Neither Celsus nor Oribasius has treated of this case of dislocation.

Rhases, Avicenna, Haly Abbas, and Albucasis agree that dislocations occur more frequently at the acromial than at the sternal end of the clavicle. Desault and Boyer, on the other hand, affirm that the accident occurs oftener at the sternal extremity; but Sir Astley Cooper's ample experience confirms the correctness of the ancient statement. Mr. Liston also agrees in stating that dislocation at the acromial end is much more frequent than at the sternal.

CXIV—ON DISLOCATION OF THE SHOULDER

The head of the arm, which is articulated with the cavity of the scapula, is often dislocated; but neither upwards, owing to the coronoid process of the scapula, which prevents it, nor often backwards, owing also to the scapula, nor forwards owing to the tendon of the biceps muscle and the acromion. Sometimes, though rarely, it is dislocated inwards and outwards, but frequently, and particularly in those who are lean, downwards. In such persons, however, as it is readily dislocated, so is it also reduced; but in those who are brawny, on the other hand, it is not readily dislocated, and is reduced with difficulty. In some cases from a blow suspicions of dislocation are formed, although none has taken place, owing to the violent inflammation which supervenes. Wherefore, dislocation downwards may be thus ascertained. The affected shoulder, when compared with the sound one, appears very different, the upper part of the arm, whence the dislocation took place, seeming hollow; and (as mentioned with regard to the sub-luxation of the acromion,) the top of the shoulder appears sharper than natural; and the dislocated head of the arm is distinctly felt in the armpit. The elbow also is removed to a distance from the ribs; or, if you attempt it, you can only bring it to the ribs with difficulty; neither can the hand be raised to the ear, owing to the stretching of the elbow; nor can any other varied motions be performed with it. In children, then, and in recent and inconsiderable displacements of the bone, it may be often reduced, as Hippocrates remarks, by the protuberant knuckle of the middle finger of the clenched hand of the surgeon, or of the sound hand of the patient, if he be not a child. But the following are more effectual modes of reduction. Having bathed the man and used relaxing affusions, let him be laid on the ground in a supine posture, and apply a moderately-sized ball, either of leather or some other soft thing to the armpit; and the surgeon being seated with his face turned to the patient upon the affected side, if the right shoulder he dislocated, let him put the heel of his right foot upon the ball previously fitted to the armpit, or if the left, that of the left foot; and seizing the hand of the affected arm, let him pull down to the feet, at the same time making counter-extension by the heel in the armpit, while an assistant, standing behind the head, pulls at the other shoulder in an opposite direction, to prevent the body from being dragged along. There is another mode of reduction, namely, by suspending the patient upon a person's shoulder. A young man taller than the patient, or standing on some elevated object, by his affected side, (the patient also being in a standing posture) is to apply his shoulder below the patient's armpit, while he stretches and pulls the patient's hand towards his own belly, so that the rest of the patient's body is suspended at the back of the person who supports him. But if the patient be light, another light child is to be suspended from him. For while the arm and the rest of the body are pulled downwards oppositely, the shoulder put under the armpit, readily replaces the dislocated limb. And the same thing may be done by means of the instrument called a pestle. It is a long piece of wood which is erected on the ground upon some other firm object. Its upper extremity, then, being rounded, and neither very thick nor thin, is applied below the armpit of the patient, who either stands or sits, according to the length of the pestle, and the hand being stretched along the pestle and pulled downwards, while the rest of the body is balanced on the opposite side and weighs downwards, the reduction takes place either spontaneously, or with the assistance of another person pulling down. And this may be done with the step of a ladder, as we described when treating of the extension for a fractured arm. Here some round body is to be fitted to the step of the ladder, such as will suit the armpit of the patient, and propel the head of the arm. But if, owing to the oldness of the accident, or the hardness of the body, we find the reduction difficult, we must have recourse to the method by the means of the instrument called ambe. The ambe is a piece of wood about two cubits in length, of the breadth of three fingers, and about two fingers' breadth in thickness, having the one extremity round and adapted for the hollow of the armpit, like the extremity of the pestle. Having then wrapped its end with linen rags, in order that it may be softer, we adjust it under the head of the humerus in the armpit, and stretching the hand along the wood, we bind it at the arm, fore-arm, and wrist; then bringing the hand with the wood over a transverse piece of wood, fastened between two erect pedestals, or again over the step of a ladder, so that the armpit may be fitted transversely to the step, we draw the hand downwards, and allow the rest of the body to hang suspended on the opposite side; for then the limb will return to its place. After the reduction, we must apply to the armpit a secure and moderately-sized ball of wool, which, if there is no inflammation present, is to be dry, but if there is inflammation, it is to be dipped in oil. Around this, the shoulder, and the other armpit, a bandage is to be put on in the form of the Greek letter X, so that the decussation may take place above the affected shoulder; and the arm is to be bound to the sides; and the elbow and hand are to be slung by the neck, so that the limb may not fall out again while the dislocation is recent. After the seventh day or later, having loosed the bandages, we must have recourse to moderate friction, so that the body being rendered firmer, the joint may become less liable to luxations. But if the limb is often dislocated, either owing to its humidity (flabbiness), or from its being long subject to the accident, we must proceed to burning, as formerly described. But since sometimes the fœtus in utero or the child, while growing, sustains a dislocation of the part which is not reduced, the flesh upon the shoulder is nothing reduced from the natural, nor is the hand obstructed in any of its operations, but the bone remains shorter, not increasing in size; and such persons are called weasel-armed. But in the case of the thigh, the bone does not grow and the limb wastes; for, not being able to sustain the weight of the body, it is not exercised. And with regard to all the other members, if they remain unreduced the parts below are greatly impaired.

Commentary. Hippocrates delivers his opinions respecting dislocations at the shoulder-joint with singular modesty and a remarkable air of truth. He says, that he had never met with a case in which the head of the humerus was not lodged in the armpit, and expresses a doubt whether in reality there be dislocations inwards or backwards. "I will not affirm," he adds, "whether or not dislocation forwards may take place, only this I can say that

I have never seen it." (De Articulis.) Galen, in his commentary on this work, mentions that he had seen five cases of the uncommon kinds of dislocation, four of which were dislocations forwards. They occurred mostly among the athletæ. In one case, of which he relates the particulars, he effected the reduction with his heel placed in the armpit. Galen states distinctly, that it is the retraction of the muscles which proves the great obstacle to reduction. (Ed. Basil, v, 585.) Hippocrates has described several methods of reduction, most of which are mentioned by our author. By the fist placed in the armpit, as described by our author. By the heel, as likewise described by him. He adds one advice not distinctly given by our author, to apply the ball placed in the armpit on the side within the head of the humerus, and not upon it. The process by suspending the patient upon the shoulder of another person is next described by him. Those by the pestle and ladder are afterwards clearly described. He then describes the ambe and the application of it to the reduction of dislocations in nearly the same terms as our author. We may here mention, by the way, that the description of the ambe given by Boyer, does not correspond exactly to the instrument recommended by Hippocrates. See drawings of Hippocrates's ambe in Heister's 'Surgery' (x, 4); in Scultet's 'Arsenal de Chirurgie' (xxii, 1); and in Littré's edition of Hippocrates (iv, 91.) Hippocrates describes other less important processes of reduction with a Thessalian chair, and a door. He remarks, that persons in a reduced habit of body are most liable to dislocations, and illustrates this position by some very acute observations on the occurrence of these accidents in cattle. After reduction, he directs that a ball of soft wool should be placed in the armpit and secured with a bandage and a sling; and he attaches great importance to well-regulated friction afterwards.

Celsus mentions two kinds of dislocation at the shoulder-joint, namely, downwards and forwards. He describes the methods of reduction by the hand, and by a wooden instrument (spathula lignea) resembling the ambe of Hippocrates. His description of the latter method is very distinct. His mode of reducing dislocations inwards merits attention. The man is to be laid on his back, and a strip of cloth or a thong of leather being placed in the armpit, its two ends are to be brought behind the patient's head and given in charge to an assistant, while another takes hold of the arm; the surgeon is then to push back the patient's head with his left hand, while with the other he raises the fore-arm and arm, and pushes the bone into its place. After reduction the armpit is to be stuffed with wool, and suitable bandages applied.

Oribasius treats of dislocations downwards, outwards, and forwards; and gives a very elaborate description of complicated machines for reducing them. Of these it is impossible to convey any correct idea without proper plates. We must be content, therefore, with referring the reader to his work. (De Machinamentis.)

Albucasis describes three kinds of dislocation at the shoulder, namely, downwards, inwards, below the pectoral muscle, and upwards, about which he expresses himself somewhat doubtful. He denies the possibility of dislocations forwards and backwards, the former being prevented by the muscles and latter by the scapula. His methods of reduction are exactly the same as those mentioned by Paulus.

Avicenna expresses himself as being doubtful whether any dislocation takes place at the shoulder except downwards, at least, he adds, he had no experience of any other case. He gives the symptoms of it very accurately, and describes all the methods of reduction mentioned by our author. He approves of the cautery to obviate the tendency to repeated dislocations.

Haly Abbas questions the occurrence of dislocations upwards, forwards, inwards, or backwards. He appears, therefore, to agree with Hippocrates in considering that downwards as the only unequivocal case of dislocation. He recommends the processes of reduction described by our author.

Rhases remarks, that owing to the shallowness of the glenoid cavity and the weakness of the ligaments the bones at the shoulder are more subject to luxations than those of any other joint. He describes the symptoms very accurately. The top of the shoulder, he says, is sharper than natural, the head of the humerus is felt in the armpit, the arm cannot be brought to the sides without pain, nor raised to the head at all. He remarks correctly that when the accident happens during delivery or in childhood, the arm does not grow to its natural size. He mentions that venesection is often of great use in reducing dislocations. He also recommends the warm bath. He denies the possibility of a dislocation in any other direction except downwards.

The ancient modes of reduction are recommended and described by Guy of Cauliac (v, 2); and Theodoricus (ii, 47.)

CXV—ON THE ELBOW

Inasmuch as the elbow-joint is more complicated than that of the shoulder, so, in like manner, are its dislocations more difficult to manage; for they are less readily occasioned, and more difficultly reduced, owing to the number of its processes and cavities. Sometimes it undergoes subluxation only, but often it is completely dislocated in every direction, and more especially forwards and backwards. It is easily recognised even by the sight, and the dislocated bone may be felt in the place to which it has been removed, while a hollow appears in the place whence it was moved. A comparison with the sound arm particularly discloses the nature of the accident. Reduction then must be made immediately before inflammation comes on, for, if this has supervened, it is difficult to cure, and some such cases become utterly irremediable, more especially if the dislocation was backwards; for of all the dislocations at the elbow-joint, that backwards is the most painful and dangerous. Small displacements then may be restored by a moderate degree of extension, the assistants keeping the hand extended, pulling, and making counter-extension at the fore-arm and arm, while the surgeon with the palm of his hand pushes the dislocated bone into its natural place. Hippocrates rectifies the dislocation forwards by bending the hand suddenly so as to force the palm straight to the shoulder of the same side; and that backwards again by frequent and strong extension; inasmuch as dislocations forwards are produced by violent extension, and those backwards by violent flexion. If the dislocation has continued long unreduced, we must have recourse to stronger extension, such in particular as that described by Hippocrates for a fractured arm, where he has recourse to the piece of wood adapted to a spade. Some of the moderns manage the matter thus: Two assistants stretching the arm as aforesaid, the one holding at the armpit, and the other below at the wrist, the surgeon, standing opposite the patient, grasps the arm with the palms of both his hands near the joint, and giving orders to bind a long folded robe or broad swathe round his hands and the arm of the patient, and to pull outwards and downwards towards the hand, whilst he, following the same course, drags the parts with his hands thus secured until they pass the articulation of the joint. The arm should be first anointed with oil, to render the part slippery and easily moved with the palms of the surgeon's hands. Thus the dislocated parts being violently pulled by the hands of the assistants will return to their proper place. After the reduction the arm is to be bent to an angular position, and treated with oblong compresses and suitable bandages.

Commentary. No author, ancient nor modern, has given so complete a view of the accidents to which the elbow-joint is subject as Hippocrates. In his works (De Fracturis, De Articulis, and Mochlicus,) he has treated of this subject with surprising accuracy and skill. He describes the following injuries of the elbow-joint: 1st. Complete luxations, laterally, anteriorly, and posteriorly. 2d. Luxations of the radius, anteriorly, posteriorly, and laterally. 3d. Fracture of the olecranon. 4th. Fracture of the apophysis of the humerus. We must give his description of the last-mentioned injury in his own words: "It sometimes happens that the head of the humerus is broken at its apophysis; and this, although it appear a more serious accident, is, in fact, less so than many other injuries of the joint." It is singular that this distinct account of a very common injury of the joint should have been overlooked or misunderstood by all his commentators and the surgical authorities down to the present day. We have often met with it in our own practice, and seen many instances in which it had been misapprehended in the practice of other surgeons. It is only within the last five or six years that it has been described in any modern work on surgery. Lateral luxation of the radius is described by him under the name of *diastasis*. (De Fracturis, 44; De Articulis, 20.) The Commentaries of Apollonius Citiensis and Galen are worth consulting although they contain no new matter. Galen remarks that in dislocations of the radius, the power of flexion and extension is often not much impaired; and this, we may add, is confirmed by modern observation. Galen's account of fractures of the olecranon is remarkable for its precision and accuracy. (Chirurg. Vet. 84.)

Celsus describes four different kinds of dislocation at the elbow, namely, forwards, backwards, and to either side. He also mentions that rare variety, in which there is a dislocation of the ulna, while the radius remains in its place. (See Sir Astley Cooper's Lectures.) The other varieties are all well described, and suitable methods of treatment recommended. When there is a dislocation forwards the arm is extended, but cannot be bent; when backwards, on the contrary, it cannot be extended, and is shorter than natural. When to either side, the arm is somewhat bent towards that side from which the bone has been moved. He lays it down as a general rule for treating all such dislocations, to extend both the members concerned in different directions, until the bones are separated from one another, and then to push them into their right position. When the dislocation is forwards, he directs us to make strong extension with the hands or with thongs, and then placing some round body upon the anterior part of the arm, to push the fore-arm over it suddenly to the shoulder. This method is well described by Hippocrates, but rather indistinctly by Paulus. In all the other cases, the best method, he says, is to make reduction in the same way that it is performed for the replacement of fractures.

Oribasius mentions the four ordinary kinds of dislocation at the elbow-joint, and describes methods of reducing them by machines. He has likewise described the separate dislocation of the radius from the humerus, and he is the only Greek authority, as far as we know, who has described the separate luxation of the ulna, but which, as stated above, had been noticed by Celsus. We need scarcely remark that a few cases of this uncommon accident have been reported of late years.

Albucasis says that the fore-arm is dislocated in all directions, but more especially backwards and forwards. His description of the mode of reduction is evidently copied from Paulus. Avicenna likewise borrows his whole account from our author.

Rhases and Haly Abbas describe the ordinary cases of complete luxation at the elbow-joint, but we believe that neither they nor any of the Arabians take notice of the dislocation of the radius from the ulna, nor the abruption of the apophysis of the humerus.

CXVI—ON DISLOCATIONS AT THE WRIST AND FINGERS

Dislocations at the wrist and fingers are attended with no difficulty, unless accompanied with a wound. This case, therefore, will be treated of under the head of dislocations with a wound. Those without a wound may be remedied by moderate extension and the anti-inflammatory plan of treatment.

Commentary. Hippocrates says that the hand is dislocated inwards and outwards, but most frequently inwards. In the former case it is found impossible to bend the fingers, and in the latter to extend them. He also makes mention of dislocations to either side. He directs us to make counter-extension upon a table, and to push down the projecting end of the bone with the hand or the heel. He also describes the separate dislocation of the radius and ulna; and, upon the whole, his account is very little different from that given by Sir Astley Cooper in his 'Lectures,' and by Mr. Liston in his 'Elements of Surgery.'

Celsus describes, in his usual elegant manner, the dislocations forwards and backwards. He denies the possibility of the lateral dislocations, and, in fact, it is now acknowledged that if ever they do occur they are incomplete. Like Hippocrates, he directs us to replace dislocations of the fingers by making extension upon a table. He does not make mention of the separate dislocation of the lower end of the radius.

Oribasius mentions the dislocations forwards and backwards, and likewise the separate dislocations of the radius and ulna. Sometimes, he says, the radius is dislocated, while the ulna remains in its place, and sometimes the ulna is dislocated while the radius remains. He describes the process of reduction with machines.

Albucasis, Avicenna, and Haly Abbas describe very accurately the dislocations forwards and backwards. They state that immediate reduction is peculiarly required in the case of this accident. Avicenna recommends a strengthening plaster to be put on the part before the splints are applied. When the joint, after reduction, is found to have lost the power of motion, Albucasis recommends us to pour hot water upon it and apply friction.

Rhases states that the ulna is more apt to be dislocated separately than the radius, which generally undergoes fracture rather than luxation. The fingers, he says, are mostly dislocated inwards.

CXVII—ON THE VERTEBRÆ OF THE SPINE

The vertebræ of the spine, when completely dislocated by accident, occasion instant death; for the spinal marrow undergoes extraordinary compression; and even when one of its nervous processes is compressed, it brings on dangerous symptoms. It often suffers sub-luxations, and when this takes place forwards it gets the name of repandation; when backwards, that of gibbosity; and when sideways, that of wry-neckedness. When there is a small sub-luxation of many vertebræ together, the distortion occasions a circular flexure of the spine, and in this case some are apt to be deceived, and take it for a complete dislocation of one spine, whereas a complete dislocation of one spinal vertebra does not produce a circular but an angular flexure of the spine, which is attended with more danger. When the dislocation is inwards, it cannot be reduced because no counter-pressure can be made on the belly. But those who imagine that they can effect anything in this case by stretching the patients upon a ladder, by apply cupping instruments, or administering sternutatories, or by producing coughing, or by inflation, are sufficiently exposed by Hippocrates. But since, often the breaking off of some of the small bones of the spine leaves a hollow appearance (as has been mentioned when treating of fractures), some have taken this for a dislocation forwards; and it being speedily healed, (for its callus is soon formed,) they have given out that a dislocation forwards is readily cured, although in fact it be wholly incurable, or difficult at least, to cure. For retention of the urine and fæces takes place, with coldness of the body; but this state is followed afterwards by an involuntary discharge of the excrements. These symptoms arise from the nerves and from muscular sympathy, and the patients soon die, more especially if the upper parts and the vertebræ of the neck be affected. But that gibbous state of the spine which mostly takes place from infancy, is a protracted affection and not speedily fatal; but, as Hippocrates has shown, it leads to disease and is incurable. But when this state occurs from an accident, the contrivances to remedy it with a ladder, suspending the patient erect, and inflation with a bladder, are altogether ridiculous. But the method of rectifying it, recommended by Hippocrates, will be alone sufficient. For, he says, a board, in length and breadth such as to contain the man, or a bench equal to it, is to be placed near a wall, being extended along the wall, and not more than a foot distant from it, and some robes are to be spread over it to prevent the body from being injured. Then the man, being bathed, is to be laid on his face along the board or bench, and a thong is to be twice passed round his breast by the armpits along the back; and the extremities of the thong are to be fastened to a pestle like a piece of wood erected on the floor at the extremity of the board or bench, and this to be given to a person standing behind the patient's head to hold, so that when the lower parts are secured oppositely, and the upper pulled towards the head, extension may be made at the proper time. Then another thong being bound round both the feet above the ankles, and again another above the loins, so that its two ends may meet upon the haunch-bone, the extremities of these thongs are to be again united together, and bound to another pestle-like piece of wood resembling that already described; and this pestle, like the former, is to be erected near the extremity of the board or bench at his feet; and then we are to order the assistants to make counter-extension by these pieces of wood. Others effect this part of the operation by what are called aselli. They are axles turned upon an erect piece of wood, which is placed at each extremity of the large board or bench, at the feet and head of the patient, and the thongs are to be wrapped round them. While the extension is thus made, we press down the prominence of the back with the palms of the hands, and if necessary we may sit upon it without apprehension. If the spine is not thus made straight, and the patient can endure pressure, we may scoop out from the adjoining wall a furrow opposite the prominence of the back, so that the length of the furrow may not be greater than a cubit, and it must be in a situation neither much higher nor lower than the patient's spine. But this furrow ought rather to be prepared beforehand, and on this account we directed the board at first to be placed near the wall. Then one extremity of a board is to be introduced into the furrow, while we press the other downward until it is clear that the spine is rectified. According to Hippocrates, extension alone without the board, and again the treatment with the board alone, is sufficient to accomplish the purpose. If this be true it will not be improper, in cases of dislocation anteriorly and laterally, to make the aforesaid extension without the compression. After the reduction, a thin piece of wood three fingers in breadth, and of such a length as to comprehend the dislocated part and some of the sound vertebræ, is to be wrapped round with a piece of linen or some flax, on account of its hardness, and applied to the spine with suitable bandages. And the patient must be kept upon a spare diet. If afterwards any remains of the protuberance are to be discovered, we must use relaxant and emollient applications, with the pressure by means of the plate. Some use a plate of lead.

Commentary. Our author's account of dislocations of the spine is entirely condensed from Hippocrates's work 'De Articulis,' and the commentary of Galen on the same. The description of the methods of reduction is so plain, that we need not take up time in illustrating it. It will be remarked that he makes mention of a mode of reducing these dislocations by means of axles or aselli. In the days of Hippocrates they were acquainted with only three of the mechanical powers, namely, the lever, the wedge, and the axis in peritrochio. The last mentioned is called by him asellus. (See De Fracturis cum Comment. Galeni.) Hippocrates makes mention of a mode of reducing dislocations of the spine, by succussion in a ladder, but expresses himself unfavorably of it as being a procedure which none but charlatans would practice. He speaks with becoming contempt of those who have recourse to ostentatious modes of performance *ad captandum vulgus*.

Celsus states very decidedly the fatal nature of dislocations of the uppermost vertebræ. Even those below the diaphragm are designated as highly dangerous. They happen either forwards or backwards. Those above the diaphragm occasion paralysis of the hands, vomitings, contractions of the tendons, difficulty of breathing, pain, and relaxation of the ears. Those below the diaphragm produce paralysis of the lower extremities, suppression of urine, or an involuntary discharge of it. Even these cases, he adds, prove fatal within three days. He says, that Hippocrates's mode of reduction by counter-extension and pressure on the part with the heel, applies only to cases of incomplete luxation.

Oribasius describes the method of reduction by means of a machine, as mentioned by our author. It will readily be understood that the whole process consisted in making counter-extension upwards and downwards, and pressing upon the part which projects with a piece of wood. (De Machinamentis.)

Albucasis explains the nature of the accident and the methods of reduction in much the same terms as our author. The patient is to be laid upon a board or bench of sufficient length, spread with some soft thing to prevent him from being hurt. Then a pole or piece of wood is to be fastened at each extremity of the bench; and a rope or swathe, being carried round the patient's body by the armpits and above his head, is to be fastened to the upper pole, which is not to be fixed firm in the ground; and another rope is to be brought round below the part affected, and fastened to the pole at his feet. Powerful counter-extension may be thus made, while the surgeon presses upon the protruded part with his hand and pushes it into its place. If these means do not succeed, he directs us to fasten a piece of wood into a hole in the wall opposite the protuberant part of the patient's back and to press down with it. Other methods are also described by him. After reduction he directs us to apply a splint with bandages, as recommended by our author.

Avicenna describes all the methods of reduction here mentioned; and in the Latin edition of his works there are plates to illustrate his descriptions. Judging from our own experience of such cases, however, we would say that such contrivances can seldom be required to reduce these dislocations, as there is much less difficulty in the reduction than in keeping the parts in place afterwards.

Haly Abbas copies the description given by Hippocrates of the mode of reduction. After the parts are restored to their place, he recommends us to apply a board (tabula lignea) three fingers broad, and of such a length as to comprehend the dislocated vertebræ and some of the adjoining ones; and to bind it firmly on to prevent a recurrence of the displacement.

The ancients were well acquainted with the curvature of the spine occasioning paralysis of the lower extremities. Alsaharavius remarks that it occurs most frequently in childhood, and arises from an inflammation or collection of humours between the vertebræ. Sometimes, he adds, it is occasioned by a gross flatus. This is the disease called *spina ventosa*. When connected with a collection of blood in the part, he recommends bleeding, clysters, and various emollient applications. When it arises from flatulence he prescribes the hermodactylus. If the usual means do not succeed he approves of the actual cautery. (Pract. xxviii, 9.)

But no ancient author has treated so fully of curvature of the spine as Rhases. He states that it occurs most frequently in childhood, and often proves fatal by occasioning pressure on the thoracic viscera. The disease, he says, may arise from a fall, a blow, an abscess, or a gross flatus contained in the vertebræ. In cases of paralysis of the lower extremities connected with this disease, he approves of applying the actual cautery to the back. (Cont. i.) He states correctly that dislocations of the upper vertebræ often prove suddenly fatal. He directs the surgeon to keep them reduced with a splint extending the whole length of the spine. (Cont. xxix.) On the spina ventosa or gibbositas, see further Serapion (v, 26.) For the cure of it, he recommends first discutient plasters, and if these do not succeed he advises recourse to the actual cautery. (v, 27.)

CXVIII—ON DISLOCATION AT THE HIP-JOINT

The other bones of the human body sometimes undergo subluxation, and sometimes complete luxation, but the articulations at the hip and the shoulder are subject only to complete luxation, more especially the hip-joint, because it has a deep and round cavity which is further strengthened by a strong brim. The limb, then, being subject to displacement from its cavity by some great violence, many differences arise according to the greater or less degree of the dislocation. Dislocation at the hip-joint takes place in four ways, or rather places; for it is dislocated either inwards, outwards, forwards, or backwards; inwards and outwards frequently, more especially inwards; but forwards and backwards very rarely. When the dislocation is inwards, the affected leg, if compared with the sound one, appears longer, the knee is more prominent, the patient cannot bend the leg at the groin, and a swelling is clearly felt in the perineum, from the head of the thigh being lodged there. When the dislocation is outwards, the symptoms are the contrary to these; for the leg appears shorter, there is a hollow in the perineum, a protuberance about the nates, the knee is turned inwards, and the leg can be bent. When the dislocation is forwards, the patient can stretch the leg without pain at the knee, but when he attempts to walk he cannot turn the foot inwards; the urine is retained, the groin is swelled, the buttocks appear wrinkled and destitute of plumpness; and in walking he supports himself upon his heel. Those who experience a dislocation backwards can neither extend the ham nor the knee, nor can they bend the limb before bending the groin also. The leg appears shorter, the groin looser, and the head of the thigh is to be felt at the buttock. When, then, from infancy, or simply, when for a length of time the limb has been neglected after being dislocated, and allowed to remain so, the cure is impracticable, callus having been already formed. But when the luxation is recent, it may be managed in the way recommended by Hippocrates. We must, then, proceed immediately to the reduction, for dislocations at the hip-joint, when allowed to remain long, are wholly irremediable. In general, then, in all the four kinds of dislocation, the reduction may be accomplished by rotating it, by bending the limb, and by extension. For if the accident be recent and the patient young, we may sometimes succeed in reducing the limb by grasping and rotating the thigh this way and that. When the dislocation is inwards we may sometimes accomplish our purpose by bending the limb at the groin inwards frequently and strongly. If the dislocation does not yield to these means we must have recourse to extension, first with the hands, certain assistants grasping the thigh and leg and pulling the limb downwards, while others grasp the body at the armpits and pull upwards. Or, if a stronger extension be required, the leg may be bound with twisted cords or thongs, above the ankle, and a little higher than the knee, lest it suffer injury; but it is not necessary to secure the breast in this manner, for, as has been said, the hands may be put under the armpits for this purpose. And the middle of a soft and strong thong is to be applied to the perineum, and brought up to the shoulders anteriorly by the groins and clavicles, and posteriorly along the back, and the two ends are to be given to an assistant to hold. Then, all pulling together so as to raise the patient's body, extension is to be thus made. This mode of extension is applicable generally in all the four varieties of dislocation. But the manner of replacement varies according to the nature of the dislocation. If the bone has been dislocated inwards, let the patient be stretched by having the middle of a thong applied to the perineum between the head of the bone and the perineum, and let the thong be brought upwards by the adjoining groin and the clavicle, and let a young man with both his arms grasp the thigh which is affected in its thickest part, and pull strongly outwards. This mode of reduction is easier than any of the others. When the limb does not thus yield we must have recourse to other contrivances more complicated but more efficacious than these. Let the man be stretched upon a large board, or bench, like that upon which we stretch those who have dislocation of the spine, and along nearly its whole length let certain gutters be scooped out, in breadth and depth not more than three fingers, and not more than four fingers distant from one another, so that the extremity of the lever being inserted into them may impel the limb wherever it is required. In the middle of the board, or bench, let another piece of wood be fastened about a foot in length, and in thickness like that which is inserted in the extremity of a spade, so that when the man is pulled along, this piece of wood may come between the perineum and the head of the thigh, so as to prevent the yielding of the body when pulled by the feet, and thereby often obviating the necessity of making counter-extension; and at the same time when the body is extended this piece of wood will push the head of the thigh outwards. The extension is to be made in the manner described above, more particularly by the foot. But if it is not thus reduced, the erect piece of wood is to be taken away, and two other pieces of wood fastened on the sides of it like posts, not more than a foot in length, and let another piece of wood be adapted to them like the step of a ladder, so that the figure of the three pieces of wood may resemble the Greek letter H; the middle piece of wood being fixed a little below the upper extremities. Then the man being laid on the sound side, we bring the sound leg between the two posts below the piece of wood corresponding to the step of a ladder, while the affected one is brought above it, so that the head of the thigh is to be adapted to it; but a folded garment is to be first wrapped about it to prevent the thigh from being bruised. Then another board of moderate breadth, and of such a length as to extend from the head of the thigh to the ankle, is to be bound along the inner side of the thigh. Then extension being made either by the pestles mentioned in treating of the dislocation of the vertebra, or some other instrument, the leg is to be pulled downwards along with the board which is fastened to it, so that by the force exerted the head of the thigh-bone may return to its proper place. There is another mode of reduction without making extension upon a board, which is much commended by Hippocrates. The patient's hands, he says, are to be bound loosely to the sides, and a soft but strong thong put round both his feet at the ankles and above the knees, four fingers distant from one another, so that the affected leg when stretched may come two inches lower down than the other. The man is afterwards to be suspended with the head two cubits distant from the ground. Then an expert young man is to seize the affected thigh in his arms, at its thickest part, where the head of the thigh is lodged, and suddenly suspend himself from the man, by which means the joint will readily return to its place. This mode of reduction is simpler than any of the others, being performed without much apparatus, but many now reprobate it as dangerous. If the dislocation is outwards, the extension is to be made as above, but the thong at the perineum is to be passed by the opposite parts, I mean the groin and clavicle. The surgeon is to propel the limb from without inwards, the lever being fastened into one of the furrows formerly prepared, and an assistant fixing the sound nates that the body may not yield. In dislocations forwards, the patient being stretched, a strong man is to apply the palm of the right hand to the affected groin, and press down with the other hand, so that the depressing force may be exerted downwards, and to the knee. In dislocations backwards, the man is not to be stretched so as to raise him up, but he is to lie upon a hard body as in dislocations outwards; and, as we mentioned with regard to dislocations of the vertebra backwards, the man is to be laid on his face upon a board or bench, and the ligatures are to be applied, not to the loins, but to the leg as mentioned a little above. But the depression, by means of a board, is to be applied at the buttocks, where the dislocated bone is lodged. And thus much respecting dislocations at the hip-joint occasioned by some external cause. But since dislocation sometimes takes place at the hip-joint, as at the shoulder, owing to a collection of humours, we must, in this case, as we mentioned in the other, have recourse to burning.

Commentary. Although the descriptions given by the medical authorities who preceded and followed our author will be found in the main exactly the same as his, we are induced to give a brief outline of them, in order to illustrate by every means in our power a subject so important as the one now on hand.

Every subsequent author is indebted to Hippocrates for his lucid and correct exposition of dislocations at the hip-joint. He says truly that the thigh-bone is dislocated in four directions, namely, inwards, which occurs frequently; outwards, the most frequently of all; backwards and forwards, both very rarely. The following are the symptoms of dislocation inwards, as described by him. The leg is longer than natural, the buttocks outwardly appear hollow; the knee, foot, and leg are turned out; the patient cannot bend his thigh at the groin; and the head of the thigh-bone occasions a tumour in the perineum. This appears evidently to be the variety described by modern surgeons as the dislocation inwards and downwards, the head of the bone being lodged near the thyroid foramen. The symptoms described by modern authors are exactly the same as those mentioned by Hippocrates. Having seen cases of it, we can bear testimony to the correctness of Hippocrates's description. The symptoms of dislocation outwards as enumerated by Hippocrates are, shortening of the limb, relaxation of the inner part of the thigh, and projection at the buttock, inclination of the knee, leg, and foot inwards, with inability to bend the limb. This case is described by modern authors as a dislocation upon the dorsum of the ilium. From personal experience we can also testify to the accuracy of the description of it given by Hippocrates. The next variety is the dislocation backwards, which, he remarks, is of rare occurrence. It is rather obscurely marked by inability to extend the leg at the hip-joint and ham, relaxation of the flesh in the groin, distension of the nates, a slight degree of shortening and inclination of the limb. He states that the head of the bone is situated below the flesh of the nates. This assuredly is the dislocation backwards upon the tuber ischii, the symptoms of which are admitted by Sir Astley Cooper to be sufficiently obscure. Hippocrates describes with great accuracy the appearance which the limb puts on afterwards when the dislocation is not reduced. (De Articulis.) Reduction, he says, may be accomplished by the hands, with a bench, or with a lever. All these modes of reduction are mentioned by our author, and therefore we shall not take up time in describing them. (Ibid. and De Vectiariis, 15.) The figure of the bench of Hippocrates, given by Littré, would appear to us excellent, and it renders the description easily understood. (Hippocrat. Op. t. iv, 44.) Littré also gives an excellent figure of the reduction by suspension. (Ib. 291.)

Apollonius Citiensis gives a most elaborate and interesting commentary on the methods of reduction recommended by Hippocrates in cases of dislocation at the hip-joint. These methods, however, may be best learned by examining the figures given in the Index Galeni, or in H. Stephens's Latin Translation of Oribasius (Ap. Med. Art. Princip.), or in Littré's Edition of Hippocrates (iii, and iv.) There is one curious passage in the commentary of Apollonius, which we must not pass by. He says that Hegetor, one of the followers of Herophilus, had maintained that dislocation of the thigh being attended with rupture of the tendon fixed into his head (ligamentum teres) it was impossible ever afterwards to keep the ball of the femur in the acetabulum. This, Apollonius correctly argues, is contrary to experience and the authority of the ancients. (Ed. Dietz, p. 35.)

Celsus describes the different modes of dislocation at the hip-joint in the following terms: "Femur in omnes quatuor partes promovetur, sæpissime in interiorem; deinde in exteriorem; raro admodum in priorem, aut posteriorem. Si in interiorem partem prolapsum est, crus longius altero et valgius est: extra enim pes ultimus spectat. Si in exteriorem, brevius varumque fit, et pes intus inclinatur; calx ingressu terram non contingit sed planta ima; meliusque id crus superius corpus, quam in priore casu, fert, minusque baculo eget. Si in priorem crus extensum est, implicarique non potest; alteri cruri ad calcem par est, sed ima planta minus in priorem partem inclinatur: dolorque in hoc casu præcipuus est, et maximè urina supprimitur. Ubi cum dolore inflammatio quievit, commodè ingrediuntur, rectusque eorum pes est. Si in posteriorem, extendi non potest erus, breviusque est; ubi consistit, calx quoque terram non contingit." His statement, however, that dislocations inwards are of most frequent occurrence of any is at issue with that of Hippocrates, who more correctly states that the dislocations outwards are the most common of all. He likewise describes clearly the methods of reduction. If the muscles of the limb be weak, it will be sufficient to make extension by means of thongs applied at the groin and the knee; but if strong, it will be better to fasten them to the upper extremities of two sticks loosely fixed in the ground, and to make counter-extension by pulling the ends of the sticks in opposite directions. A more powerful method is by stretching the limb upon a board having axles at both ends with thongs fastened to them, by turning which such powerful extension could be made as would be sufficient even to break the muscles and tendons. When these are stretched, if the bone is dislocated forwards, some round body is to be placed in the groin, and the knee is to be suddenly carried over it, for the same reason and in the same manner as in dislocations at the shoulder. In the other cases the surgeon is directed to push the bone towards its place, while an assistant propels the hip-joint.

Oribasius mentions the four varieties of dislocation at the hip-joint. In three of them, he says, the leg is extended and cannot be bent; but in the dislocation backwards, it is bent and cannot be extended. He has described the method of reducing these dislocations by machines, of which he gives plates.

Albucasis describes the four varieties of dislocation and the methods of reduction in much the same terms as Paulus. His modes of reducing them are: 1st. By rotating the limb in all directions. 2d. By making extension and counter-extension with the aid of two assistants. 3d. By suspending the patient, and getting a strong assistant to grasp the affected leg and swing himself by it. 4th. By making extension with ropes fastened to two sticks or pieces of wood as recommended for dislocations of the spine. When the dislocation is forwards, the surgeon is to press down the prominent part with his hands; but if backwards, a board is to be used in the manner described by our author.

Avicenna agrees with Hippocrates, in opposition to Celsus, that dislocation outwards (on the dorsum of the ilium) is of more frequent occurrence than the dislocation inwards (on the foramen ovale.) His description of the modes of reduction is evidently taken from Paulus.

Haly Abbas describes the four varieties mentioned by Hippocrates, and recommends much the same treatment. The account of them given by Rhases is exactly the same.

The earlier modern writers on surgery, describe the four varieties of dislocation at the hip-joint in the same terms as the ancients. They evidently follow the Arabians. See Theodoricus (ii, 51); Guido de Cauliaco (v, 2, 7.) From the contents of this section it will be clearly seen how erroneous is the statement made by the late Sir Astley Cooper, that the profession was entirely ignorant of the nature of these accidents until within these last few years.

CXIX—ON DISLOCATION AT THE KNEE

The knee is dislocated in three ways: inwards, outwards, and towards the ham; for it is prevented by the patella from being dislocated forwards. Using, then, the same modes of extension, sometimes by the hands alone, and sometimes by cords, we must have recourse to suitable bandages, and the other suitable treatment, the part being in particular preserved free from motion.

Commentary. Hippocrates, like our author, mentions three directions in which the bones of the knee-joint may be dislocated: namely, inwards, outwards, and backwards. He has not noticed the dislocation forwards, which is, in fact, a very rare case. Celsus mentions, however, that Meges had related a case of dislocation forwards, which was successfully treated by him. But most of the other authorities, he says, have denied the possibility of such an occurrence. He directs the surgeon to reduce dislocations at the knee upon general principles, by making extension and counter-extension. Hippocrates represents dislocations at the knee as being of more frequent occurrence, but less dangerous, than those of the elbow.

Oribasius, like our author, treats only of three kinds of dislocation at the knee. Albucasis denies the possibility of a dislocation forwards. He directs the surgeon, in making reduction, to turn his back to the patient, and take the limb out between his knees; then while an assistant makes extension at the foot, he is to replace the bones with his hands. This seems a very proper method of reduction.

Avicenna likewise mentions only three modes of dislocation. He has described dislocation of the patella, a case omitted by our author. He directs us after making reduction, to fill the hollows with compresses, and then to apply splints and bandages. He says that the knee is often dislocated in walking. He must surely allude to a species of sub-luxation first well described by the late Mr. Hey, of Leeds; for a complete luxation is a very rare occurrence, and is never occasioned but by great violence.

Haly Abbas and Rhases describe only three kinds of dislocation at the knee, and deny the possibility of a dislocation forwards. Both evidently copy from our author.

The earlier modern surgeons, as usual, adopt the views of the Arabians, and accordingly deny the possibility of a dislocation forwards. See Theodoricus (ii, 52.) They would appear to have been wholly unacquainted with the works of Celsus, and to have derived all their information from the Arabians.

Dislocations at the knee-joint are now found to be of much rarer occurrence than they are represented to be by the ancient authorities. In fact only a very few cases have been reported in modern times. We would beg, therefore, to refer our readers to a case related in the 'Medical Gazette,' Dec. 16, 1842, by the author of this Commentary. It is necessary to remark, however, that several typographical mistakes occur in the Report, which are partly corrected in a subsequent number of the same periodical.

CXX—ON DISLOCATION AT THE ANKLE, AND ALSO OF THE TOES

The articulation at the ankle, if but a little displaced, is remedied by moderate extension; but if completely dislocated, it requires greater force. We may endeavour therefore, in this case, to make strong extension by the hands; but if reduction does not take place, having stretched the man on the ground in a supine posture, we are to fasten into the floor a long and strong peg, between his two thighs, so as to prevent the body from yielding to the extension by the foot; or rather let the peg be fastened before the man is laid down; or if we have the large board at hand on the middle of which, as we said, a wooden peg a foot long is fastened, we may make the extension upon it. An assistant then grasping the thigh, and making counter-extension, another assistant is to pull the foot with his hands or by a thong, and the surgeon is to rectify the dislocation with his hands, while some other person keeps the other foot down below. After the reduction it is to be bound carefully, some folds of the bandage being carried along the front of the foot, and some towards the ankle; but we must take care not to include the posterior tendon which is inserted into the heel. And the man is to be kept from walking for forty days; for those who attempt to walk before the cure is completed impair the actions of the part. If from a leap, as commonly happens, the bone of the heel is moved from its place, or if any inflammatory state is brought on, it is to be remedied by gentle extension and reduction, anti-inflammatory embrocations and secure bandages, the man being kept also in a quiet state until the part is restored. And dislocation of the toes, as we said with regard to the fingers, may be remedied without difficulty by moderate extension. In all these luxations and sub-luxations, after the reduction, and rest for a suitable number of days, any inflammation or swelling which may remain in the joints, and occasion a protracted impairment of the function thereof, is to be cured by emollient applications, the materials of which must be known to every one who is conversant with the matters relative to our art.

Commentary. Hippocrates states that dislocation at the ankle is generally produced by leaping from a great height. He remarks that the accident gives rise to excessive swelling of the part. When the parts have been reduced, he directs us to apply a bandage to retain them properly in position, which, he says, it requires some address to perform in a suitable manner. He recommends us to reduce dislocations of the toes and of the bones of the foot like those of the hand. His account of dislocations of the astragalus and of the os calcis is curious, but there is some difficulty in clearly apprehending his views. We need scarcely say that it is a subject still requiring elucidation.

According to Celsus, dislocations at the ankle-joint may take place in all directions. He recommends us to reduce them with the hands, by making extension and counter-extension. He advises us to make the patient lie in bed longer than in ordinary cases.

Oribasius makes mention of only three modes of dislocation at the ankle; namely, inwards, outwards, and backwards.

According to Albucasis, dislocation at the ankle can only take place inwards or outwards. When the bones of the tarsus are displaced, he directs us to restore them by making the patient put his foot upon the ground; and the surgeon, by placing his foot upon it and standing erect, is to push them into their place. After reduction, a splint is to be put under the sole, and secured with bandages. Rhases, Avicenna, and Haly Abbas evidently copy from our author. They give the same account as Hippocrates of dislocation of the astragalus.

Luxations of the tarsal bones are described in Sir Astley Cooper's 'Surgical Lectures,' and other modern works. Modern authors are agreed that dislocations may take place in all directions, and that they may be complete or incomplete. It will be remarked that Paulus makes mention of sub-luxations.

This is the place where we shall be expected to give some account of the knowledge possessed by the ancients of the nature and treatment of

Club-foot. It is singular that Hippocrates is almost the only ancient author who has treated of the subject in an interesting manner, and of him one need have little hesitation in affirming, that he displays more practical acquaintance with it than any other writer until the time of Stromeyer. He states that there are more than one variety of this *impediment*; that it is not, properly speaking, a *dislocation*, but a *declination* of the foot from its natural position; and that most cases of congenital club-foot admit of cure, if it be attempted before the limb is much wasted. He gives minute directions for restoring the limb to its proper shape by the fingers, and for securing it with waxed bandages and compresses, above which a piece of stout leather or a plate of lead is to be bound. Over all a leaden boot, like the Chian shoes, may be applied if necessary. By these means, he does not hesitate to declare that the deformity may be generally overcome more readily than one would have believed, "without cutting or burning, or any other complex mode of treatment." (De Articulis, 62.) Galen's commentary on this chapter is of use in illustrating the text of Hippocrates, but supplies no additional information for any practical purpose. (v, 642, ed. Basil.)

CXXI—ON DISLOCATIONS WITH A WOUND

In the case of dislocations with a wound the utmost discretion is required. For these, if reduced, occasion the most imminent danger, and sometimes death, the surrounding nerves and muscles being inflamed by the extension, so that strong pains, spasms, and acute fevers are produced, more particularly in the case of the elbows, knees, and joints above, for the nearer that they are to the vital parts the greater is the danger they induce. Wherefore, Hippocrates, by all means, forbids us to apply reduction and strong bandaging to them, and directs us to use only anti-inflammatory and soothing applications to them at the commencement, for that by this treatment life may sometimes be preserved. But what he recommends for the fingers alone, we would attempt to do for all the other joints: at first, and while the part remains free from inflammation, we would reduce the dislocated joint by moderate extension, and if we succeed in our object we may persist in using the anti-inflammatory treatment only. But if inflammation, spasm, or any of the afore-mentioned symptoms come on, we must dislocate it again if it can be done without violence. If, however, we are apprehensive of this danger (for perhaps if inflammation should come on it will not yield,) it will be better to defer the reduction of the greater joints at the commencement; and when the inflammation subsides, which happens about the seventh or ninth day, then, having foretold the danger from reduction, and explained how, if not reduced, they will be mutilated for life, we may try to make the attempt without violence, using also the lever to facilitate the process. We are to apply the same treatment to the ulcer as recommended for fractures with a wound.

Commentary. Hippocrates, as stated by our author, was decidedly averse to immediate reduction in cases of dislocation complicated with an external wound. Hence, in compound dislocations at the ankle, he forbids us to interfere at first, as attempts at reduction will certainly bring on convulsions or gangrene. Modern experience agrees with that of the father of medicine as to the danger attending these accidents. Compound luxations at the wrist, he says, prove fatal if reduced, but if let alone they generally get better. (De Artic. 64.) Compound dislocations at the knee are said to be particularly dangerous. (Ibid. 66.)

Celsus follows the line of practice recommended by Hippocrates. In cases of compound dislocations at the shoulder and hip-joint, he states that the danger is great if they are left unreduced, but pronounces death to be certain if they are reduced. Like Hippocrates, he approves of immediate reduction only in dislocations of the bones of the feet and hands. Even these, however, are not to be interfered with while the parts are in an inflamed state. He approves of bleeding, a spare diet, and rest. When a naked bone protrudes and cannot be got restored to its place, he advises it to be sawed off. (viii, 25.)

Galen gives his unqualified sanction to the practice of Hippocrates. See his commentary on the work 'De Articulis' and 'Nicetæ Collectio.'

Albucasis, like our author, recommends gentle attempts at reduction before swelling and inflammation come on, and soothing treatment afterwards.

The practice of Haly Abbas differs nothing in principle from that of our author and Albucasis. If reduction has not been performed early, he forbids it until the inflammation has subsided.

Rhases appears to have copied his rules of treatment from our author. He recommends us, if possible, to replace the parts before inflammation comes on, but forbids it while they are in that state, for fear of occasioning convulsions and death.

CXXII—ON DISLOCATION COMPLICATED WITH FRACTURE

If a dislocation be attended with fracture without a wound we must apply the common extension, and replacement by the hands, as described for simple fractures. But if complicated with a wound, we must apply the suitable treatment from what has been said of fractures with a wound, and dislocations in particular.

Commentary. Haly Abbas says that when a wound, a fracture, and a dislocation are combined in one case, each is to be treated upon general principles.

Albucasis directs us to remove any spiculæ of bone which may protrude in such cases. He exhorts the surgeon to act cautiously but confidently, as such conduct will prove most pleasing in the sight of his Creator, and redound to his own glory.